# Respiratory Medicine

Respiratory Medicine offers clinical and research-oriented resources for pulmonologists and other practitioners and researchers interested in respiratory care. Spanning a broad range of clinical and research issues in respiratory medicine, the series covers such topics as COPD, asthma and allergy, pulmonary problems in pregnancy, molecular basis of lung disease, sleep disordered breathing, and others. The series editors are Sharon Rounds, MD, Professor of Medicine and of Pathology and Laboratory Medicine at the Alpert Medical School at Brown University, Anne Dixon, MD, Professor of Medicine and Director of the Division of Pulmonary and Critical Care at Robert Larner, MD College of Medicine at the University of Vermont, and Lynn M. Schnapp, MD, George R. And Elaine Love Professor and Chair of Medicine at the University of Wisconsin-Madison School of Medicine and Public Health.

More information about this series at http://www.springer.com/series/7665

Kathleen O. Lindell • Sonye K. Danoff
Editors

# Palliative Care in Lung Disease

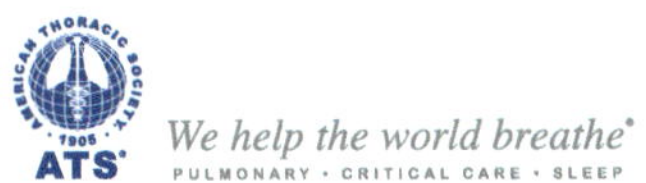


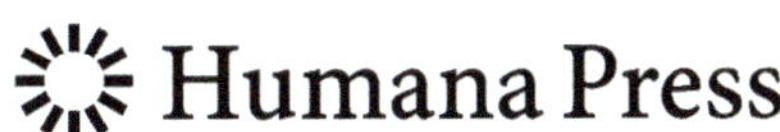

*Editors*
Kathleen O. Lindell
College of Nursing
Medical University of South Carolina
Charleston, SC
USA

Sonye K. Danoff
Department of Medicine
Johns Hopkins University
Baltimore, MD
USA

ISSN 2197-7372 ISSN 2197-7380 (electronic)
Respiratory Medicine
ISBN 978-3-030-81790-9 ISBN 978-3-030-81788-6 (eBook)
https://doi.org/10.1007/978-3-030-81788-6



This Humana imprint is published by the registered company Springer Nature Switzerland AG
The registered company address is: Gewerbestrasse 11, 6330 Cham, Switzerland

# Foreword

Some 45 years ago, when I was thinking about specializing in pulmonary medicine, word on the street about the specialty was not inviting: "There's nothing you can do about chronic lung disease." Common respiratory conditions such as COPD, lung cancer, cystic fibrosis, pulmonary fibrosis, pulmonary hypertension, and the pneumoconioses were considered largely untreatable. Beyond a dose of albuterol, theophylline, or codeine, dyspnea and cough were symptoms to be endured. Young physicians seeking glamor in the field settled for whatever prestige could be extracted from fiberoptic bronchoscopy, thoracentesis, and mechanical ventilation.

Since that time, extraordinary advances in cause-and-cure research have given rise to wondrous disease-modifying therapies for several chronic respiratory diseases. Vigorous efforts at disease prevention have greatly reduced occupational respiratory diseases and are favorably impacting the prevalence of tobacco-related conditions; yet, the global burden of lung disease remains profound.

Much to the benefit of those who suffer from chronic lung disease, a second mode of therapy beyond disease modification is taking hold within pulmonology and is even considered glamorous in some quarters. Lofty definitions have been written for palliative medicine. I think of palliative care as the best achievable response of a clinician when patients suffering from chronic disease plead for help to be more comfortable, remain in control of their lives, and die in peace.

Palliative pulmonary care starts at the time of diagnosis of advanced lung disease and accelerates as the disease progresses and medical options become limited.

People suffering from advanced lung disease are likely to complain to a clinician about one or more of four particularly distressing experiences using words that may resemble these: "I lose my breath and struggle to catch it"; "This cough is killing me"; "I can't do anything"; and "I am terrified of what will come." Full-service pulmonary clinicians learn how to layer on top of disease-modifying treatment useful guidance and assistive tools to help people live better in the face of such complaints.

Regrettably, many clinicians hearing those complaints reach primarily for prescription drugs to ameliorate distressing symptoms. Opioids, benzodiazepines, and antidepressants flow freely. Expertise in prescribing these symptom-modifying drugs is essential to current practice of palliative pulmonary medicine. However, much of the magic of palliative care derives from artful application of nonpharmacological therapies, including attentive listening; cognitive behavioral therapy to help people cope; education on physical conditioning and getting things done; and selective application of physical assistive devices.

Application of these non-drug strategies need not consume exhaustive amounts of time. Here are examples of quick guidance clinicians can offer to help people live better with advanced lung disease:

> You set out walking like a sprightly 30-year-old: then you stop, get disgusted, and turn back. Instead, try walking more slowly and keep going just within the limits of your tolerance for breathlessness. You'll go farther faster.

> Insist that your husband walk a half step behind instead of 10 steps ahead so you can set the pace instead of struggling to keep up with him.

> You need never fear that you will suffocate to death. When the time comes, we can help to take away your hunger for air and allow you to pass calmly with dignity.

Here are examples of often-overlooked assistive devices that can improve the daily experience and functional independence of individuals who are disabled by advanced lung disease:

- For mobility—a power scooter or power chair
- For clearance of respiratory secretions—a nebulizer for delivery of hypertonic saline and a nasal rinse kit
- For orthopnea—an adjustable-position bed frame
- For intermittent dyspnea at rest—a hand-held or desktop fan or as-needed use of noninvasive ventilation to ease the work of breathing

One form of respiratory distress remains almost as intractable as ever. Nonproductive cough plagues some people with chronic lung disease and others with no apparent underlying respiratory disorder. However, progress is coming. Chronic, nonbeneficial cough is increasingly understood as a neuropathic disorder. Therapeutic trials currently underway of drugs that target a hypersensitive cough reflex offer new hope to those who suffer terribly from this commonly underappreciated form of respiratory distress.

Even though palliative respiratory medicine remains a young field, there is now so much to know relative to what I learned during my pulmonary fellowship. This book, sponsored by the American Thoracic Society and edited by two clinician masters of palliative medicine, Kathleen Lindell, PhD, RN, and Sonye Danoff, MD, PhD, assembles current knowledge of palliative care for advanced lung disease.

Clinicians who master the insights and skills detailed in this book will never think or say, "There's nothing more I can do for you" when addressing a lung disease patient in distress. Instead, they will be well prepared to abide by the immortal punch line in the physician's Oath of Maimonides: "May I approach every patient like a fellow creature in pain."

John Hansen-Flaschen
Paul F. Harron Jr., Family Emeritus Professor of Medicine
Pulmonary, Allergy, and Critical Care Division
University of Pennsylvania
Philadelphia, PA, USA

# Preface

If we have learned anything from the COVID-19 pandemic, it is that serious illness is often accompanied by both physical and emotional suffering and that palliative care can be critical in alleviating these symptoms. Our vision for this book is to provide the compelling argument for why palliative care is so important in lung disease and to highlight the wide variety of work being done around the world to promote quality of life for patients with lung disease and their caregivers.

The foreword provides a historical perspective of palliative care and the important role it can play for patients with advancing lung disease and their caregivers.

The first part offers a background about what palliative care is, what constitutes advanced lung disease, and what current research shows as inadequacies in providing palliative care for these patients.

The second part describes effectively evaluating patient experience in advancing lung disease including the importance of keeping the patient at the center of care; assessing quality of life, breathlessness, preparatory grief, anxiety, and depression; as well as best practices to address symptom management and communication with patients and caregivers.

The third part discusses the role of palliative care in specific lung diseases including chronic obstructive lung disease (COPD), interstitial lung disease (ILD), lung cancer, neuromuscular disease, pulmonary arterial hypertension (PAH), and pediatric lung disease.

And, lastly, the fourth part addresses ways to improve access to palliative care. There is description of a specialty palliative care program for patients with ILD, and advice on how to address policy that promotes palliative care. This part finishes with the experience of palliative care delivery during a pandemic.

We hope that we convey our passion for reducing suffering and promoting quality of life for the patients we are privileged to provide care for and that you, too, become passionate regarding the importance of palliative care delivery in lung disease.

Charleston, SC, USA — Kathleen Oare Lindell
Baltimore, MD, USA — Sonye K. Danoff

# Contents

# Contributors

**Kathleen M. Akgün MD, MS** Department of Medicine, Section of Pulmonary, Critical Care and Sleep Medicine (PCCSM), VA Connecticut Healthcare System, West Haven, CT, USA

Department of Internal Medicine, Section of PCCSM, Yale University School of Medicine, New Haven, CT, USA

**Alice M. Boylan, MD** Medical University of South Carolina, Division of Pulmonary and Critical Care, Mt Pleasant, SC, USA

**Jared Chiarchiaro, MD, MS** Division of Pulmonary Allergy and Critical Care Medicine, Oregon Health & Science University, Portland, OR, USA

**David Christiansen, MD** Section of Respiratory Medicine, Department of Medicine, University of Manitoba, Winnipeg, MB, Canada

**Sonye K. Danoff, MD, PhD** Division of Pulmonary & Critical Care Medicine, Johns Hopkins University School of Medicine, Baltimore, MD, USA

**Marianne de Visser, MD, PhD** Department of Neurology, Amsterdam University Medical Centers, University of Amsterdam, Amsterdam Neuroscience, Amsterdam, Netherlands

**Elisabeth Potts Dellon, MD, MPH** Department of Pediatrics, Division of Pulmonology, University of North Carolina School of Medicine, Chapel Hill, NC, USA

**Shelli Feder, PhD, APRN, FNP-C, ACHPN** Yale School of Nursing, New Haven, CT, USA; Palliative Care Service, VA Connecticut Healthcare System, West Haven, CT, USA

**Betty Ferrell, RN, PhD, MA, FAAN, FPCN, CHPN** Division of Nursing Research and Education, City of Hope National Medical Center, Duarte, CA, USA

**Rebecca Anna Gersten, MD** Johns Hopkins University School of Medicine, Baltimore, MD, USA

**Annie Rhea Harrington, MD** Southern California Permanente Medical Group, Pulmonary & Critical Care Medicine, Anaheim, CA, USA

**Irene J. Higginson, FMed Sci PhD** Cicely Saunders Institute of Palliative Care, Policy and Rehabilitation, King's College London, London, UK

**Anand S. Iyer, MD, MSPH** Division of Pulmonary, Allergy, and Critical Care Medicine, Birmingham, AL, USA

Department of Medicine, University of Alabama at Birmingham, Birmingham, AL, USA

Lung Health Center, Department of Medicine, University of Alabama at Birmingham, Birmingham, AL, USA

Center for Palliative and Supportive Care, Division of Gerontology, Geriatrics, and Palliative Care, University of Alabama at Birmingham, Birmingham, AL, USA

**Renea Jablonski, MD** University of Chicago, Department of Medicine, Section of Pulmonary and Critical Care Medicine, Chicago, IL, USA

**Meena Kalluri, MD, FCCP** Division of Pulmonary Medicine, Department of Medicine, University of Alberta, Edmonton, AB, Canada

Alberta Health Services, Edmonton, AB, Canada

**Dina Khateeb, DO** Berks Schuylkill Respiratory Specialists, Wyomissing, PA, USA

**Matthew Koslow, MD** Interstitial Lung Disease Program, Department of Medicine, National Jewish Health, Denver, CO, USA

**Michael Kreuter, MD** Center for Interstitial and Rare Lung Diseases, Pneumology and Respiratory Critical Care Medicine, Thoraxklinik, University Hospital of Heidelberg, German Center for Lung Research (DZL), Heidelberg, Germany

**Taylor Lincoln, MD, MS** Department of Internal Medicine, Division of Pulmonary, Critical Care, and Sleep Medicine, University of Pittsburgh School of Medicine, Pittsburgh, PA, USA

**Matthew Maddocks, PhD** Cicely Saunders Institute of Palliative Care, Policy and Rehabilitation, King's College London, London, UK

**Catharina C. Moor, MD, PhD** Academic Centre of Excellence for Interstitial Lung Diseases and Sarcoidosis, Department of Respiratory Medicine, Erasmus MC, University Medical Centre Rotterdam, Rotterdam, Netherlands

**Evan Orlikow, MD** Section of Respiratory Medicine, Department of Medicine, University of Manitoba, Winnipeg, MB, Canada

**Mary G. Prieur, PhD** Departments of Psychiatry and Pediatrics, University of North Carolina School of Medicine, Chapel Hill, NC, USA

**Charles C. Reilly, PhD** Cicely Saunders Institute of Palliative Care, Policy and Rehabilitation, King's College London, London, UK

Department of Physiotherapy, King's College Hospital NHS Foundation Trust, London, UK

**Lynn F. Reinke, PhD** Department of Veterans Affairs, Puget Sound Health Care System, Health Services R&D, Seattle, WA, USA

University of Washington, School of Nursing, Department of Biobehavioral Nursing and Health Informatics, Seattle, WA, USA

**Anne Marie Russell, PhD, APRN, RHV, PGCE, ATSF** University of Exeter College of Medicine and Health, Royal Devon and Exeter NHS Trust Clinical Academic Unit, Exeter, UK

**Lesley Ann Saketkoo, MD, MPH** New Orleans Scleroderma and Sarcoidosis Patient Care and Research Center, New Orleans, LA, USA

University Medical Center – Comprehensive Pulmonary Hypertension Center and Interstitial Lung Disease Clinic Programs, New Orleans, LA, USA

Family First Medical and Well-Being Clinics, Post-COVID (Long and Multi-system) Patient Care Center, New Orleans/Kenner, LA, USA

Delricht Research Center, New Orleans, LA, USA

Louisiana State University and Tulane University Schools of Medicine, New Orleans, LA, USA

**Debra G. Sandford, B Psych, M Psych, PhD Candidate** The University of Adelaide, Adelaide Medical School, Adelaide, SA, Australia

The Royal Adelaide Hospital, Department of Thoracic Medicine, Adelaide, SA, Australia

**Dena Schulman-Green, PhD** New York University Rory Meyers College of Nursing, New York, NY, USA

**Mary Strek, MD** University of Chicago, Department of Medicine, Section of Pulmonary and Critical Care Medicine, Chicago, IL, USA

**Donald R. Sullivan, MD, MA, MCR** Division of Pulmonary and Critical Care Medicine, Department of Medicine, Oregon Health & Science University, Portland, OR, USA

Center to Improve Veteran Involvement in Care, Portland VA Healthcare System, Portland, OR, USA

**Jeffrey Swigris, DO, MS** Interstitial Lung Disease Program, Department of Medicine, National Jewish Health, Denver, CO, USA

**Matthias Villalobos, MD** Department of Thoracic Oncology, Thoraxklinik, University Hospital of Heidelberg, Translational Lung Research Center Heidelberg (TLRC-H), German Center for Lung Research (DZL), Heidelberg, Germany

**Jason Weatherald, MD** Section of Respirology, Department of Medicine, University of Calgary, Calgary, AB, Canada

**Marlies S. Wijsenbeek, MD, PhD** Academic Centre of Excellence for Interstitial Lung Diseases and Sarcoidosis, Department of Respiratory Medicine, Erasmus MC, University Medical Centre Rotterdam, Rotterdam, Netherlands

# Chapter 1
# Palliative Care in Lung Disease

**Betty Ferrell and Annie Rhea Harrington**

## "I'm Out of Breath"

This phrase, commonly voiced by a patient to a clinician, demands pause and deep exploration. These words often begin a conversation that is fraught with challenges for both the clinician and the suffering patient. Assessing the patient's concerns, diagnosing the etiology of the complaint, developing a care plan, and providing ongoing support through the continuum of what may turn out to be a severe and fatal respiratory condition can be difficult for even the most expert practitioner. With these daunting challenges of serious pulmonary disease, both patients and clinicians can find ways to "breathe easier" through the integration of palliative care into pulmonary medicine.

Respiratory symptoms can be caused by a wide variety of physical, mental, social, and environmental factors [1–4]. Primary pulmonary problems, extrapulmonary diseases that directly or indirectly impact the lungs and airways, as well as psychological conditions can all lead to complaints of trouble breathing. In the most benign cases, "running out of breath" represents a limitation to otherwise healthy physical exertion, a signal that despite normal physiology, someone is not able to reach the level of functioning that they desire and deem necessary for quality of life. In the most severe cases, being truly without breath is followed shortly by being

B. Ferrell (✉)
Division of Nursing Research and Education, City of Hope National Medical Center, Duarte, CA, USA
e-mail: bferrell@coh.org

A. R. Harrington
Southern California Permanente Medical Group, Pulmonary & Critical Care Medicine, Anaheim, CA, USA
e-mail: Annie.R.Harrington@kp.org





K. O. Lindell, S. K. Danoff (eds.), *Palliative Care in Lung Disease*, Respiratory Medicine, https://doi.org/10.1007/978-3-030-81788-6_1

without life. Pulmonary disease is for many a constant reminder of the possibility of death.

Respiratory disease and the end of life are healthcare experiences that are universally a part of the human condition. While virtually everyone has had a minor upper respiratory infection with mild respiratory symptoms, others develop advanced pulmonary diseases with severe symptoms that impact quality of life and ultimately limit one's life span. Heart disease, cancer, chronic lower respiratory disease, and respiratory infection comprise four of the top ten causes of death in the United States [5], and all cause respiratory symptoms. Worldwide, primary respiratory tract cancers and tuberculosis also enter the top ten causes of death, extending the prevalence of chronic respiratory concerns around the globe [6]. While modern medicine has been able to reduce morbidity and mortality in many respiratory conditions, the COVID-19 pandemic has presented yet another pulmonary disease challenge worldwide. Whether caring for a patient in the clinic or at the ICU bedside, the combined efforts of those trained in both pulmonary medicine and palliative care can improve both quality of life and the quality of death.

Palliative care has evolved as a model of health care focused on quality of life concerns in serious illness [7]. It builds on the foundation of hospice care, focused on the end of life, and extends the principles of this care across the trajectory of disease from the time of diagnosis. Palliative care began with a focus on cancer and late-stage disease, but it has rapidly expanded to include chronic illnesses such as heart failure, renal disease, neurological diseases, and dementia. As described below, there are many characteristics of pulmonary disease that make it an ideal target for palliative care, with the ultimate aim of improving quality of life for patients and families [8–10].

As palliative care has developed and expanded its focus across many diseases, there are common characteristics identified, or key domains that apply across serious illnesses. These are reflected in the National Consensus Project for Quality Palliative Care, Clinical Practice Guidelines [7]. These guidelines, now in the fourth edition, have guided the field through the eight domains of care, including Structure and Processes of Care; Physical, Psychological and Psychiatric, Social, and Spiritual, Religious, and Existential Aspects of Care; Cultural Aspects of Care; Care of the Patient Nearing the End of Life; and Ethical and Legal Aspects of Care [7].

Table 1.1 depicts these domains with application to pulmonary disease. There are many features of pulmonary disease that make these domains of care even more relevant. Pulmonary diseases are associated with high symptom burden, with often severe respiratory symptoms but also many other associated physical symptoms such as fatigue and cachexia. Psychological symptoms are also common including anxiety and depression. A common feature of these patients is concurrent chronic illnesses such as cardiac disease, adding to the symptom burden and quality of life impact.

The guideline domain of social aspects of care is very relevant given the family caregiver demands in pulmonary disease, including managing multiple respiratory treatments and medications, oxygen, and care by multiple clinicians. The Spiritual domain is important for patients with severe illness, as they face their mortality and often reflect on religious, spiritual, or existential concerns.

**Table 1.1** Palliative care domains applied to care of patients with pulmonary disease

| Domain | Application to pulmonary disease |
|---|---|
| Domain 1: Structure and Processes of Care | Challenges in prognostication for chronic pulmonary diseases<br>Pulmonary diseases often have prolonged, unpredictable courses and acute, life-threatening exacerbations<br>Coordination of inpatient, outpatient, and ICU care<br>Determining the role of pulmonary clinicians as primary providers of palliative care |
| Domain 2: Physical Aspects of Care | Managing respiratory symptoms such as dyspnea, cough, wheezing<br>Managing other symptoms such as pain, fatigue, and cachexia |
| Domain 3: Psychological and Psychiatric Aspects of Care | Uncertainty of prognosis in chronic pulmonary disease<br>Managing anxiety, depression, insomnia<br>Suffering associated with a chronic, life-altering disease with significant morbidity |
| Domain 4: Social Aspects of Care | Pulmonary disease impacts relationships, intimacy, and work<br>Family caregiver burden associated with chronic and advanced pulmonary disease<br>Greater social isolation as compared to other chronic illnesses<br>Social biases and stigma associated with smoking-related diseases<br>Family caregivers are often older with chronic illnesses of their own |
| Domain 5: Spiritual, Religious, and Existential Aspects of Care | Spiritual/existential distress associated with a debilitating illness<br>Overall physical and psychological burden of pulmonary disease leads to suffering |
| Domain 6: Cultural Aspects of Care | As with all chronic and serious illnesses, pulmonary disease is influenced by cultural factors and health beliefs |
| Domain 7: Care of the Patient Nearing the End of Life | Deaths often occur following acute exacerbations or crisis in chronic pulmonary illness<br>Respiratory and related symptoms may be exacerbated as diseases advance and at the end of life |
| Domain 8: Ethical and Legal Aspects of Care | Decisions regarding ventilation support, withdrawal of mechanical ventilation, and lung transplant<br>Early advanced care planning and goals of care conversations are needed |

The Cultural domain, described in more detail later in this chapter, is increasingly important as the population becomes more diverse and as clinicians recognize the influence of cultural factors on patient and family values, beliefs, and healthcare decisions.

The seventh domain, Care of the Patient Nearing the End of Life, has important implications for patients with pulmonary disease. Extensive literature has documented issues central to this population such as ventilator withdrawal, control of dyspnea in the final hours, and the many issues specific to care in the ICU setting [1–4].

The final domain, Ethical and Legal Aspects of Care, is relevant in all serious illnesses but also particularly relevant in pulmonary disease where conflicts often arise related to withdrawal of life support, lung transplant decisions, code status, or chronic respiratory management.

In the chapters to come in this text, the reader can apply these domains through the individual patient's clinical course: from initial assessment, to diagnosis, to symptom management, through the end of life. The concluding chapters of this book expand these domains from the individual level to broader societal impact and healthcare policy, including future directions, and contemporary challenges, including the COVID-19 pandemic.

## "I Need Air": Palliative Care Assessment in Lung Disease

The initial evaluation of a patient with respiratory symptoms can be a daunting task. The American Thoracic Society defines dyspnea as "a term used to characterize a subjective experience of breathing discomfort that is comprised of qualitatively distinct sensations that vary in intensity. The experience derives from interactions among multiple physiological, psychological, social, and environmental factors, and may induce secondary physiological and behavioral responses" [11]. Similarly, other common symptoms of respiratory disease including cough, fatigue, pain, depression, anxiety, insomnia, and anorexia can each have multifactorial causes, with complex exacerbating and alleviating factors. In 1 study of 85 patients presenting to a pulmonary unit with a complaint of chronic dyspnea, the initial impression of the etiology of dyspnea based upon the patient history alone was correct in only 66 percent of cases [12]. Classically, the primary care or pulmonary clinician will use history, physical exam, laboratory results, imaging studies, and cardiopulmonary function tests to reach an initial diagnosis and then determine a disease-focused treatment plan. As symptoms progress, clinicians struggle further to understand refractory symptoms and prognosticate heterogenous diseases. Integrating palliative care into pulmonary disease assessment from initial presentation through the course of illness can help both the patient and clinician through this challenging process. Chapters 1, 2, 3, 4, 5, 6, and 7 of this textbook provide an outstanding resource for navigating patient symptoms, needs, and outcomes, with tools to evaluate and improve quality of life for patients and families with lung disease.

Integrating palliative care consultation also provides an interdisciplinary, whole person assessment. The initial evaluation by a palliative care social worker or nurse may add tremendous insight about the patient and family needs. One strong point of agreement across sources is the critical need to implement palliative care early in the course of the disease [3, 13–16].

## "From One Breath to the Next": Palliative Care Approaches to Diverse Pulmonary Diseases

Practitioners in pulmonary medicine encounter many patients with similar initial presentations but ultimately different diagnoses and courses of care. Pulmonary diseases are often divided into broad categories such as obstructive lung disease, restrictive lung disease, pulmonary vascular disease, and lung cancer, with unique pathophysiologic processes defining distinct pulmonary diagnoses within each group. Clinicians can use these diagnostic categories to not only guide disease and treatment but also symptom management, communication, and advanced care planning within specific patient populations. The disease trajectory of chronic lung diseases is often uncertain. For example, patients with chronic obstructive pulmonary disease (COPD) usually decline gradually, whereas patients with pulmonary fibrosis have an unpredictable disease course with median survival less than 4 years. For both patients, the decline can be more rapid if the patient's underlying lung disease worsens or if the patient has other comorbid conditions. In the SUPPORT, data showed that 5 days prior to death, patients with lung cancer were predicted to have a <10% chance of surviving for 6 months while patients with COPD were predicted to have a >50% chance of this survival [17, 18].

Chapters 8, 9, 10, 11, 12, 13, 14, 15, and 16 of this textbook focus on the unique needs within special chronic lung disease patient populations, including those with COPD, interstitial lung disease, lung cancer, neuromuscular disease, pulmonary arterial hypertension, and pediatric pulmonary disease. While these diseases vary in many aspects, the domains of palliative care apply as they reflect universal concerns. Pulmonary diseases are also, in many ways, similar to other serious illnesses such as heart failure, end-stage renal disease, advanced cancer, or late-stage dementia. There are also unique aspects of lung disease including the profound impact of lung diseases on patient function and QOL. People living with lung disease also face social and cultural issues such as the blame associated with smoking-related diseases and the isolation often imposed on those with oxygen dependence.

## "Clearing the Air": Contemporary Challenges and Future Directions for Palliative Care in Pulmonary Disease

The twenty-first century has brought astounding advances as well as staggering challenges to pulmonary disease care. Advances in pharmacologic therapies for lung cancer, idiopathic pulmonary fibrosis, and pulmonary hypertension have impacted patient experiences with varied outcomes. Non-small cell lung cancer mortality in men decreased by 6.3% annually from 2013 through 2016, while lung cancer-specific survival increased from 26% for men diagnosed in 2001 compared to 35% who were diagnosed in 2014 [19]. This analysis based on SEER data showed improvement in survival across racial and ethnic groups and was thought to be in large part due to the development of targeted therapies.

Idiopathic pulmonary fibrosis, a subtype of interstitial lung disease, has a notoriously poor median survival of 3 years. The development of two new anti-fibrotic medications, pirfenidone and nintedanib, both approved by the US FDA in 2014 for treatment of idiopathic pulmonary fibrosis, has been shown to slow progression of the disease, though has not shown an improvement in mortality [17, 20].

Pulmonary arterial hypertension research has led to the development of multiple new medications targeting three pathways of the disease [21]. However, patients continue to have progression of disease with significant symptom burden and high rates of healthcare resource utilization. Despite numerous advances in basic science and clinical pulmonary medicine over the last two decades, there remains a need for improved patient care through focus on quality of life, symptom management, and advanced care planning which palliative care can provide.

Furthermore, pulmonary diseases are more prevalent in populations with decreased access to health care and increased environmental exposures contributing to disease. Care is increasingly provided to an aging population, in outpatient settings, by telehealth and care is dependent on family caregivers. Many of these family caregivers are also elderly with their own chronic illnesses, often with pulmonary diseases. Healthcare systems are keenly interested in models of care which can increase patient and family satisfaction, reduce hospital admissions, and provide the most cost-efficient care [22, 23]. As is true with all serious illnesses, there is a need to devote attention to underserved communities and minority populations who are especially vulnerable to inadequate care, late diagnosis, and limited access to supportive care [23].

The year 2020 has brought issues of public health crisis, healthcare justice, and racial disparities to the forefront of pulmonary disease. In December 2019 the severe acute respiratory syndrome coronavirus 2 (SARS-CoV-2) was first recognized in Wuhan, China. By January 2020, the virus was declared a public health emergency of international concern by the WHO, and in March 2020 it was recognized as a pandemic. As workgroups came together to diagnose and manage the profound pulmonary disease associated with this virus, palliative care practitioners assumed a central role in helping with bedside patient care, remote family communication, and end-of-life preparation. Key tenets of palliative care, including advanced care planning to ensure goal-concordant care, decision-making regarding life-prolonging treatments, and ethical/legal issues regarding chronic ventilator support, have been essential in the management of critically ill patients with COVID-19 infection [24].

Furthermore, palliative care team members have brought important skills to aid healthcare system management, including ethical distribution of healthcare resources, and use of alternative care environments outside of traditional healthcare settings such as home care. The COVID-19 pandemic has been perhaps the greatest healthcare challenge in a century; that challenge has been met at the front lines by both pulmonary medicine and palliative care providers working side by side.

During this time of pandemic, a domestic crisis also occurred. On May 25, 2020, a video captured an African-American man, George Floyd, and his words "I can't breathe" shortly before his death in police custody. His death ignited an international Black Lives Matter movement, not only focusing on racial injustice involving police brutality but also extending the discussion of racial and ethnic inequalities throughout society. Advocacy groups including White Coats for Black Lives have highlighted the passion that healthcare providers have in recognizing and addressing racism, inequality, and diversity in health care. Palliative care practitioners bring a strong foundation focused on social, cultural, and spiritual aspects of health care.

Chapters 16, 17, and 18 of this textbook discuss multidisciplinary models and healthcare policies for improving palliative care in advanced lung disease through the current pandemic and beyond. Pulmonary disease, as all other chronic illnesses, is greatly impacted by social factors and changes in healthcare delivery.

## "Breathing Easier": A Collaborative Future for Palliative Care in Lung Disease

The field of pulmonary medicine continues to make significant advances in diagnosing, managing, and treating lung disease. Similarly, the field of palliative care has a growing evidence base demonstrating effectiveness in symptom management, psychosocial and spiritual support, as well as enhanced survival [25–28] and cost implications of aggressive care at the end of life [24, 29, 30]. This textbook could not be timelier in bringing together the fields of pulmonary disease and palliative care. The chapters in the text address the key experiences of patients living with a broad range of pulmonary diseases and their daily challenges of breathlessness, anxiety, diminished function, and uncertainty, from initial assessment through end of life. The chapters represent common factors across pulmonary diseases, as well as those unique to specific diagnosis of COPD, lung cancer, interstitial lung disease (ILD), pulmonary hypertension (PH), and many others.

There is an expanding body of literature specifically addressing the benefits of palliative care in pulmonary disease [31–37], including better symptom management [38]. Extensive additional work is needed to test models of palliative care delivery across pulmonary diseases [2, 4, 39–43].

## References

1. Janssen K, Rosielle D, Wang Q, Kim HJ. The impact of palliative care on quality of life, anxiety, and depression in idiopathic pulmonary fibrosis: a randomized controlled pilot study. Respir Res. 2020;21(1):2. Published 2020 Jan 3. https://doi.org/10.1186/s12931-019-1266-9.
2. Ruggiero R, Reinke LF. Perspective, palliative care in advanced lung diseases: a void that needs filling. Ann Am Thorac Soc. 2018;15(11): 1265–1268. PubMed: 30134117. https://doi.org/10.1513/AnnalsATS.201805-347HP. www.atsjournals.org.
3. Reinke LF, Jansen DJA, Curtis JR. Palliative care for adults with nonmalignant chronic lung disease. Uptodate, April 2020. https://www.uptodate.com/contents/palliative-care-for-adults-with-nonmalignant-chronic-lung-disease.
4. Lindell K, Raghu G. Palliative care for patients with pulmonary fibrosis: symptom relief is essential. Eur Respir J. 2018;52(6):1802086. https://doi.org/10.1183/13993003.02086-2018.
5. Center for Disease Control, National Center for Health Statistics, Leading Causes of Death, Data for the US, Deaths: leading causes for 2017, table 1. https://www.cdc.gov/nchs/fastats/leading-causes-of-death.htm.
6. World Health Organization, Global Health Observatory (GHO) data, 2018. https://www.who.int/gho/mortality_burden_disease/causes_death/top_10/en/.

7. National Consensus Project for Quality Palliative Care. Clinical practice guidelines for quality palliative care. 4th ed. Richmond: National Coalition for Hospice and Palliative Care; 2018. https://www.nationalcoalitionhpc.org/ncp.
8. Maddocks M, Lovell N, Booth S, Man WD, Higginson IJ. Palliative care and management of troublesome symptoms for people with chronic obstructive pulmonary disease. Lancet. 2017;390:988–1002.
9. Smith LE, Moore E, Ali I, et al. Prognostic variables and scores identifying the end of life in COPD: systematic review. Int J Chron Obstruct Pulmon Dis. 2017;12:2239–56.
10. Curtis JR. Palliative and end-of-life care for patients with severe COPD. Eur Respir J. 2008;32:796–803.
11. American Thoracic Society, Patient resources, dyspnea. https://www.thoracic.org/patients/patient-resources/dyspnea.php.
12. Pratter MR, Curley FJ, Dubois J, Irwin RS. Cause and evaluation of chronic dyspnea in a pulmonary disease clinic. Arch Intern Med. 1989;149(10):2277.
13. Temel JS, Sloan J, Zemla T, et al. Multisite, randomized trial of early integrated palliative and oncology care in patients with advanced lung and gastrointestinal cancer: alliance A221303. J Palliat Med. Published Online:7 Feb 2020. https://doi.org/10.1089/jpm.2019.0377.
14. Sullivan DR, Chan B, Lapidus JA, et al. Association of early palliative care use with survival and place of death among patients with advanced lung cancer receiving care in the Veterans Health Administration [published online September 19, 2019]. JAMA Oncol. https://doi.org/10.1001/jamaoncol.2019.3105.
15. Scheerens C, Chambaere K, Pardon K, et al. Development of a complex intervention for early integration of palliative home care into standard care for end-stage COPD patients: a phase 0-I study. PLoS One. 2018;13(9):e0203326. https://doi.org/10.1371/journal.pone.0203326. eCollection 2018.PMID: 30231042.
16. Hoerger M, Greer JA, Jackson VA, et al. Defining the elements of early palliative care that are associated with patient-reported outcomes and the delivery of end-of-life care. J Clin Oncol. 2018;36(11):1096–102. https://doi.org/10.1200/JCO.2017.75.6676. PMID: 29474102. Epub 2018 Feb 23.
17. King T, Bradford WZ, Castro-Bernardini S, Fagan EA, Glaspole I, Glassberg MK, Gorina M, Hopkins PM, Kardatzke D, Lancaster L, Lederer DJ, Nathan SJ, Pereira CA, Sahn SA, Sussman R, Swigris JJ, Noble, PW for the ASCEND Study Group. A phase 3 trial of pirfenidone in patients with idiopathic pulmonary fibrosis. N Engl J Med. 2014;370:2083–92.
18. Claessens MT, Lynn J, Xhong Z, et al. Dying with lung cancer or chronic obstructive pulmonary disease: insights from SUPPORT. J Am Geriatr Soc. 2000;48(suppl)S146–S153. First published 2015. https://doi.org/10.1111/j.1532-5415.2000.tb03124.x.
19. Howlader N, Forjaz G, Mooradian MJ, et al. The effect of advances in lung-cancer treatment on population mortality. N Engl J Med. 2020;383:640–9. https://doi.org/10.1056/NEJMoa1916623.
20. Richeldi L, du Bois RM, Raghu G, Azuma A, Brown KK, Costabel U, Cottin V, Flaherty KR, Hansell DM, Inoue Y, Kim DS, Kolb M, Nicholson AG, Noble PW, Selman M, Taniguchi H, Brun M, Le Maulf F, Girard M, Stowasser S, Schlenker-Herceg R, Disse B, Collard HR. For the INPULSIS Trial Investigators. Efficacy and safety of nintedanib in idiopathic pulmonary fibrosis. N Engl J Med. 2014;370:2071–82.
21. Mayeux JD, Pan IZ, Dechand J, Jacobs JA, Jones TL, McKellar SH, Beck E, Hatton ND, Ryan JJ. Management of pulmonary arterial hypertension. Curr Cardiovasc Risk Rep. 2021;15(1):2. https://doi.org/10.1007/s12170-020-00663-3. Epub 2020 Nov 18. PMID: 33224405; PMCID: PMC7671829.
22. Rocker GM, Simpson AC, Horton R. Palliative care in advanced lung disease: the challenge of integrating palliation into everyday care. Chest. 2015;148:801.
23. Smallwood N, Currow D, Booth S, Spathis A, Irving L, Philip J. Attitudes to specialist palliative care and advance care planning in people with COPD: a multi-national survey of pal-

liative and respiratory medicine specialists. BMC Palliat Care. 2018;17(1):115. https://doi.org/10.1186/s12904-018-0371-8.
24. Ritchey K, Foy A, McArdel E, Gruenewald DA. Reinventing palliative care delivery in the era of COVID-19: how telemedicine can support end of life care. Am J Hosp Palliat Med. 2020;37(11):992–7.
25. Brown CE, Jecker NS, Curtis JR. Inadequate palliative care in chronic lung disease. An issue of health care inequality. Ann Am Thorac Soc. 2016;13:311.
26. Resnick MJ. Association of early palliative care use with survival and place of death among patients with advanced lung cancer receiving care in the Veterans Health Administration. J Urol. 2020;204(1):176–7. https://doi.org/10.1097/JU.0000000000001051.01.
27. Parker J. Palliative care linked to survival in lung cancer. Hospice News. 2019, Sept 25. https://hospicenews.com/author/jparker/.
28. Bennett C. Timing of palliative care linked to better lung cancer survival lung cancer, Lung Cancer Awareness Month, News. October 9, 2019. https://www.cancernetwork.com/lung-cancer/timing-palliative-care-linked-better-lung-cancer-survival.
29. Brown CE, Engelberg RA, Nielsen EL, Curtis JR. Palliative care for patients dying in the intensive care unit with chronic lung disease compared with metastatic cancer. Ann Am Thorac Soc. 2016;13:684.
30. Rush B, Hertz P, Bond A, et al. Use of palliative care in patients with end-stage COPD and receiving home oxygen: national trends and barriers to care in the United States. Chest. 2017;151:41.
31. Lindell KO, et al. Palliative care and location of death in decedents with idiopathic pulmonary fibrosis. Chest. 2015;147(2):423–9.
32. Zou RH, Kass DJ, Gibson KF, et al. The role of palliative care in reducing symptoms and improving quality of life for patients with idiopathic pulmonary fibrosis: a review. Pulm Ther. 2020;6:35–46. https://doi.org/10.1007/s41030-019-00108-2.
33. Maddocks M, Lovell N, Booth S, et al. Palliative care and management of troublesome symptoms for people with chronic obstructive pulmonary disease. Lancet. 2017;390:988–102. https://doi.org/10.1016/S0140-6736(17)32127-X.
34. Hui D, Bruera E. Integrating palliative care into the trajectory of cancer care. Nat Rev Clin Oncol. 2016;13:159–71.
35. Cullen GT, Fontes G. Integrating palliative care in COPD treatment. Fed Pract. 2016;33(8):40–2.
36. Henson LA, Maddocks M, Evans C, Davidson M, Hicks S, Higginson IJ. Palliative care and the management of common distressing symptoms in advanced cancer: pain, breathlessness, nausea and vomiting, and fatigue. J Clin Oncol. 2020;38(9):905–14. https://doi.org/10.1200/JCO.19.00470. Epub 2020 Feb 5.PMID: 32023162.
37. Iyer AS, Dionne-Odom JN, Khateeb DM, et al. A qualitative study of pulmonary and palliative care clinician perspectives on early palliative care in Chronic Obstructive Pulmonary Disease. J Palliat Med. 2020;23(4):513–26. https://doi.org/10.1089/jpm.2019.0355. Epub 2019 Oct 29. PMID: 31657654.
38. Smallwood N, Moran T, Thompson M, Eastman P, Le B, Philip J. Integrated respiratory and palliative care leads to high levels of satisfaction: a survey of patients and carers. BMC Palliat Care. 2019;18(1):7. https://doi.org/10.1186/s12904-019-0390-0. PMID: 30660204.
39. Halpin D. Palliative care for Chronic Obstructive Pulmonary Disease. Signs of progress, but still a long way to go. Am J Respir Crit Care Med. 2018;198(11). https://doi.org/10.1164/rccm.201805-0955ED. PubMed: 29889550.
40. Weiss A, Porter S, Rosenberg D, et al. Chronic obstructive pulmonary disease: a palliative medicine review of the disease, its therapies, and drug interactions. J Pain Symptom Manage. 2020;S0885-3924(20)30061-0. https://doi.org/10.1016/j.jpainsymman.2020.01.009. Online ahead of print. PMID: 32004618.
41. Scheerens C, Deliens L, Van Belle S, Joos G, Pype P, Chambaere K. "A palliative end-stage COPD patient does not exist": a qualitative study of barriers to and facilitators for early integra-

tion of palliative home care for end-stage COPD. NPJ Prim Care Respir Med. 2018;28(1):–23. https://doi.org/10.1038/s41533-018-0091-9.PMID. 29925846.
42. Narsavage GL, Chen Y-J, Korn B, Elk R. The potential of palliative care for patients with respiratory diseases. Breathe. 2017;13:278–89. https://doi.org/10.1183/20734735.014217.
43. Bowman B, Meier DE. Palliative care for respiratory disease: an education model of care. Chron Respir Dis. 2018;15(1):36–40. www.ncbi.nlm.nih.gov › pmc › articles › PMC5802661. Published online 2017 Jul 20. https://doi.org/10.1177/1479972317721562.

# Chapter 2
# An Introduction to Advanced Lung Disease

**Renea Jablonski and Mary Strek**

## Introduction

Chronic lung diseases are a leading cause of morbidity and mortality, resulting in an estimated four million premature deaths worldwide each year [1]. As the population ages, chronic pulmonary disease will only become more prevalent in light of the growing recognition of the link between aging and the development of lung disease [2]. Currently, diseases of the respiratory tract are three of the ten leading causes of death worldwide: chronic obstructive pulmonary disease (COPD) is third, acute lower respiratory tract infections are fourth, and cancers of the pulmonary system are sixth [3]. Tens of millions of others suffer from other advanced lung diseases (ALDs) which together are responsible for over 10% of disability-adjusted life years [4], a metric that approximates the amount of life and productivity lost due to disease. While less common ALDs, such as interstitial lung disease (ILD) or pulmonary arterial hypertension (PAH), affect a smaller number of patients overall than COPD or lung cancer, they often result in a high symptom burden in affected patients.

While death from chronic respiratory failure is frequently the common final pathway across the spectrum of ALD, the burdens patients face and the trajectories to that endpoint vary across disease processes. This chapter will explore the natural history and symptom burden of various chronic lung diseases in order to introduce the need for early, thoughtful symptom management in these patients.

R. Jablonski · M. Strek (✉)
University of Chicago, Department of Medicine, Section of Pulmonary and Critical Care Medicine, Chicago, IL, USA
e-mail: reneaj@medicine.bsd.uchicago.edu; mstrek@medicine.bsd.uchicago.edu





K. O. Lindell, S. K. Danoff (eds.), *Palliative Care in Lung Disease*, Respiratory Medicine, https://doi.org/10.1007/978-3-030-81788-6_2

## Chronic Obstructive Pulmonary Disease

COPD is a process that affects both the airways and the lung parenchyma. Increasingly, exposures to noxious gases and particles from tobacco smoking, biomass fuel/indoor cooking, and some occupational exposures are recognized as major risk factors for disease development [5–7]. Additional risk factors include hereditary alpha-1 antitrypsin deficiency and processes that limit the ability to attain peak adult lung function such as premature birth, severe pulmonary infections in childhood, and uncontrolled childhood asthma [8]. Patients with COPD have chronic respiratory symptoms that may include dyspnea, cough with or without sputum production, chest tightness, and wheezing. Airflow obstruction on spirometry is required for the diagnosis, and computed tomography (CT) imaging of the chest may show emphysema, gas trapping, or airway wall thickening [5, 8]. COPD is variably progressive, though not uniformly fatal. There is evidence that systemic inflammation and associated chronic comorbid illnesses increase the morbidity and mortality associated with a COPD diagnosis. Some patients are prone to acute exacerbations of their underlying obstructive lung disease that may require hospitalization and intensive care unit admission and contribute to patient and healthcare costs. Despite the use of inhaled bronchodilator therapy, which is the cornerstone of medical management in COPD, daily symptom burden is high and often not systematically or effectively addressed.

Since 2001, the Global Initiative for Chronic Obstructive Lung Disease (GOLD) has published an expert panel report on the prevention, diagnosis, and management of COPD which is regularly updated [5]. It recommends the regular assessment of the type and severity of patient symptoms using standardized tools. Initially measuring breathlessness by the Modified British Medical Research Council (mMRC) Questionnaire [9] was considered an adequate assessment of symptoms in COPD as it correlated with measures of health and predicted mortality [10–12]. Recent updates to the GOLD recommendations include the addition of the COPD Assessment Test (CAT) and COPD Control Questionnaire which allow for assessment of symptoms across multiple domains [5, 13]. Based on a patient's degree of symptoms and history of exacerbations, therapy consisting of single or multiple long-acting bronchodilators with or without inhaled corticosteroids is used [5]. Mainstays of treatment including referral to pulmonary rehabilitation, which improves dyspnea and quality of life in patients with COPD [14], provision of supplemental oxygen, and tobacco cessation apply to all patients with COPD regardless of disease severity.

The Evaluation of COPD Longitudinally to Identify Predictive Surrogate Endpoints (ECLIPSE) study was designed to identify factors that predict disease progression and COPD endotypes and identify clinically useful biomarkers [15]. While the presence and degree of airflow obstruction was related to breathlessness, health status, reduced 6-minute walk distance (6MWD), and number of exacerbations, it did not completely capture the heterogeneity in symptoms across GOLD stages and reinforces the importance of global symptom assessment regardless of the severity of airflow limitation [16]. Mortality risk in COPD can be predicted using the body mass index (BMI), obstruction, dyspnea, and exercise (BODE) index which integrates BMI, forced expiratory volume in 1 second (FEV1), mMRC dyspnea scale score, and 6MWD to predict both mortality from respiratory disease and all-cause mortality [17]. A newer version of the BODE mortality assessment tool uses age, mMRC dyspnea scale, and airflow obstruction as measured by the FEV1 (Age, Dyspnea, Airflow Obstruction or ADO index) to predict 2-year mortality using clinical variables that are easily obtained in clinic [18].

There is accumulating evidence that COPD is not confined to the lung but rather is a systemic process with the metabolic syndrome, systemic inflammation, hormonal imbalance, and hypoxia contributing to an increased symptom burden and numerous comorbid conditions [5, 8]. Signs and symptoms beyond the respiratory tract include weight loss, skeletal muscle weakness with limb muscle dysfunction, anxiety, and depression [14, 19]. Medical comorbid or associated conditions in COPD include anemia, coronary artery disease, hypertension, heart failure, gastroesophageal dysfunction with microaspiration, osteoporosis, and hypoxia. In addition, COPD has been noted to overlap with a variety of other chronic lung diseases including asthma, bronchiectasis, ILD, lung cancer, and obstructive sleep apnea which may further increase symptom burden and negatively affect outcomes [5, 8, 20].

Acute worsening of pulmonary symptoms not related to other illnesses or conditions and requiring additional therapy defines an acute exacerbation of COPD (AE-COPD) [5]. Symptoms of AE-COPD usually consist of worsening dyspnea, increased cough, or a change in sputum character. They are most often caused by viral infections of the respiratory tract with bacterial infection and environmental pollution acting as potential contributing factors. AE-COPD results in increased symptoms, decreased lung function, poorer health status and quality of life, increased hospitalization and risk of hospital readmission, higher risk of COPD progression, and mortality [8, 21, 22]. A single AE-COPD that results in hospitalization is associated with increased risk of future exacerbations [23], and thus strategies for future exacerbation risk reduction should be explored at the time of each event.

There is evidence in the literature and clinical practice that symptoms and burden of disease in COPD are considerable and remain under-evaluated and poorly addressed. A recent research letter analyzed data from a Swedish national registry-based cohort of COPD patients on long-term oxygen therapy who were also enrolled in the Swedish Register of Palliative Care and died from COPD compared with those enrolled who died of cancer during the same time period [24]. Patients with COPD had greater symptoms including breathlessness and anxiety and lower rates of complete relief of dyspnea and anxiety during the last week of life [24]. Importantly, despite the high symptom burden in COPD, prescription of as-needed medications for symptom relief was lower in COPD patients as compared to the group with cancer confirming previous observations that patients with COPD at the end of life frequently have unaddressed symptoms that may be greater than those with cancer.

## Interstitial Lung Disease

Interstitial lung diseases (ILDs) are a heterogeneous group of conditions characterized by expansion of the interstitial compartment of the lung by fibrosis, inflammation, or a combination of the two. ILD may be idiopathic or secondary to an identified cause including connective tissue disease, occupational exposure (e.g., asbestos), hypersensitivity to an inhaled antigen (e.g., chronic hypersensitivity pneumonitis), and medications. Idiopathic pulmonary fibrosis (IPF) is characterized by inexorable progression of lung fibrosis with limited therapeutic options and is the prototypical example of an ILD. A detailed history, physical examination, and serological assessment are critical components of the evaluation for suspected or diagnosed ILD [25] as identification of the underlying etiology dictates therapy. In situations where exposures drive ILD development, environmental modification may play a key role in mitigating progression of symptoms [26]. In addition to exposure mitigation, immunosuppressive therapy, often employing corticosteroids and steroid-sparing agents, may be used in the treatment of some non-IPF ILDs.

Recently, the approval and adoption of two novel antifibrotic therapies [27, 28] is changing the natural history of this disease before our eyes. IPF patients receiving antifibrotic therapy have a reduced rate of lung function decline and may survive longer [29] or be at lower risk for acute exacerbations of IPF [30], a major cause of morbidity and mortality in IPF. Recognition of a progressive fibrotic phenotype across ILDs has led many in the field to call for a "lumping" together of diseases with similar features of advanced radiographic or pathologic fibrosis and parallel clinical trajectories that may benefit from a shared therapeutic approach targeting pro-fibrotic processes in the lungs. A recently published analysis of antifibrotic therapy in progressive fibrotic ILD (PF-ILD) demonstrated the value of treatment based on disease behavior across multiple disease classifications [31], and the use of antifibrotic therapy is now approved by the US Food and Drug Administration for other forms of PF-ILD. Although current therapies may slow the loss of lung function, they do not stop the decline or restore lost lung function, and additional medications are an urgent and unmet need in the field of IPF and other fibrosing ILDs.

Historically, patients diagnosed with IPF had a median life expectancy of 3–5 years from the time of diagnosis [32], a survival worse than many cancers. Clinicians caring for patients with IPF or other PF-ILDs recognize, however, that these diseases may have a heterogeneous course with up to a quarter of IPF patients surviving 10 years after diagnosis [33]. Easily identifiable markers of disease progression, including worsening respiratory symptoms, a 10% or greater decline in forced vital capacity (FVC) over a 6- to 12-month period, and hospital admission for an acute exacerbation [34, 35], can predict short-term mortality in IPF. More granular detail on prognosis can be provided by the validated gender, age, and physiology (GAP) indexes which integrate ILD subtype, age, gender, FVC, and diffusing capacity for carbon monoxide (DLCO) to predict 1-, 3-, and 5-year survival [36, 37]. Unfortunately there is no current widely accepted biomarker that can be used at the time of ILD diagnosis to predict disease trajectory, and this remains an active and exciting area of ongoing research in this patient population [38].

One major life-limiting complication that patients with all forms of PF-ILD are at risk of is acute exacerbation (AE) of their ILD. In IPF, an AE is defined as a clinically significant decline with worsening dyspnea usually lasting less than a month in duration associated with new radiographic ground glass opacities and/or consolidation that is not completely explained by heart failure [39]. The annual incidence for AE-IPF is estimated to be 4–20% per year [39]. Triggers for AE-IPF are often unknown, but the increased incidence in winter months [40] and increased bacterial burden in the BAL fluid of patients with AE-IPF [41] suggest that infections play an important role. Surgery is a potentially overlooked risk factor with AE-IPF occurring after both thoracic [42] and extrathoracic surgical procedures [43]. All patients with ILD may benefit from evaluation of the risk-benefit ratio of any procedure as well as discussion of goals of care and end of life planning prior to surgery. Development of AE-IPF is more frequent in patients with worse lung function and is associated with a 50% in-hospital mortality [44], rising to over 90% in patients who require mechanical ventilation [45]. Increasingly the presence of AE with similarly poor outcomes is recognized in other fibrotic ILDs [46]. A recent consensus definition of AE in IPF will hopefully facilitate research into the etiology and treatment of this devastating complication [39].

The goal of living well with ILD requires a multidisciplinary approach and fluidity as a patient's needs often change as their disease progresses [47]. Regardless of the underlying etiology of ILD, patients experience a high symptom burden and reduced quality of life. Importantly, although antifibrotics attenuate the loss of lung function and may reduce the incidence of AE-IPF, they are not associated with decreased pulmonary symptoms or improved healthcare-related quality of life [27, 28]. Side effects of medications commonly used for ILDs, including immunosuppressive therapy and antifibrotics, may even add to symptom burden and compound the development of frailty leading to further reductions in quality of life. Common symptoms across PF-ILDs include cough, anxiety, and breathlessness, which may be more common than in patients with advanced stages of lung cancer [48]. In addition to physical symptoms, patients with an ILD diagnosis can experience significant psychic distress regarding treatment options and prognosis, which may be magnified by the significant amount of disinformation present on the internet [49]. Comorbidities including cardiac disease, pulmonary hypertension, emphysema, and sleep-disordered breathing should be aggressively managed due to their impacts on quality and quantity of life [50]. Transition to the use of long-term oxygen therapy in ILD may serve as a trigger to consider palliative care referral [48], with one nationwide registry analysis demonstrating a mean survival of 8.4 months from the time of oxygen initiation.

## Lung Cancer

Lung cancer continues to be the leading cause of cancer death worldwide [51]. In the United States, lung cancer is projected to be responsible for 12.7% of new cancer diagnoses and 22.4% of all cancer deaths in the year 2020 [52]. The diagnosis and management of lung cancer has become increasingly complex as we expand our understanding of driver mutations in lung cancer and employ complementary genotype-targeted therapy for treatment. Regardless of the intent of treatment (curative or palliative), side effects associated with cancer therapy are common and can include fatigue, anorexia and weight loss, nausea, bone marrow toxicity, increased susceptibility to infections, and increasingly immune-related adverse events due to checkpoint inhibitor therapy.

The International Association for the Study of Lung Cancers (IASLC) International Staging Project recently updated the guidance for lung cancer staging in both non-small cell lung cancer (NSCLC) [53] and small-cell lung cancer (SCLC) [54]. Appropriate lung cancer staging involves initial radiographic staging using CT imaging, whole body positron emission technology (PET), or integrated PET-CT to assess tumor size, enlargement of mediastinal lymph nodes, and survey for distant metastases. Tissue sampling allows for confirmation of cancer diagnosis, evaluation of underlying cell type, and molecular profiling for driver mutations that may allow for the use of targeted therapies. Integration of the data acquired from clinical or pathologic staging allows a patient to be provided with accurate prognostic information and identification of appropriate treatment plans. Prognosis varies by stage, ranging from an anticipated 92% survival at 60 months in patients with stage 1A NSCLC [53] to 1–2% for patients diagnosed with extensive-stage disease in SCLC [55].

Although lung cancer incidence and mortality are slowly decreasing due to the implementation of lung cancer screening and higher rates of tobacco cessation [51], the overall percentage of patients diagnosed with advanced or metastatic disease remains unchanged [56]. Regardless of stage, patients with lung cancer suffer from a high symptom burden [57]. Common symptoms reported by patients with lung cancer include cough, dyspnea, fatigue, pain, and nausea/vomiting with nearly all patients – 93.5% in one nationwide analysis – reporting at least one symptom in the prior month [57]. Interestingly, there appears to be discordance between patients and their medical team on the assessment of symptom intensity [58], which could potentially result in undertreatment and reduced quality of life for lung cancer patients despite calls for early initiation of palliative care in this population. Emotional problems, including anxiety, depression, and psychic distress, are associated with increased symptom burden and reduced quality of life [59].

## Neuromuscular Disease

Weakness of the respiratory muscles is common among patients with chronic neuromuscular disease. These processes may show waxing and waning disease activity over time (e.g., multiple sclerosis, myasthenia gravis) or may be characterized by progressive respiratory failure with few effective therapies (e.g., muscular dystrophy, amyotrophic lateral sclerosis).

Neuromuscular diseases affecting the respiratory system can manifest in multiple ways. Bulbar dysfunction can lead to cough and dysphonia, increase the risk of chronic aspiration and aspiration pneumonia, and result in unintentional weight loss due to decreased oral intake. Patients may have a weak cough leaving them susceptible to infections and mucus plugging of the lower airways. Alveolar hypoventilation may result in symptoms of dyspnea and orthopnea and result in arterial hypoxemia or hypercarbia and increased accessory muscle use. Nocturnal hypoventilation can cause headaches, daytime hypersomnolence, and impaired cognition. Critically, the degree of respiratory muscle involvement may not track with the presence of skeletal muscle weakness and requires separate assessment which can be done using spirometry and testing of respiratory muscle strength. Regular screening of patients at risk for pulmonary complications of their chronic neuromuscular disease is a necessary component of their care and should be part of the routine multidisciplinary evaluation in neuromuscular disease clinics.

Respiratory muscle function is a key determinant of quality of life in patients with ALS [60], with deaths in ALS patients most often due to respiratory failure. The ability to provide prognostic information to patients suffering from chronic neuromuscular disease is unfortunately limited. Recently, a validated model to predict survival free from tracheostomy or chronic noninvasive mechanical ventilation (>23 hours per day) was published which allows patients to be stratified into five groups based on anticipated time from symptom onset to the survival outcome [61]. Another predictive score attempted to use common clinically available data to predict respiratory insufficiency within 6 months of presentation to an adult ALS clinic [62]. Regardless of trajectory, early implementation of nocturnal noninvasive ventilation in ALS patients has been shown to prolong survival (by 205 days [63] in one study) and can be employed in concert with nutritional support, assistive devices for cough, and therapies targeting excess salivation, spasticity, and emotional lability to improve quantity and quality of life. Notably, the development of cognitive dysfunction, including frontotemporal dementia [64], is common in ALS. All patients with progressive neuromuscular disease have the potential to progress to a point where they can no longer communicate their preferences for care, highlighting the importance for ongoing discussions regarding long-term care preferences in this population.

## Pulmonary Arterial Hypertension

Pulmonary hypertension (PH) is a disease characterized by elevations in the pulmonary artery pressure. Based on the World Health Organization (WHO) classification system, PH can be divided into five categories based on etiology [65]. WHO group I, classified as pulmonary arterial hypertension (PAH), is a rare disease affecting an estimated 5–15 persons per one million adults [66, 67]. In contrast to the other processes discussed in this chapter, patients with PAH tend to be younger with females more affected than males.

With improved disease awareness and implementation of appropriate pulmonary vasodilator therapy [68], both hospital admissions and mortality appear to be decreasing [69, 70]. Even with treatment, PAH carries a high mortality with an estimated 5-year survival of only 65% [71]. Factors associated with a poorer prognosis in PAH include male sex, age over 50 years, the failure to improve to a lower WHO functional class with vasodilator therapy, and the presence of right ventricular failure. Patients with PH secondary to chronic lung disease (WHO group 2) have a poorer prognosis with a 5-year survival of only 38%, whereas patients with PH secondary to cardiac disease (WHO group 3) have a similar life expectancy as patients with PAH [72].

Symptomatically, patients with PH present with dyspnea, fatigue, and exercise limitation. Patients with PH secondary to other processes, such as those in WHO group 2 or 3, may also present with symptoms of chronic lung or cardiovascular disease. As the disease progresses and right heart failure develops, patients may suffer from exertional chest pain due to subendocardial hypoperfusion, pre-syncope, and syncope due to an inadequate rise in cardiac output with activity or reflex bradycardia and abdominal pain and decreased appetite secondary to passive hepatic congestion and/or ascites. As with all patients with chronic lung disease, patients should be treated with appropriate supportive care including supplemental oxygen, diuresis, and pulmonary rehabilitation which improves both exercise capacity and quality of life [73]. The primary cause of death in patients with PAH is thought to be acute right ventricular failure leading to complete cardiopulmonary collapse occurring secondary to anesthesia, infection, intravascular volume depletion, or interruption of pulmonary vasodilator therapy.

## Cystic Fibrosis and Pediatric Pulmonary Disease

Cystic fibrosis (CF) is a hereditary disorder due to mutations in the gene coding for the cystic fibrosis transmembrane regulator (CFTR) protein. Dysfunction of the CFTR protein results in impaired ion transport across the epithelial cell surface in multiple organ systems including the sinuses, lungs, and pancreas [74]. While clinical severity is variable, depending in part on the underlying CFTR mutation and residual CFTR protein function, there have been significant advances in therapy for patients with CF over the past decade. Despite increasing implementation of CFTR modulator therapy, CF remains an illness associated with decreased life expectancy. The greatest morbidity is from progressive bronchiectasis and recurrent pulmonary infections; mortality in CF is primarily due to respiratory failure [75–77]. The symptom burden is high with recurrent sinus disease, chronic daily cough which is frequently productive of copious volumes of sputum, pancreatic insufficiency with weight loss from exocrine pancreatic dysfunction, and development of insulin-dependent diabetes mellitus from endocrine pancreatic dysfunction which are present in many patients with CF [74, 78]. CF is associated with acute worsening in pulmonary symptoms, also known as CF exacerbations, some of which require prolonged hospitalization and/or home administration of intravenous antibiotics. The combined burden of acute and chronic morbidity leads to a reduced quality of life with associated anxiety and depression that has been described in numerous studies [79–81].

Women have been shown to have worse outcomes than men with CF [76, 82]. A decline in lung function as measured by the FEV1 has been associated with mortality and weight loss, while diabetes and chronic pulmonary infection with *Pseudomonas aeruginosa* are linked to ongoing loss of lung function [77]. The development of CFTR modulators that correct chloride channel and ion transport dysfunction results in improved symptoms and lung function, weight gain, and reduced pulmonary exacerbations [74]. It is expected that children born with CF, identified by newborn screening and appropriately treated with CFTR modulator therapy before a significant decline in lung function, may approach a more normal life expectance albeit with the physical and psychological burdens secondary to having a lifelong illness that requires a commitment to intensive daily therapies [83]. The improved outcomes have resulted in more adults than children with CF; thus successful transition of care from pediatric to adult providers has become of great importance as discussed below [74, 77].

In addition to CF, serious pediatric lung diseases include childhood ILD (chILD), neuromuscular weakness, PAH, and bronchopulmonary dysplasia (BPD) [84–87]. These conditions may be associated with chronic respiratory symptoms and increased mortality. Neuromuscular weakness may require home-assisted ventilation. In all cases where children with chronic lung disease approach adulthood, the transition from the pediatric to the adult pulmonary care setting requires a thoughtful and structured approach to assist the adolescent in this important step and engage the parents who are accustomed to being the primary care providers [88, 89]. It is a process that should begin early and address the many barriers that might prevent a successful transition [89] including communication failures and lack of planning while utilizing a standardized process to facilitate the independence of the adolescent and comfort of the parent.

## Lung Transplantation

Although lung transplantation (LT) can be considered as a curative treatment for some ALDs (e.g., idiopathic pulmonary fibrosis, PAH) and a palliative therapy for others (e.g., COPD), the median life expectancy for patients undergoing LT is approximately 6.7 years [90]. Following successful LT, a major cause of morbidity and mortality remains chronic rejection of the allograft, which is termed chronic lung allograft dysfunction (CLAD). According to the largest registry of LT recipients worldwide, CLAD affects nearly half of living LT recipients at 5 years and more than 75% of survivors at 10 years post-transplant [90, 91]. Unfortunately, CLAD frequently leads to recurrence of the same symptoms for which a patient sought LT including dyspnea, cough, and progressive respiratory failure. Clearly even patients with ALDs transplanted with "curative" intent are at risk of recurrent, limiting pulmonary symptoms necessitating palliative care.

## Conclusion

For most of us, the act of breathing occurs without thought approximately 20,000 times per day. Patients with ALDs are therefore constantly reminded of their disease. Over 90% of patients with ALDs suffer from dyspnea, with chronic cough another frequent and potentially stigmatizing symptom. The so-called disability spiral, where symptoms including breathlessness and exercise intolerance restrict ongoing activity and consequently result in progression of deconditioning, is all too common in patients with ALDs. All patients with ALDs deserve equal emphasis on maintenance of quality of life while disease-modifying therapies attempt to prolong survival. Frequent, patient-centered reassessment of symptom burden should be integrated into the routine care of patients with chronic pulmonary disease from the time of their diagnosis through the end of life.

## References

1. Societies FIR. The global impact of respiratory diseases - second edition. Sheffield: European Respiratory Society; 2017.
2. Thannickal VJ, Murthy M, Balch WE, Chandel NS, Meiners S, Eickelberg O, et al. Blue journal conference. Aging and susceptibility to lung disease. Am J Respir Crit Care Med. 2015;191(3):261–9. https://doi.org/10.1164/rccm.201410-1876PP.
3. Collaborators GMaCoD. Global, regional, and national life expectancy, all-cause mortality, and cause-specific mortality for 249 causes of death, 1980-2015: a systematic analysis for the Global Burden of Disease Study 2015. Lancet. 2016;388(10053):1459–544. https://doi.org/10.1016/S0140-6736(16)31012-1.
4. Collaborators GDaH. Global, regional, and national disability-adjusted life-years (DALYs) for 315 diseases and injuries and healthy life expectancy (HALE), 1990-2015: a systematic analysis for the Global Burden of Disease Study 2015. Lancet. 2016;388(10053):1603–58. https://doi.org/10.1016/S0140-6736(16)31460-X.
5. Global strategy for the diagnosis, management, and prevention of chronic obstructive pulmonary disease (2020 report); 2020.
6. Blanc PD, Annesi-Maesano I, Balmes JR, Cummings KJ, Fishwick D, Miedinger D, et al. The occupational burden of nonmalignant respiratory diseases. An official American Thoracic Society and European Respiratory Society statement. Am J Respir Crit Care Med. 2019;199(11):1312–34. https://doi.org/10.1164/rccm.201904-0717ST.
7. Salvi SS, Barnes PJ. Chronic obstructive pulmonary disease in non-smokers. Lancet. 2009;374(9691):733–43. https://doi.org/10.1016/S0140-6736(09)61303-9.
8. Riley CM, Sciurba FC. Diagnosis and outpatient management of chronic obstructive pulmonary disease: a review. JAMA. 2019;321(8):786–97. https://doi.org/10.1001/jama.2019.0131.
9. Fletcher C. Standardised questionnaire on respiratory symptoms: a statement prepared and approved by the MRC Committee on the Aetiology of Chronic Bronchitis (MRC breathlessness score). BMJ. 1960;2:1665.

10. Bestall JC, Paul EA, Garrod R, Garnham R, Jones PW, Wedzicha JA. Usefulness of the Medical Research Council (MRC) dyspnoea scale as a measure of disability in patients with chronic obstructive pulmonary disease. Thorax. 1999;54(7):581–6. https://doi.org/10.1136/thx.54.7.581.
11. Sundh J, Janson C, Lisspers K, Ställberg B, Montgomery S. The Dyspnoea, Obstruction, Smoking, Exacerbation (DOSE) index is predictive of mortality in COPD. Prim Care Respir J. 2012;21(3):295–301. https://doi.org/10.4104/pcrj.2012.00054.
12. Nishimura K, Izumi T, Tsukino M, Oga T. Dyspnea is a better predictor of 5-year survival than airway obstruction in patients with COPD. Chest. 2002;121(5):1434–40. https://doi.org/10.1378/chest.121.5.1434.
13. Jones PW, Harding G, Berry P, Wiklund I, Chen WH, Kline LN. Development and first validation of the COPD Assessment Test. Eur Respir J. 2009;34(3):648–54. https://doi.org/10.1183/09031936.00102509.
14. Maltais F, Decramer M, Casaburi R, Barreiro E, Burelle Y, Debigaré R, et al. An official American Thoracic Society/European Respiratory Society statement: update on limb muscle dysfunction in chronic obstructive pulmonary disease. Am J Respir Crit Care Med. 2014;189(9):e15–62. https://doi.org/10.1164/rccm.201402-0373ST.
15. Vestbo J, Anderson W, Coxson HO, Crim C, Dawber F, Edwards L, et al. Evaluation of COPD longitudinally to identify predictive surrogate end-points (ECLIPSE). Eur Respir J. 2008;31(4):869–73. https://doi.org/10.1183/09031936.00111707.
16. Agusti A, Calverley PM, Celli B, Coxson HO, Edwards LD, Lomas DA, et al. Characterisation of COPD heterogeneity in the ECLIPSE cohort. Respir Res. 2010;11:122. https://doi.org/10.1186/1465-9921-11-122.
17. Celli BR, Cote CG, Marin JM, Casanova C, Montes de Oca M, Mendez RA, et al. The body-mass index, airflow obstruction, dyspnea, and exercise capacity index in chronic obstructive pulmonary disease. N Engl J Med. 2004;350(10):1005–12. https://doi.org/10.1056/NEJMoa021322.
18. Puhan MA, Garcia-Aymerich J, Frey M, ter Riet G, Antó JM, Agustí AG, et al. Expansion of the prognostic assessment of patients with chronic obstructive pulmonary disease: the updated BODE index and the ADO index. Lancet. 2009;374(9691):704–11. https://doi.org/10.1016/S0140-6736(09)61301-5.
19. Yohannes AM, Kaplan A, Hanania NA. Anxiety and depression in chronic obstructive pulmonary disease: recognition and management. Cleve Clin J Med. 2018;85(2 Suppl 1):S11–S8. https://doi.org/10.3949/ccjm.85.s1.03.
20. Budhiraja R, Siddiqi TA, Quan SF. Sleep disorders in chronic obstructive pulmonary disease: etiology, impact, and management. J Clin Sleep Med. 2015;11(3):259–70. https://doi.org/10.5664/jcsm.4540.
21. Wedzicha JA, Seemungal TA. COPD exacerbations: defining their cause and prevention. Lancet. 2007;370(9589):786–96. https://doi.org/10.1016/S0140-6736(07)61382-8.
22. Seemungal TA, Donaldson GC, Paul EA, Bestall JC, Jeffries DJ, Wedzicha JA. Effect of exacerbation on quality of life in patients with chronic obstructive pulmonary disease. Am J Respir Crit Care Med. 1998;157(5 Pt 1):1418–22. https://doi.org/10.1164/ajrccm.157.5.9709032.
23. Rothnie KJ, Müllerová H, Smeeth L, Quint JK. Natural history of chronic obstructive pulmonary disease exacerbations in a general practice-based population with chronic obstructive pulmonary disease. Am J Respir Crit Care Med. 2018;198(4):464–71. https://doi.org/10.1164/rccm.201710-2029OC.
24. Ahmadi Z, Lundström S, Janson C, Strang P, Emtner M, Currow DC, et al. End-of-life care in oxygen-dependent COPD and cancer: a national population-based study. Eur Respir J. 2015;46(4):1190–3. https://doi.org/10.1183/09031936.00035915.
25. Raghu G, Remy-Jardin M, Myers JL, Richeldi L, Ryerson CJ, Lederer DJ, et al. Diagnosis of idiopathic pulmonary fibrosis. An official ATS/ERS/JRS/ALAT clinical practice guideline. Am J Respir Crit Care Med. 2018;198(5):e44–68. https://doi.org/10.1164/rccm.201807-1255ST.

26. Fernández Pérez ER, Swigris JJ, Forssén AV, Tourin O, Solomon JJ, Huie TJ, et al. Identifying an inciting antigen is associated with improved survival in patients with chronic hypersensitivity pneumonitis. Chest. 2013;144(5):1644–51. https://doi.org/10.1378/chest.12-2685.
27. King TE, Bradford WZ, Castro-Bernardini S, Fagan EA, Glaspole I, Glassberg MK, et al. A phase 3 trial of pirfenidone in patients with idiopathic pulmonary fibrosis. N Engl J Med. 2014;370(22):2083–92. https://doi.org/10.1056/NEJMoa1402582.
28. Richeldi L, du Bois RM, Raghu G, Azuma A, Brown KK, Costabel U, et al. Efficacy and safety of nintedanib in idiopathic pulmonary fibrosis. N Engl J Med. 2014;370(22):2071–82. https://doi.org/10.1056/NEJMoa1402584.
29. Nathan SD, Albera C, Bradford WZ, Costabel U, Glaspole I, Glassberg MK, et al. Effect of pirfenidone on mortality: pooled analyses and meta-analyses of clinical trials in idiopathic pulmonary fibrosis. Lancet Respir Med. 2017;5(1):33–41. https://doi.org/10.1016/S2213-2600(16)30326-5.
30. Richeldi L, Cottin V, du Bois RM, Selman M, Kimura T, Bailes Z, et al. Nintedanib in patients with idiopathic pulmonary fibrosis: combined evidence from the TOMORROW and INPULSIS(®) trials. Respir Med. 2016;113:74–9. https://doi.org/10.1016/j.rmed.2016.02.001.
31. Flaherty KR, Wells AU, Cottin V, Devaraj A, Walsh SLF, Inoue Y, et al. Nintedanib in progressive fibrosing interstitial lung diseases. N Engl J Med. 2019;381(18):1718–27. https://doi.org/10.1056/NEJMoa1908681.
32. Raghu G, Collard HR, Egan JJ, Martinez FJ, Behr J, Brown KK, et al. An official ATS/ERS/JRS/ALAT statement: idiopathic pulmonary fibrosis: evidence-based guidelines for diagnosis and management. Am J Respir Crit Care Med. 2011;183(6):788–824. https://doi.org/10.1164/rccm.2009-040GL.
33. Nathan SD, Shlobin OA, Weir N, Ahmad S, Kaldjob JM, Battle E, et al. Long-term course and prognosis of idiopathic pulmonary fibrosis in the new millennium. Chest. 2011;140(1):221–9. https://doi.org/10.1378/chest.10-2572.
34. Paterniti MO, Bi Y, Rekić D, Wang Y, Karimi-Shah BA, Chowdhury BA. Acute exacerbation and decline in forced vital capacity are associated with increased mortality in idiopathic pulmonary fibrosis. Ann Am Thorac Soc. 2017;14(9):1395–402. https://doi.org/10.1513/AnnalsATS.201606-458OC.
35. Ley B, Bradford WZ, Weycker D, Vittinghoff E, du Bois RM, Collard HR. Unified baseline and longitudinal mortality prediction in idiopathic pulmonary fibrosis. Eur Respir J. 2015;45(5):1374–81. https://doi.org/10.1183/09031936.00146314.
36. Ley B, Ryerson CJ, Vittinghoff E, Ryu JH, Tomassetti S, Lee JS, et al. A multidimensional index and staging system for idiopathic pulmonary fibrosis. Ann Intern Med. 2012;156(10):684–91. https://doi.org/10.7326/0003-4819-156-10-201205150-00004.
37. Ryerson CJ, Vittinghoff E, Ley B, Lee JS, Mooney JJ, Jones KD, et al. Predicting survival across chronic interstitial lung disease: the ILD-GAP model. Chest. 2014;145(4):723–8. https://doi.org/10.1378/chest.13-1474.
38. Campo I, Zorzetto M, Bonella F. Facts and promises on lung biomarkers in interstitial lung diseases. Expert Rev Respir Med. 2015;9(4):437–57. https://doi.org/10.1586/17476348.2015.1062367.
39. Collard HR, Ryerson CJ, Corte TJ, Jenkins G, Kondoh Y, Lederer DJ, et al. Acute exacerbation of idiopathic pulmonary fibrosis. An international working group report. Am J Respir Crit Care Med. 2016;194(3):265–75. https://doi.org/10.1164/rccm.201604-0801CI.
40. Collard HR, Richeldi L, Kim DS, Taniguchi H, Tschoepe I, Luisetti M, et al. Acute exacerbations in the INPULSIS trials of nintedanib in idiopathic pulmonary fibrosis. Eur Respir J. 2017;49(5). https://doi.org/10.1183/13993003.01339-2016.
41. Molyneaux PL, Cox MJ, Wells AU, Kim HC, Ji W, Cookson WO, et al. Changes in the respiratory microbiome during acute exacerbations of idiopathic pulmonary fibrosis. Respir Res. 2017;18(1):29. https://doi.org/10.1186/s12931-017-0511-3.
42. Sakamoto S, Homma S, Mun M, Fujii T, Kurosaki A, Yoshimura K. Acute exacerbation of idiopathic interstitial pneumonia following lung surgery in 3 of 68 consecutive patients: a retrospective study. Intern Med. 2011;50(2):77–85. https://doi.org/10.2169/internalmedicine.50.3390.

43. Ghatol A, Ruhl AP, Danoff SK. Exacerbations in idiopathic pulmonary fibrosis triggered by pulmonary and nonpulmonary surgery: a case series and comprehensive review of the literature. Lung. 2012;190(4):373–80. https://doi.org/10.1007/s00408-012-9389-5.
44. Song JW, Hong SB, Lim CM, Koh Y, Kim DS. Acute exacerbation of idiopathic pulmonary fibrosis: incidence, risk factors and outcome. Eur Respir J. 2011;37(2):356–63. https://doi.org/10.1183/09031936.00159709.
45. Al-Hameed FM, Sharma S. Outcome of patients admitted to the intensive care unit for acute exacerbation of idiopathic pulmonary fibrosis. Can Respir J. 2004;11(2):117–22. https://doi.org/10.1155/2004/379723.
46. Suzuki A, Kondoh Y, Brown KK, Johkoh T, Kataoka K, Fukuoka J, et al. Acute exacerbations of fibrotic interstitial lung diseases. Respirology. 2020;25(5):525–34. https://doi.org/10.1111/resp.13682.
47. Kreuter M, Bendstrup E, Russell AM, Bajwah S, Lindell K, Adir Y, et al. Palliative care in interstitial lung disease: living well. Lancet Respir Med. 2017;5(12):968–80. https://doi.org/10.1016/S2213-2600(17)30383-1.
48. Ahmadi Z, Wysham NG, Lundström S, Janson C, Currow DC, Ekström M. End-of-life care in oxygen-dependent ILD compared with lung cancer: a national population-based study. Thorax. 2016;71(6):510–6. https://doi.org/10.1136/thoraxjnl-2015-207439.
49. Goobie GC, Guler SA, Johannson KA, Fisher JH, Ryerson CJ. YouTube videos as a source of misinformation on idiopathic pulmonary fibrosis. Ann Am Thorac Soc. 2019;16(5):572–9. https://doi.org/10.1513/AnnalsATS.201809-644OC.
50. King CS, Nathan SD. Idiopathic pulmonary fibrosis: effects and optimal management of comorbidities. Lancet Respir Med. 2017;5(1):72–84. https://doi.org/10.1016/S2213-2600(16)30222-3.
51. Bray F, Ferlay J, Soerjomataram I, Siegel RL, Torre LA, Jemal A. Global cancer statistics 2018: GLOBOCAN estimates of incidence and mortality worldwide for 36 cancers in 185 countries. CA Cancer J Clin. 2018;68(6):394–424. https://doi.org/10.3322/caac.21492.
52. SEER Database; 2020.
53. Goldstraw P, Chansky K, Crowley J, Rami-Porta R, Asamura H, Eberhardt WE, et al. The IASLC lung cancer staging project: proposals for revision of the TNM stage groupings in the forthcoming (eighth) edition of the TNM classification for lung cancer. J Thorac Oncol. 2016;11(1):39–51. https://doi.org/10.1016/j.jtho.2015.09.009.
54. Nicholson AG, Chansky K, Crowley J, Beyruti R, Kubota K, Turrisi A, et al. The International Association for the Study of Lung Cancer Lung Cancer Staging Project: proposals for the revision of the clinical and pathologic staging of small cell lung cancer in the forthcoming eighth edition of the TNM classification for lung cancer. J Thorac Oncol. 2016;11(3):300–11. https://doi.org/10.1016/j.jtho.2015.10.008.
55. Lassen U, Osterlind K, Hansen M, Dombernowsky P, Bergman B, Hansen HH. Long-term survival in small-cell lung cancer: posttreatment characteristics in patients surviving 5 to 18+ years--an analysis of 1,714 consecutive patients. J Clin Oncol. 1995;13(5):1215–20. https://doi.org/10.1200/JCO.1995.13.5.1215.
56. Howlader N, Forjaz G, Mooradian MJ, Meza R, Kong CY, Cronin KA, et al. The effect of advances in lung-cancer treatment on population mortality. N Engl J Med. 2020;383(7):640–9. https://doi.org/10.1056/NEJMoa1916623.
57. Walling AM, Weeks JC, Kahn KL, Tisnado D, Keating NL, Dy SM, et al. Symptom prevalence in lung and colorectal cancer patients. J Pain Symptom Manage. 2015;49(2):192–202. https://doi.org/10.1016/j.jpainsymman.2014.06.003.
58. Iyer S, Roughley A, Rider A, Taylor-Stokes G. The symptom burden of non-small cell lung cancer in the USA: a real-world cross-sectional study. Support Care Cancer. 2014;22(1):181–7. https://doi.org/10.1007/s00520-013-1959-4.
59. Morrison EJ, Novotny PJ, Sloan JA, Yang P, Patten CA, Ruddy KJ, et al. Emotional problems, quality of life, and symptom burden in patients with lung cancer. Clin Lung Cancer. 2017;18(5):497–503. https://doi.org/10.1016/j.cllc.2017.02.008.

60. Bourke SC, Shaw PJ, Gibson GJ. Respiratory function vs sleep-disordered breathing as predictors of QOL in ALS. Neurology. 2001;57(11):2040–4. https://doi.org/10.1212/wnl.57.11.2040.
61. Westeneng HJ, Debray TPA, Visser AE, van Eijk RPA, Rooney JPK, Calvo A, et al. Prognosis for patients with amyotrophic lateral sclerosis: development and validation of a personalised prediction model. Lancet Neurol. 2018;17(5):423–33. https://doi.org/10.1016/S1474-4422(18)30089-9.
62. Ackrivo J, Hansen-Flaschen J, Wileyto EP, Schwab RJ, Elman L, Kawut SM. Development of a prognostic model of respiratory insufficiency or death in amyotrophic lateral sclerosis. Eur Respir J. 2019;53(4). https://doi.org/10.1183/13993003.02237-2018.
63. Bourke SC, Tomlinson M, Williams TL, Bullock RE, Shaw PJ, Gibson GJ. Effects of non-invasive ventilation on survival and quality of life in patients with amyotrophic lateral sclerosis: a randomised controlled trial. Lancet Neurol. 2006;5(2):140–7. https://doi.org/10.1016/S1474-4422(05)70326-4.
64. Phukan J, Elamin M, Bede P, Jordan N, Gallagher L, Byrne S, et al. The syndrome of cognitive impairment in amyotrophic lateral sclerosis: a population-based study. J Neurol Neurosurg Psychiatry. 2012;83(1):102–8. https://doi.org/10.1136/jnnp-2011-300188.
65. Simonneau G, Montani D, Celermajer DS, Denton CP, Gatzoulis MA, Krowka M, et al. Haemodynamic definitions and updated clinical classification of pulmonary hypertension. Eur Respir J. 2019;53(1). https://doi.org/10.1183/13993003.01913-2018.
66. Humbert M, Sitbon O, Chaouat A, Bertocchi M, Habib G, Gressin V, et al. Pulmonary arterial hypertension in France: results from a national registry. Am J Respir Crit Care Med. 2006;173(9):1023–30. https://doi.org/10.1164/rccm.200510-1668OC.
67. Ling Y, Johnson MK, Kiely DG, Condliffe R, Elliot CA, Gibbs JS, et al. Changing demographics, epidemiology, and survival of incident pulmonary arterial hypertension: results from the pulmonary hypertension registry of the United Kingdom and Ireland. Am J Respir Crit Care Med. 2012;186(8):790–6. https://doi.org/10.1164/rccm.201203-0383OC.
68. Galiè N, Humbert M, Vachiery JL, Gibbs S, Lang I, Torbicki A, et al. 2015 ESC/ERS guidelines for the diagnosis and treatment of pulmonary hypertension: the Joint Task Force for the Diagnosis and Treatment of Pulmonary Hypertension of the European Society of Cardiology (ESC) and the European Respiratory Society (ERS): endorsed by: Association for European Paediatric and Congenital Cardiology (AEPC), International Society for Heart and Lung Transplantation (ISHLT). Eur Respir J. 2015;46(4):903–75. https://doi.org/10.1183/13993003.01032-2015.
69. Anand V, Roy SS, Archer SL, Weir EK, Garg SK, Duval S, et al. Trends and outcomes of pulmonary arterial hypertension-related hospitalizations in the United States: analysis of the nationwide inpatient sample database from 2001 through 2012. JAMA Cardiol. 2016;1(9):1021–9. https://doi.org/10.1001/jamacardio.2016.3591.
70. Stein PD, Matta F, Hughes PG. Scope of problem of pulmonary arterial hypertension. Am J Med. 2015;128(8):844–51. https://doi.org/10.1016/j.amjmed.2015.03.007.
71. Benza RL, Miller DP, Barst RJ, Badesch DB, Frost AE, McGoon MD. An evaluation of long-term survival from time of diagnosis in pulmonary arterial hypertension from the REVEAL Registry. Chest. 2012;142(2):448–56. https://doi.org/10.1378/chest.11-1460.
72. Gall H, Felix JF, Schneck FK, Milger K, Sommer N, Voswinckel R, et al. The Giessen pulmonary hypertension registry: survival in pulmonary hypertension subgroups. J Heart Lung Transplant. 2017;36(9):957–67. https://doi.org/10.1016/j.healun.2017.02.016.
73. Morris NR, Kermeen FD, Holland AE. Exercise-based rehabilitation programmes for pulmonary hypertension. Cochrane Database Syst Rev. 2017;1:CD011285. https://doi.org/10.1002/14651858.CD011285.pub2.
74. Ratjen F, Bell SC, Rowe SM, Goss CH, Quittner AL, Bush A. Cystic fibrosis. Nat Rev Dis Primers. 2015;1:15010. https://doi.org/10.1038/nrdp.2015.10.
75. MacKenzie T, Gifford AH, Sabadosa KA, Quinton HB, Knapp EA, Goss CH, et al. Longevity of patients with cystic fibrosis in 2000 to 2010 and beyond: survival analysis of the Cystic Fibrosis Foundation patient registry. Ann Intern Med. 2014;161(4):233–41. https://doi.org/10.7326/M13-0636.

76. Dodge JA, Lewis PA, Stanton M, Wilsher J. Cystic fibrosis mortality and survival in the UK: 1947-2003. Eur Respir J. 2007;29(3):522–6. https://doi.org/10.1183/09031936.00099506.
77. Kerem E, Viviani L, Zolin A, MacNeill S, Hatziagorou E, Ellemunter H, et al. Factors associated with FEV1 decline in cystic fibrosis: analysis of the ECFS patient registry. Eur Respir J. 2014;43(1):125–33. https://doi.org/10.1183/09031936.00166412.
78. Goss CH, Edwards TC, Ramsey BW, Aitken ML, Patrick DL. Patient-reported respiratory symptoms in cystic fibrosis. J Cyst Fibros. 2009;8(4):245–52. https://doi.org/10.1016/j.jcf.2009.04.003.
79. Sawicki GS, Rasouliyan L, McMullen AH, Wagener JS, McColley SA, Pasta DJ, et al. Longitudinal assessment of health-related quality of life in an observational cohort of patients with cystic fibrosis. Pediatr Pulmonol. 2011;46(1):36–44. https://doi.org/10.1002/ppul.21325.
80. Smith BA, Modi AC, Quittner AL, Wood BL. Depressive symptoms in children with cystic fibrosis and parents and its effects on adherence to airway clearance. Pediatr Pulmonol. 2010;45(8):756–63. https://doi.org/10.1002/ppul.21238.
81. Riekert KA, Bartlett SJ, Boyle MP, Krishnan JA, Rand CS. The association between depression, lung function, and health-related quality of life among adults with cystic fibrosis. Chest. 2007;132(1):231–7. https://doi.org/10.1378/chest.06-2474.
82. Nick JA, Chacon CS, Brayshaw SJ, Jones MC, Barboa CM, St Clair CG, et al. Effects of gender and age at diagnosis on disease progression in long-term survivors of cystic fibrosis. Am J Respir Crit Care Med. 2010;182(5):614–26. https://doi.org/10.1164/rccm.201001-0092OC.
83. Sawicki GS, Sellers DE, Robinson WM. High treatment burden in adults with cystic fibrosis: challenges to disease self-management. J Cyst Fibros. 2009;8(2):91–6. https://doi.org/10.1016/j.jcf.2008.09.007.
84. Cleveland RH, Lee EY. Pediatric interstitial (diffuse) lung disease. Imag Pediatr Pulmonol. 2019(September):145–97.
85. Panitch HB. Respiratory implications of pediatric neuromuscular disease. Respir Care. 2017;62(6):826–48. https://doi.org/10.4187/respcare.05250.
86. Ivy D. Pulmonary hypertension in children. Cardiol Clin. 2016;34(3):451–72. https://doi.org/10.1016/j.ccl.2016.04.005.
87. Michael Z, Spyropoulos F, Ghanta S, Christou H. Bronchopulmonary dysplasia: an update of current pharmacologic therapies and new approaches. Clin Med Insights Pediatr. 2018;12:1179556518817322. https://doi.org/10.1177/1179556518817322.
88. Quittner AL, Goldbeck L, Abbott J, Duff A, Lambrecht P, Solé A, et al. Prevalence of depression and anxiety in patients with cystic fibrosis and parent caregivers: results of The International Depression Epidemiological Study across nine countries. Thorax. 2014;69(12):1090–7. https://doi.org/10.1136/thoraxjnl-2014-205983.
89. Willis LD. Transition from pediatric to adult care for young adults with chronic respiratory disease. Respir Care. 2020;65(12):1916–22. https://doi.org/10.4187/respcare.08260.
90. Chambers DC, Cherikh WS, Harhay MO, Hayes D, Hsich E, Khush KK, et al. The International Thoracic Organ Transplant Registry of the International Society for Heart and Lung Transplantation: thirty-sixth adult lung and heart-lung transplantation Report-2019; Focus theme: donor and recipient size match. J Heart Lung Transplant. 2019;38(10):1042–55. https://doi.org/10.1016/j.healun.2019.08.001.
91. Kulkarni HS, Cherikh WS, Chambers DC, Garcia VC, Hachem RR, Kreisel D, et al. Bronchiolitis obliterans syndrome-free survival after lung transplantation: an International Society for Heart and Lung Transplantation Thoracic Transplant Registry analysis. J Heart Lung Transplant. 2019;38(1):5–16. https://doi.org/10.1016/j.healun.2018.09.016.

# Chapter 3
# Inadequate Palliative Care in Lung Disease

**Matthias Villalobos and Michael Kreuter**

Chronic lung disease affects millions of individuals, their relatives, and the respective healthcare services worldwide with steadily increasing prevalence. Patients are living longer but nonetheless suffering from a high and complex symptom burden that comprises physical, psychosocial, and spiritual needs. Various guidelines recommend the integration of palliative care in the disease trajectory. Still, numerous barriers hinder the adequate provision of this specialized care in chronic lung disease. The goal of this chapter is to highlight these barriers to understand what is needed to improve the provision of palliative care for patients with lung disease. To deliver a comprehensive view on these barriers, all relevant levels (patient and family caregiver/healthcare professionals/healthcare system) will be addressed.

## Barriers to Communication: Telling the Truth

"…Is palliative care not solely a euphemism for dying soon…."

"…I do not want to be labelled as a doomed man – that's why I do not like to be sent to palliative care…."

"…I fear it to some extent because I don't know exactly what it means…."

M. Villalobos (✉)
Department of Thoracic Oncology, Thoraxklinik, University Hospital of Heidelberg, Translational Lung Research Center Heidelberg (TLRC-H), German Center for Lung Research (DZL), Heidelberg, Germany
e-mail: matthias.villalobos@med.uni-heidelberg.de

M. Kreuter
Center for Interstitial and Rare Lung Diseases, Pneumology and Respiratory Critical Care Medicine, Thoraxklinik, University Hospital of Heidelberg, German Center for Lung Research (DZL), Heidelberg, Germany
e-mail: kreuter@uni-heidelberg.de



K. O. Lindell, S. K. Danoff (eds.), *Palliative Care in Lung Disease*, Respiratory Medicine, https://doi.org/10.1007/978-3-030-81788-6_3

"...I would appreciate if somebody would talk to me about it...."

These statements of patients affected by advanced lung disease [38] illustrate the challenges of communicating what palliative care means and does. Good communication is of central importance and additionally one of the most complex tasks in palliative care. Most barriers for the adequate provision and integration relate to the lack of the necessary communication skills when it comes to telling the truth to those affected with advanced disease. An antiquated but still existent perception of the patient-physician relationship is that of a protective and omniscient doctor who decides by him-/herself what might be the best medical choice for the patient by even deliberately withholding the truth. In the last decades, the patient's wish for truthful information and consequently the emphasis on patient involvement and shared decision-making has grown steadily. Patients have a right to information and clinicians should support and respect their autonomy to make their own choices. Different preferences in regard to the patient's cultural, religious, and social background should be included in the approach [56]. To adequately address these issues, professionals have to be highly skilled communicators.

During the course of chronic lung disease, shared decision-making between physician and patient on different interventions with a potential for temporary benefit but not cure is challenging [48]. Patients' hope for improvement while being confronted with possible deterioration and worst-case scenarios including end-of-life decision-making constitutes a continuous and strenuously challenging balancing act for the clinician. In this context, breaking bad news is considered to be one of the most difficult tasks, and most physicians find it stressful [52] as they feel poorly prepared [9]. Clinicians often fear that telling the truth may destroy hope in the patient or that discussing palliative care may even lead to the feeling of being abandoned. On the contrary, studies demonstrate that patients want open and honest discussions and that these do not affect hope [29]. As medical training still focusses on restorative and curative therapies, many clinicians lack the skills to talk about palliative therapy goals and feel uncomfortable with it. This reluctance may be perceived by patients with chronic lung disease as frustrating because issues concerning advance care planning (ACP) and other patient-centered goals are left unaddressed [5, 53].

Disclosure of prognosis plays a central role when breaking bad news in advanced disease. Most of the evidence and experience about prognosis communication were developed in cancer care. The setting is much more uncertain in nonmalignant diseases [6]. Over the years, several oncological studies have led to the development of prognostic models that help to predict survival time [49]. For sure, accurate prognostication is much more challenging in chronic lung disease. This can be illustrated by results from the SUPPORT (Study to Understand Prognoses and Preferences for Outcomes and Risks of Treatments) study. Using the available data, prognostic model calculation for lung cancer patients showed a median 6-month survival estimate of 20% in the last week before death that declined to nearly 0% on the day before. COPD patients, however, had median 6-month survival estimates of 40% or more in 5 of the last 7 days before death [16]. Because of this uncertainty and inaccuracy in predicting prognosis, it is understandable that fewer patients are referred in time to a palliative care service particularly as long as clinicians equate palliative care with end-of-life care [10]. The uncertainty that clinicians feel because of insufficient knowledge or awareness has to be differentiated from the uncertainty that is inherent to the context of prognostication. This may complicate the decision-making process, too.

Shared decision-making and associated tools such as decision aids can help patients and healthcare providers to better deal with this uncertainty. It enables patients to orient themselves in the available evidence and decision options. Ideally the process integrates their values and preferences. Decision aids, for example, specifically developed fact boxes, may be helpful to support risk literacy. But nonetheless, residual uncertainty may persist and it should be addressed and coped with. As wishes and preferences may vary over time, patients and clinicians should continuously revisit options if information and circumstances change. Goals of care should be adapted respectively [8].

Ideally, the decision-making process should be started early in the course of disease or even before becoming ill. This is the goal of advance care planning. Unfortunately, most patients with chronic lung disease report that their doctors have not discussed advance directives or end-of-life care with them [18, 53]. Nonetheless, patients with interstitial lung disease (ILD), including idiopathic pulmonary fibrosis, report a desire to engage in these discussions, but this wish is generally unmet [5]. The European Association for Palliative Care (EAPC) defined that "advance care planning enables individuals to define goals and preferences for future medical treatment and care, to discuss these goals and preferences with family and healthcare providers, and to record and review these preferences if appropriate" [47]. In an extended definition, it underlines the importance of identifying values and reflecting upon the possible consequences of scenarios of serious illness and deterioration. ACP must be understood as a complex communication process that includes personal reflection and discussion with relatives and clinicians about values, preferences, and wishes. The focus should be broader than the physical domain alone, including concerns across psychological, social, and spiritual domains. Consequently, ACP represents more than the sole completion of an advance care directive, even if this is for certain one of the goals in the process. An individualized approach is recommended that adapts to the patient's willingness and pace, always respecting and tailoring the strategy to whether or not the patient wants to engage in these discussions. Additionally, ACP should be adapted to local legal and cultural circumstances. By this means, ACP can improve the quality of patient-physician communication, reduce aggressive care at the end of life, increase the use of palliative care, and strengthen goal-concordant care [11].

In summary, high-quality communication plays a fundamental role in supporting, coping, and adapting to the realities of illness throughout the whole course of disease. Continuous communication about prognosis, preferences, and individual goals of care is vital to foster advance care planning and timely integration of palliative care. A continuous adaptation to the patient's and relatives' pace and coping strategies is necessary. If clinicians engage in open and empathetic discussions and train for needed communication skills, they may support hope even when giving honest information. To discuss patient-centered goals may help offering palliative care that exactly meets those goals while continuing to provide medically appropriate restorative therapies [31, 41].

## Barriers to Adequate Medical Treatment: The Opioid Myth

Symptom control is one of the pillars of palliative care. It is important to mention that the indication for medical treatment may occur at different stages of serious illness irrespective of diagnosis and prognosis [37]. The research and implementation of palliative symptom control has mainly focused on oncological patients. But even in cancer care, not all patients receive the appropriate medical treatment. Despite advances, in patients with other conditions including chronic lung disease, implementation is largely behind. Patients with chronic lung disease often experience higher symptom burden and worse quality of life compared to patients with cancer [61]. Thus, the palliative care needs of patients with chronic lung disease are frequently unmet [40, 50]. In COPD those needs increase over time as the disease advances. Exacerbations occur more and more frequently and often unpredictably. This is frightening and often accompanied with helplessness. The functional decline progresses and along with it the social isolation. The central symptom is breathlessness that often is poorly controlled because of its complexity and association with fear or even panic attacks that may evolve into a vicious circle. Several studies support the use of opioids for relieving dyspnea in advanced COPD. Still, surveys suggest that there is significant reluctance in physicians to using opioids for other than terminal stages or even then. Also in patients the mention of opioids is often received with rejection due to unfounded fears of addiction or associations with dying [59]. When asking clinicians about barriers to prescription, they acknowledge that opioid therapy might be beneficial, but they also describe discomfort because of insufficient knowledge and lack of appropriate training. Professionals often worry about providing opioids as well as benzodiazepines because of fear of respiratory depression or addiction. Studies confirm just the opposite. Systematic reviews of randomized trials conclude that low-dose opioids are safe and effective in patients with advanced COPD for decreasing refractory dyspnea and improving quality of life [44]. The concerns that many clinicians have could not be confirmed as there was no increase in adverse events, such as respiratory depression or death. Even studies evaluating palliative sedation show mostly no evidence of hastening death when using opioids adequately [15, 58]. Despite this data, clinicians remain hesitant to prescribe these drugs [1]. As an avoidable consequence, patients with chronic lung disease unjustly suffer from burdensome symptoms as breathlessness, cough, pain, and anxiety.

## Barriers to Coordination and Continuity of Care: Working in Multidisciplinary Settings

The care of patients suffering from chronic lung disease is complex, and the majority of patients are exposed to multiple healthcare providers and multidisciplinary settings hazarding the continuum of care. Particularly in those patients with advanced disease, the disruptive provision of care should be avoided.

A central element in the provision of palliative care is interprofessional collaboration. Oncological studies incorporating interprofessional involvement (notably physicians and nurses) showed more consistent results regarding the positive effects of early integration of palliative care [30]. Reasons for this may arise from the different perspectives of the involved professions toward care needs and goals. Thus, healthcare delivery may be enriched and become more holistic. But interprofessional collaboration remains challenging. Differences between healthcare professions include organizational, procedural, and relational factors. These differences may evolve from educational aspects including the socialization process. It is important to consider that there exist even different "cultures" in each profession that include values, beliefs, attitudes, and, even, jargon. Other influential factors involve gender and social class issues, and also historic factors. But, as in all cultural aspects, it is important to state that these are not static but may change flexibly over time. In current practice we observe that these differences may even be reinforced through the increasing specialization as this leads to more profound immersion in the own professions' culture, strengthening common beliefs and attitudes. All these aspects may challenge or even hinder effective interprofessional collaboration. To overcome these barriers, innovative educational strategies have implemented interprofessional modules early in the training of healthcare providers [26]. Various aspects of professional practice may facilitate good interprofessional collaboration in a multidisciplinary setting: a transparent communication network between service providers (e.g., by sharing common electronic documentation platforms) and regular team meetings, including voluntary agencies and family caregivers in the communication network, having a key individual (keyworker) to facilitate continuity and coordination of care to reduce fragmentation [3, 17]. Specialized nurses may play this very central role as keyworkers in continuity and navigation through the healthcare system and the illness trajectory. Although evidence is still limited, for COPD several studies suggest that nurse-led interventions may have a beneficial impact on health and quality of life of patients [25].

When addressing continuity in care, it is important to understand the most likely illness trajectories as they differ between oncological and non-oncological diseases [43]. This understanding helps to improve the patient-clinician relationship as it is an important basis for honest communication. When patients suffering from advanced disease and their relatives ask about prognosis, the best approach is offering to talk about best- and worst-case scenarios. This includes possible patterns of decline as this is often an unspoken question. Helping to foresee probable complications allows a more realistic understanding of the situation and facilitates advance care planning and end-of-life decision-making. It also ensures timely integration of other health and social service providers and earlier detection of probable needs. To have this knowledge may help patients and their relatives to be in better control of their situation and to empower them to deal with its demands. The wish of dying at home that is expressed by the vast majority of patients may then be discussed earlier in the course of disease [39, 60]. This allows better preparation and improves, as in other aspects of care, the concordance of care with patients' goals. As important as it is for professionals to keep in mind the disease-specific trajectories, flexibility and regular review is necessary. The addressed trajectories relate to the physical condition. Other trajectories may exist regarding psychosocial or spiritual dimensions. Spiritual well-being may be affected at different times of disease unrelated to physical symptoms. This may differ between cancer and nonmalignant disease but, of course, also individually. Nonetheless, strong similarities exist during the dying phase of patients with cancer and those with chronic lung disease.

## Internal Barriers: Recognizing Stigma

Stigmatization in patients with chronic lung disease may happen in different ways. Most prominently, smoking as a well-known risk factor and the visibility of anti-smoking campaigns can lead to a sense of guilt. Patients with a smoking-related disease as COPD and lung cancer often realize this stigma and feel responsible for being affected. In addition to this self-blame, they may be actively confronted with the blame assigned by others. Feeling and being stigmatized may affect COPD patients significantly, contributing to their social isolation (including job-related discrimination), depression, and loss of quality of life. Another factor that can aggravate the isolation is the fear of embarrassment. In everyday social life, COPD patients may feel ashamed because of productive and disruptive coughing and attacks of breathlessness. They may even identify their disease as a dirty one. Also someone nearby witnessing this behavior may feel uncomfortable leading to more negative social reactions and burden. Other visual triggers for stigmatization are inhalers and supplement oxygen that identify the individual immediately as someone affected by the disease. As a consequence patients start to withdraw from social activities to avoid unpleasant situations. In turn, this leads to further adverse emotional reactions, such as loss of self-esteem and feelings of uselessness. Mood disturbances like depression and anxiety often associated with COPD may in part result in withdrawing from social life. As this situation includes self-blaming, patients may be more reluctant than others to ask for help, not wanting to burden others. Unfortunately, relatives and strangers may feel irritated or even repulsed by symptoms like coughing and breathlessness, distancing from the affected. As COPD may be seen as a self-imposed disease [55], they may even feel little sympathy and less impulse of helping. The patients' reluctance to ask for help may include the assistance offered from health and social care services. But also here stigma influences the relationship. Healthcare providers know the association between COPD and smoking, which possibly affects their responses to the patient. Some may even feel negative reactions that can have major implications for the patient's care [7].

As a consequence of this stigmatization by healthcare providers and the implicit bias, palliative care may not be adequately offered and integrated in the care of patients with smoking-related chronic lung disease as COPD. The bias may not be openly expressed. Nonetheless, it can be perceived by the patient [23]. A few studies show that clinicians are less willing to offer palliative care when they know that the patient suffers from a smoking-related disease [27, 34]. The benefit of palliative care may be even questioned if the patient continues smoking. Importantly, it must be emphasized that professional treatment or its withdrawal resulting from bias is inappropriate even if not intended [33].

Healthcare systems often discriminate against patients from vulnerable populations as ethnic minorities and people from lower socioeconomic status and education. Complicating this, symptom burden is often higher in these populations [20]. A significant proportion of COPD patients are socioeconomically disadvantaged and have lower levels of education. If healthcare providers and patients differ in their system of values, this may lead to inconsistencies and unfairness in allocation and delivery of care [57]. In the worst case, these inconsistencies may even be related, conscious or unconsciously, to prejudice and discrimination toward a vulnerable group that is already underserved. Clinicians should be aware of this bias and offer palliative care equally to patients with smoking-related chronic lung disease and refrain from interjecting personal values if the patient continues smoking. Further, they should acknowledge that this patient population is affected by discrimination or bias because of their smoking history even if it is unintentionally.

## Barriers to Implementation: Talking About Education and Policy

Lack of knowledge and lack of expertise among healthcare providers about how to recognize a patient in need of palliative care and how to engage in the corresponding discussions are important barriers in the provision of this care. The widespread misconception that palliative care equals end-of-life care and, thus, should only be offered to terminal patients hinders the provision of this specialized care to patients with chronic lung disease [36]. Despite advances in training, many clinicians caring for patients with chronic lung disease still lack the knowledge and communication skills to effectively offer palliative care when referral is appropriate. When analyzing the factors that contribute to this deficit, medical education plays a pivotal role. Still, training focuses mainly on restorative and curative therapies despite improvements in the medical curricula [24]. Consequently, physicians feel poorly prepared in the communication skills necessary for aspects of palliative care such as breaking bad news. Published communication models like SPIKES deliver a framework and have been successfully incorporated into the medical curriculum [4]. Still, learned communication skills often fail to be transferred into practice, and limited evidence exists about the sustainability over time [42]. Various studies have shown that medical students have insufficient to no training at all in palliative care and thus do not feel confident to handle situations that involve palliative care issues. In a study that asked medicine residents, many reported that referrals to palliative care services were most commonly carried out when the patient was terminally ill as opposed to earlier in the course of disease. In addition, the most common barrier identified was discrepancies in goals of care between medical professionals and patients [35]. Another qualitative study analyzing barriers for referral to palliative care showed the need for structured education across disciplinary lines to overcome misconceptions and improve communication techniques [21]. The challenges regarding communication skills grow constantly. For example, evidence from the last years has shown the positive effects of early integration of palliative care. This leaves the clinician, on the one hand, with the additional task of addressing palliative care early in the course of disease, adding to the emotional burden of these conversations. On the other hand, the development of new treatment options in modern medicine pushes patients' expectations, putting more emotional pressure on the physician [45]. Strategies for dealing with this balancing act are still not taught sufficiently or at all, leaving the physician alone in this everyday struggle during consultations.

An additional barrier for successful implementation of palliative care services constitutes the inadequate size of trained workforce (physicians, nurses, social workers, physiotherapists, and other professions). The underrepresentation of palliative care physicians is shown by the following numbers from the USA: there are approximately 1 cardiologist for every 70 persons with a heart attack and 1 oncologist for every 140 newly diagnosed cancer patients but only 1 palliative care physician for every 1200 persons living with advanced illness. 80% of programs report that they lack funding to hire staff [2]. In addition, even when funds are available, several services complain about difficulties in recruiting adequately trained and qualified professionals.

Another barrier is the substantial challenge of identifying and referring patients appropriately and at the right time. The needs of patients are best exemplified in a survey of patients with advanced cancer. It showed that more than 60% of patients have unmet needs, primarily characterized as psychosocial/emotional or symptom-specific. This was associated with a self-perceived need for palliative care services. Many patients were open to try palliative care if it was recommended by their physicians. Still, many physicians behave passively, leaving the initiative to discuss end-of-life questions to the patient. This has the risk that important aspects of care remain unaddressed. From an ethical perspective, a proactive stance is recommended [45].

Another detected obstacle is the misconception to equate "palliative care" and "hospice care." The latter is meant for patients that have stopped disease-modifying treatment, are not expected to recover from their condition, and generally have a life expectancy of less than 6 months. This misleading association and the taboo that talking about dying represents may lead to strong distress when using the term "palliative." One study decided to analyze the effect of changing the service name from "palliative care" to "supportive care." Most providers in the study found the term "supportive care" more helpful as, in their perception, it would not reduce hope and stated that they would more likely refer a patient to a service with this name. As a result, the name change at this specific institution led to a significant increase in referrals [19]. Even if the strategy was successful, it may not seem the ultimate or only solution for the barriers related to the misconception of palliative care as related solely to dying. Adding to the uncertainty concerning what palliative care means and does, there is no consensus about which active treatment may be included in the care of patients with advanced disease. For example, some services only admit patients who have stopped all life-sustaining treatment (e.g., chemotherapy and radiation for cancer patients) and have completed advance directives, whereas others show less requirements or restrictions.

Additional economic policy-related issues also constitute a systematic barrier that hinders adequate provision of palliative care. Most of the time, healthcare payment systems reward more medical interventions and the volume of medical procedures than long-term services that are needed for people with chronic and serious illness. Complex and possibly lengthy conversations as we find in prognosis discussions, end-of-life decision-making, or goals-of-care conferences are normally not adequately paid. In most healthcare systems, technical devices and elaborate interventions are rewarded more generously than communication and person-oriented care. Consequently, lack of effective reimbursement coupled with limited time for good communication and coordination of care leaves healthcare providers with insufficient incentives to engage in effective palliative care discussions with their patients and their relatives [28].

An additional financial disparity concerns research. A report from the UK (2006–2010) showed that only 0.2% of total grants awarded by the NIH were related to palliative care research [2]. Nonetheless, in the last decade, research in palliative care has steadily increased even demonstrating that it lowers costs by goal-oriented care that improves quality of life and reduces futile interventions and medical treatment.

When analyzing institutional and political barriers that hinder the adequate access and delivery of palliative care in chronic lung disease, two major principles have to be mentioned: the principle of sufficiency and the principle of justice [13]. The principle of sufficiency demands that the delivery of palliative care should not be based on diagnosis or prognosis, but guided by medical needs. These needs demand a comprehensive approach because they comprise physical, psychosocial, and spiritual issues. This complexity is often not represented or addressed in the responsible healthcare services. As described before, the burden is often higher in patients with chronic lung disease and stretches out over longer periods of time than in patients with lung cancer [61]. Unfortunately, it is often underappreciated by healthcare professionals leading to lower quality of life because of inefficient use of services. Referrals to palliative care services are less likely than for cancer patients. This leaves several needs untreated. On the other hand, disregard of palliative care aspects fosters the use of futile, aggressive treatment even at the end of life.

Consequently, palliative symptom control is unsatisfying. Because of reluctance in the prescriptions of opioids and benzodiazepines, the adequate relief of dyspnea as a central symptom of chronic lung disease is neglected. It is also important to evaluate what happens when patients with advanced lung disease receive intensive care. One study showed that patients dying in the intensive care unit with COPD received fewer elements of palliative care on average compared to cancer patients and had longer lengths of stay [12]. Patients with COPD were more likely to receive cardiopulmonary resuscitation 1 hour before death, and patients with ILD were less likely to have documentation of pain assessment in the last days of life. Both patients with COPD and ILD were less likely to have a do-not-resuscitate order in place at the time of death and were also less likely to have documentation of discussions of prognosis. In theory, as hospital stays were in general longer, more opportunities for offering the lacking elements should have been given.

Concerning psychosocial needs, the prevalence of depression and anxiety is as high as or higher than in cancer patients. Still, patients with chronic lung disease are less frequently treated for these symptoms. The burden of family caregivers is underrepresented, too [51, 54]. Relatives from patients with breathlessness often suffer from lower quality of life leading to higher risks for their psychological health and poorer quality of patient's care. Despite increasing attention in implementing support services for family members of patients with cancer, family members of patients with chronic lung disease are more often overlooked and lack equal access to such resources [22].

It relates to the ethical principle of justice that similar cases must be treated similarly. Not offering palliative care to patients with chronic lung disease that suffer from an equal or even higher symptom burden compared to other diseases is thus ethically unjust. Unfortunately, evidence shows that palliative care is still provided unequally. Justice also concerns fairness in allocating healthcare resources [14]. Adequate palliative care is in its essence part of basic health care and should be available to everyone with medical need [32, 46]. There should be no disparities in care between patients with different diagnoses if the palliative care needs are similar. As there still is no standardized palliative care approach for patients with chronic lung disease, the care is provided inconsistently, too late, or not at all. Even if patients do not experience explicit discrimination, this inadequate implementation signals implicit rationing. To achieve equal implementation compared to patients with cancer, practice standards are necessary. Improving education and training professionals is necessary to reach the evidence-based recommendations that patients with chronic lung disease should receive palliative care as standard of care.

## In the End: A Global Perspective

Worldwide estimates show that approximately 40 million people are in need of palliative care each year, but only about 14% receive it [63]. Nearly 80% of the population in need live in low- and middle-income countries. It is to expect that these numbers will grow constantly as a result of the ageing population and the increase of noncommunicable diseases and their life expectancy. COPD plays a prominent role as the prevalence is steadily increasing and it is the third leading cause of death in 2019 [62].

One policy issue that hinders adequate provision of palliative care is in many cases the unnecessarily restrictive regulations for opioids. This contradicts international conventions on access to essential drugs. Some national health policies still do not include palliative care at all. There is still insufficient awareness about palliative care in policy-makers, healthcare providers, and the public in general. The training for professionals in palliative care is often insufficient or nonexistent. Education must deliver information about what palliative care is, including modern models of early integration. Benefits for patients but also for the healthcare system should be demonstrated. Misconceptions about palliative care, such as that it is only meant for patients with cancer or only indicated for the last weeks of life, should be actively addressed and corrected, as well as fears and prejudices concerning morphine and addiction. Special cultural, religious, and social aspects concerning beliefs about death and dying should be detected and included. Still, the implementation lags behind in many countries and regions. WHO data from 2019 show that funding for palliative care was available in 68% of countries, with only 40% of countries reporting that the services reached at least half of patients in need. Concerning the responsibility of national health policies, the WHO has included the following aspects as a minimum: "health system policies that integrate palliative care services into the structure and financing of national health-care systems at all levels of care; policies for strengthening and expanding human resources, including training of existing health professionals, embedding palliative care into the core curricula of all new health professionals, as well as educating volunteers and the public; and a medicines policy which ensures the availability of essential medicines for managing symptoms, in particular opioid analgesics for the relief of pain and respiratory distress." Further, the WHO states that "palliative care needs to be provided in accordance with the principles of universal health coverage. All people, irrespective of income, disease type or age, should have access to a nationally determined set of basic health services, including palliative care. Financial and social protection systems need to take into account the human right to palliative care for poor and marginalized population groups. A sustainable, quality and accessible palliative care system needs to be integrated into primary health care, community and home-based care, as well as supporting care providers such as family and community volunteers. Most importantly, providing palliative care should be considered an ethical duty for all health professionals."

## References

1. Ahmadi Z, Bernelid E, Currow DC, Ekström M. Prescription of opioids for breathlessness in end-stage COPD: a national population-based study. Int J Chron Obstruct Pulmon Dis. 2016;11:2651–7.
2. Aldridge MD, Hasselaar J, Garralda E, van der Eerden M, Stevenson D, McKendrick K, Centeno C, Meier DE. Education, implementation, and policy barriers to greater integration of palliative care: a literature review. Palliat Med. 2016;30:224–39.

3. Ansa BE, Zechariah S, Gates AM, Johnson SW, Heboyan V, De Leo G. Attitudes and behavior towards interprofessional collaboration among healthcare professionals in a large academic medical center. Healthcare (Basel). 2020;8(3):323.
4. Baile WF, Buckman R, Lenzi R, Glober G, Beale EA, Kudelka AP. SPIKES: a six-step protocol for delivering bad news: application to the patient with cancer. Oncologist. 2000;5(4):302–11.
5. Bajwah S, Higginson IJ, Ross JR, Wells AU, Birring SS, Riley J, Koffman J. The palliative care needs for fibrotic interstitial lung disease: a qualitative study of patients, informal care-givers and health professionals. Palliat Med. 2013;27:869–76.
6. Bellou V, Belbasis L, Konstantinidis AK, Tzoulaki I, Evangelou E. Prognostic models for outcome prediction in patients with chronic obstructive pulmonary disease: systematic review and critical appraisal. BMN. 2019;367:I5358. https://doi.org/10.1136/bmj.I5358.
7. Berger BE, Kapella MC, Larson JL. The experience of stigma in chronic obstructive pulmonary disease. West J Nurs Res. 2011;33:916–32.
8. Berger Z. Navigating the unknown: shared decision-making in the face of uncertainty. J Ge Intern Med. 2014;30:675–8.
9. Bharmal A, Morgan T, Kuhn I, Wee B, Barclay S. Palliative and end-of-life care and junior doctors': a systematic review and narrative synthesis. BMJ Support Palliat Care. 2019. https://doi.org/10.1136/bmjspcare-2019-001954.
10. Boland J, Martin J, Wells AU, Ross JR. Palliative care for people with non-malignant lung disease: a summary of current evidence and future direction. Palliat Med. 2013;27:811–6.
11. Brinkman-Stoppelenburg A, Rietjens JA, van der Heide A. The effects of advance care planning on end-of-life care: a systematic review. Palliat Med. 2014;28:1000–25.
12. Brown CE, Engelberg RA, Nielsen EL, Curtis JR. Palliative care for patients dying in the ICU with chronic lung disease compared with metastatic cancer. Ann Am Thorac Soc. 2016;13:684–9.
13. Brown CE, Jecker NS, Curtis JR. Inadequate palliative care in chronic lung disease. Ann Am Thorac Soc. 2016;13:311–6.
14. Carter D, Gordon J, Watt AM. Competing principles for allocating health care resources. J Med Philos. 2016;41(5):558–83.
15. Cherny NI, Radbruch L. European Association for Palliative Care (EAPC) recommended framework for the use of sedation in palliative care. Palliat Med. 2009;23:581–93.
16. Claessens MT, Lynn J, Zhong Z, Desbiens NA, Phillips RS, Wu AW, Harrell FE Jr, Connor AF Jr, Study to Understand Prognoses and Preferences for Outcomes and Risks of Treatments. Dying with lung cancer or chronic obstructive pulmonary disease: insights from SUPPORT. J Am Geriatr Soc. 2000;48:146–53.
17. Cowley S, Bliss J, Mathew A, Mc VG. Effective interagency and interprofessional working: facilitators and barriers. Int J Palliat Nurs. 2002;8:30–9.
18. Curtis JR, Engelberg R, Young JY, Vig LK, Reinke LF, Wenrich MD, McGrath B, McCown E, Back AL. An approach to understanding the interaction of hope and desire for explicit prognostic information among individuals with severe chronic obstructive pulmonary disease or advanced cancer. J Palliat Med. 2008;11(4):610–20.
19. Dalal S, Palla HD, Nguyen L, Chacko R, Li Z, Fadul N, Scott C, Thornton T, Coldman B, Amin Y, Bruera E. Association between a name change from palliative care to supportive care and the timing of patient referrals at comprehensive cancer center. Oncologist. 2011;16:105–11.
20. Eisner MD, Blanc PD, Omachi TA, Yelin EH, Sidney S, Katz PP, Ackerson LM, Sanchez G, Tolstykh I, Iribarren C. Socioeconomic status, race and COPD health outcomes. J Epidemiol Community Health. 2011;65:26–34.
21. Enguidanos S, Cardenas V, Wenceslao M, Hoe D, Mejia K, Lomeli S, Rahman A. Health care providers barriers to patient referral to palliative care. Am J Hosp Palliat Care. 2020. https://doi.org/10.1177/1049909120973200.
22. Figueiredo D, Gabriel R, Jacome C, Cruz J, Marques A. Caring for relatives with chronic obstructive pulmonary disease: how does the disease severity impact on family carers? Aging Ment Health. 2014;18:385–93.

23. FitzGerald C. A neglected aspect of conscience: awareness of implicit attitudes. Bioethics. 2014;28:24–32.
24. Fitzpatrick D, Heah R, Patten S, Ward H. Palliative care in undergraduate medical education – how far have we come? Am J Hosp Palliat Med. 2017;34(8):762–73.
25. Fletcher MJ, Dahl BH. Expanding nurse practice in COPD: is it key to providing high quality, effective and safe care? Prim Care Respir J. 2013;22:230–3.
26. Fox L, Onders R, Hermansen-Kobulnicky CJ, Nguyen TN, Myran L, Linn B, Hornecker J. Teaching interprofessional teamwork skills to health professional students: a scoping review. J Interprf Care. 2018;32(2):127–35.
27. Fusi-Schmidhauser T, Frogatt K, Preston N. Living with advanced chronic obstructive pulmonary disease: a qualitative interview study with patients and informal carers. COPD. 2020;17(4):410–8.
28. Herrmann A, Carey ML, Zucca AC, Boyd LA, Roberts BJ. Australian GP's perceptions of barriers and enablers to best practice palliative care: a qualitative study. BMC Palliat Care. 2019;18(1):90.
29. Holland AE, et al. Be honest and help me prepare for the future: what people with interstitial lung disease want from education in pulmonary rehabilitation. Chron Respir Dis. 2015;12(2):93–101.
30. Hui D, Bruera E. Integrating palliative care into the trajectory of cancer care. Nat Rev Clin Oncol. 2016;13:159–71.
31. Jain N, Bernacki RE. Goals of care conversations in serious illness: a practical guide. Med Clin North Am. 2020;104(3):375–89.
32. Jecker NS, Pearlman RA. An ethical framework for rationing health care. J Med Philos. 1992;17:79–96.
33. Jecker NS. Caring for "socially undesirable" patients. Camb Q Healthc Ethics 1996;5:500–10.
34. Johnson JL, Campbell AC, Bowers M, Nichol AM. Understanding the social consequences of chronic obstructive lung disease: the effects of stigma and gender. Proc Am Thorac Soc. 2007;4:680–2.
35. Kamel G, Paniagua M, Uppalapati A. Palliative care in the intensive care unit: residents well trained to provide optimal care to critically ill patients? Am J Hosp Palliat Care. 2014. https://doi.org/10.1177/1049909114536979.
36. Kavalieratos D, Mitchell EM, Carey TS, Dev S, Biddle AK, Reeve BB, Abernethy AP, Weinberger M. "Not the grim reaper service": an assessment of provider knowledge, attitudes, and perceptions regarding palliative care referral barriers in heart failure. J Am Heart Assoc. 2014;3:e000544.
37. Kelley AS, Morrison RS. Palliative care for the seriously ill. N Engl J Med. 2015;373:747–55.
38. Kreuter M, Bendstrup E, Russel A-M, Bajwah S, Lindell K, Adir Y, Brown CE, Calligaro G, Cassidy N, Corte TJ, Geissler K, Hassan AA, Johannson KA, Kairall R, Kolb M, Kondoh Y, Quadrelli S, Swigris J, Udwadia Z, Wells A, Wijsenbeek M. Palliative care in interstitial lung disease: living well. Lancet Respir Med. 2017;5:968–80.
39. Lindell K, Liang Z, Hoffman L, Rosenzweig M, Saul M, Pilewski J, Gibson K, Kaminski N. Palliative care and location of death in decedents with idiopathic pulmonary fibrosis. Chest. 2015;147(2):423–9.
40. Maddocks M, Lovell N, Booth S, Man WDC, Higginson IJ. Palliative care and management of troublesome symptoms for people with chronic obstructive pulmonary disease. Lancet. 2017;390(10098):988–1002.
41. Meehan E, Sweeney C, Folwy T, Lehane E, Kelleher AB, Hally RM, Shanagher D, Korn B, Rabbitte M, Detering KM, Cornally N. Advance care planning in COPD: guidance development for healthcare professionals. BMJ Support Palliat Care. 2019. https://doi.org/10.1136/bmjspcare-2019-002002.
42. Moore PM, Rivera Mercado S, Grez Artiques M, Lawrie TA. Communication skills training for healthcare professionals working with people who have cancer. Cochrane Database Syst Rev. 2013;3:CD003751.

43. Murray SA, Kendall M, Boyd K, Sheikh A. Illness trajectories and palliative care. BMJ. 2005;330:1007–11.
44. Nici L, Mammen MJ, Charbek E, Alexander PE, Au DH, Boyd CM, Criner GJ, Donaldson GC, Dreher M, Fan VS, Gershon AS, Han MK, Krishnan JA, Martinez FJ, Meek PM, Morgan M, Polkey MI, Puhan MA, Sadatsafavi M, Sin DD, Washko GR, Wedzicha JA, Aaron SD. Pharmacological management of chronic obstructive pulmonary disease. An official American Thoracic Society clinical practice guideline. Am J Respir Crit Care Med. 2020;201(9):e56–69.
45. Pfeil TA, Laryionava K, Reiter-Theil S, Hiddemann W, Winkler EC. What keeps oncologists from addressing palliative care early on with incurable cancer patients? An active stance seems key. Oncologist. 2015;20:56–61.
46. Quill TE, Abernethy AP. Generalist plus specialist palliative care – creating a more sustainable model. N Engl J Med. 2013;368:1173–5.
47. Rietjens JAC, Sudore RL, Connolly M, van Velden JJ, Drickamer MA, Droger M, van der Heide A, Heyland DK, Houttekier D, Janssen DJA, Orsi L, Payne S, Seymour J, Jox RJ, Korfage IJ, on behalf of the European Association for Palliative Care. Definition and recommendations for advance care planning: an international consensus supported by the European Association for Palliative Care. Lancet Oncol. 2017;18:e543–51.
48. Rocker GM, Simpson AC, Horton R. Palliative care in advanced lung disease: the challenge of integrating palliation into everyday care. Chest. 2015;148(3):801–9.
49. Salpeter SR, Malter DS, Luo EJ, Lin AY, Stuart B. Systematic review of cancer presentations with a median survival of six months or less. J Palliat Med. 2012;15:175–85.
50. Schroedl CJ, Yount SE, Szmuilowicz E, Hutchinson PJ, Rosenberg SR, Kalhan R. A qualitative study of unmet healthcare needs in chronic obstructive pulmonary disease: a potential role for specialist palliative care? Ann Am Thorac Soc. 2014;11:1433–8.
51. Shah RJ, Collard HR, Morisset J. Burden, resilience and coping in caregivers of patients with interstitial lung disease. Heart Lung J Acute Crit Care. 2018;47(3):264–8.
52. Shanafelt T, Dyrbye L. Oncologist burnout: causes, consequences, and responses. J Clin Oncol. 2012;30:1235–41.
53. Sorensen AR, Marsaa K, Prior TS, Bendstrup E. Attitude and barriers in palliative care and advance care planning in nonmalignant chronic lung disease: results from a Danish national survey. J Palliat Care. 2020;35(4):232–5. https://doi.org/10.1177/0825859720936012.
54. Strang S, Osmanovic M, Hallberg C, Strang P. Family caregivers' heavy and overloaded burden in advanced chronic obstructive pulmonary disease. J Palliat Med. 2018;21(12):1768–72.
55. Stuber J, Galea S, Link BG. Smoking and the emergence of a stigmatized social status. Soc Sci Med. 2008;67:420–30.
56. Surbone A. Telling the truth to patients with cancer: what is the truth? Lancet Oncol. 2006;7:944–50.
57. Van Boekel LC, Brouwers EP, van Weeghel J, Garretsen HF. Stigma among health professionals towards patients with substance use disorders and its consequences for health care delivery: systematic review. Drug Alcohol Depend. 2013;131:23–35.
58. Verberkt CA, van den Beuken-van Everdingen MHJ, Schols JMGA, Datla S, Dirksen CD, Johnson MJ, van Kuijk SMJ, Woulters EFM, Janssen DJA. Respiratory adverse effects of opioids for breathlessness: a systematic review and meta-analysis. Eur Respir J. 2017;50(5):1701153. https://doi.org/10.1183/13993003.01153-2017.
59. Verberkt CA, van den Beuken-van Everdingen MHJ, Wouters EFM, Janssen DJA. Attitudes of patients with chronic breathlessness towards treatment with opioids. Eur Respir J. 2020;55:1901752. https://doi.org/10.1183/13993003.01752-2019.
60. Vidal M, Rodriguez-Nunez A, Hui D, Allo J, Williams JL, Park M, Liu D, Bruera E. Place-of-death preferences among patients with cancer and family caregivers in inpatient and outpatient palliative care. BMJ Support Palliat Care. 2020. https://doi.org/10.1136/bmjspcare-2019-002019.

61. Weingaertner V, Scheve C, Gerdes V, Schwarz-Eywill M, Prenzel R, Bausewein C, Higginson IJ, Voltz R, Herich L, Simon ST, PAALiativ Project. Breathlessness, functional status, distress, and palliative care needs over time in patients with advanced chronic obstructive pulmonary disease or lung cancer: a cohort study. J Pain Symptom Manage. 2014;48(4):569–81.
62. WHO. 2020. https://www.who.int/health-topics/chronic-respiratory-diseases.
63. WHO. 2020. https://www.who.int/news-room/fact-sheets/detail/palliative-care.

# Chapter 4
# Patient-Centredness and Patient-Reported Measures (PRMs) in Palliation of Lung Disease

**Anne Marie Russell and Lesley Ann Saketkoo**

## Introduction

The use of patient-reported outcomes (PROs) – in contrast to other non-patient-focused healthcare quantifications such as operational outputs, revenue and population statistics – is long established. Florence Nightingale, over 100 years ago, suggested a simple three-point health-related outcome assessment for her patients: relieved; unrelieved; and dead [1]. Since this time, alongside a phenomenal evolution in scientific and medical technology fuelling the prevention, diagnosis and treatment

"Dr Russell is a National Institute for Health Research (NIHR) 70@70 Senior Research Fellow. The views expressed in this article are those of the author(s) and not necessarily those of the NIHR, or the Department of Health and Social Care."

A. M. Russell (✉)
University of Exeter College of Medicine and Health, Royal Devon and Exeter NHS Trust Clinical Academic Unit, Exeter, UK
e-mail: a.russell4@exeter.ac.uk

L. A. Saketkoo
New Orleans Scleroderma and Sarcoidosis Patient Care and Research Center, New Orleans, LA, USA

University Medical Center – Comprehensive Pulmonary Hypertension Center and Interstitial Lung Disease Clinic Programs, New Orleans, LA, USA

Family First Medical and Well-Being Clinics, Post-COVID (Long and Multi-system) Patient Care Center, New Orleans/Kenner, LA, USA

Delricht Research Center, New Orleans, LA, USA

Louisiana State University and Tulane University Schools of Medicine, New Orleans, LA, USA
e-mail: lsaketk@tulane.edu


K. O. Lindell, S. K. Danoff (eds.), *Palliative Care in Lung Disease*, Respiratory Medicine, https://doi.org/10.1007/978-3-030-81788-6_4

of disease and prolonged survival attempts to measure the impact of the healthcare outputs on patients' health and well-being progressed at a much slower pace.

PROs reflect one component of a patient-focused umbrella of outcomes called clinical outcome assessments (COAs), i.e. outcomes directly relevant to the patient and their condition. COAs may assess biologic changes or changes in the patient's health condition as observed by the patient, clinician or non-clinician observer. Overall, patient-centred concepts encompass the biopsychosocial perspective, both the patient and clinician being persons sharing power in decision-making, responsibility and knowledge through a therapeutic alliance [2–4] essentially driven by respect for the patient. Truly patient-centred care motivates and empowers patients with a voice and sense of control despite the burden of a life-limiting health condition.

Though 'patient-centredness', sometimes referred to as '*person*-centredness', has become a buzzword for healthcare excellence, the patient has not always been at the centre of these approaches. Despite growing efforts in science, healthcare policy and research, patient-centred models continue to struggle against a revenue-centred healthcare industry, whereby myopic analytics diminish the value and resources of patients and care team members, leaving patients vulnerable and support teams exhausted.

Beyond clinical care, patient-centred concepts have become integrated into research designs and methodological approaches, and instrument development. Enlisting patient partners, for example, in co-designing scientific studies is one such approach to enhance trial feasibility [6, 7]. In regard to research and policy-making, 'nothing about us, without us' is becoming more of a reality with the strengthening patient voice and participation [5].

Patient-centred outcomes research (PCOR), an emerging field, strives to meet these challenges in optimising patient-centred healthcare. PCOR investigates prevention, diagnostic, treatment or healthcare delivery strategies as informed by strategies that integrate patient perspectives, priorities, preferences, beliefs and values and crossed with patient-valued outcomes and long-term fiscal health.

Palliative care epitomises the values and principles of patient-centred care: palliating symptom distress, accommodating for impairment and optimising health-related quality of life (HRQoL). Palliative care demands continually refreshing our awareness and frame of reference as patients' preferences and values change in response to their changing experience of their fluctuating health condition and life circumstances. Patient-centred strategies and COAs provide tools to gauge and respond to these changes.

We offer a framework, albeit not exhaustive, for understanding, discriminating between and enhancing the meaningful selection of patient-centred strategies and assessment instruments to optimise all avenues of effort in palliative care in lung disease. These efforts might include design and development of healthcare delivery models, clinical care protocols, clinical research and implementation of responsive patient-directed care. This framework reviews a scope of various types of patient-reported measures (PRMs) that gauge diverse queries in palliative care such as outcomes, lived experience, motivation or treatment preference. Further, this chapter is designed to support the content of the subsequent chapters of this textbook.

## Patient-Centredness

The concept of patient-centredness originated in the 1960s when focus shifted towards seeing each patient as a unique human being [8] with more than their biological processes being relevant to the health equation, namely, the psychosocial context [9]. The ideal of an egalitarian clinician-patient relationship progressively became tenable [2]. Over time a greater consistency rather than divergence in defining the principles of patient-centred care [10] took hold. However, the academic=perspective emphasis of patient-centredness might shift in relation to disease-specific factors (diagnosis per se; comorbidities; disease stage; symptom intensity) or cultural, socio-economic or psychological contexts. For example, patient-centred focus in oncology is driven heavily by enhanced communication as a learnt skill [11], whereas respiratory care may initially be more directed towards symptom, treatment and general information [12].

Patient-centredness is becoming a mainstay of clinical research and an influencer of health services policy and provision. The National Health Service England (NHSE) places a strong emphasis on personalisation, coordination and enablement in healthcare [13]. In the USA, the FDA commissioned a 'Voice of the Patient' series as part of the Patient-Focused Drug Development initiative to gather patients' perspectives on their condition and on therapies potentially available to treat their condition [6, 7, 14].

Increasing value is being placed on the patient as an expert and decision-making partner. A range of instruments exist to support both patient and clinician in these processes. These are described in detail later and include patient-reported outcome measures (PROMs) that capture changes in symptoms, health status perception or HRQoL; patient-reported experience measures (PREMs) that identify patient-experienced strengths and weakness of healthcare delivery systems; patient activation or patient engagement measures (PAMs/PEMs) that identify areas where patients may need supportive intervention in self-management skills such as disease or medication knowledge and lifestyle awareness; and patient preference measures that assist in patient decision-making or support value-based health economic choices.

Patient-centredness has gathered momentum and permeates approaches to care. While there is some variance in terminology, overarching patient-centred concepts include:

- Biopsychosocial perspective
- Patient as person
- Clinician as person
- Sharing power, responsibility and knowledge
- A bi-directional therapeutic alliance [2–4]

The Picker Institute has defined eight interrelated principles essential to patient-centred care [15] which have been modified and integrated into the NHS Patient Experience Framework (Fig. 4.1).

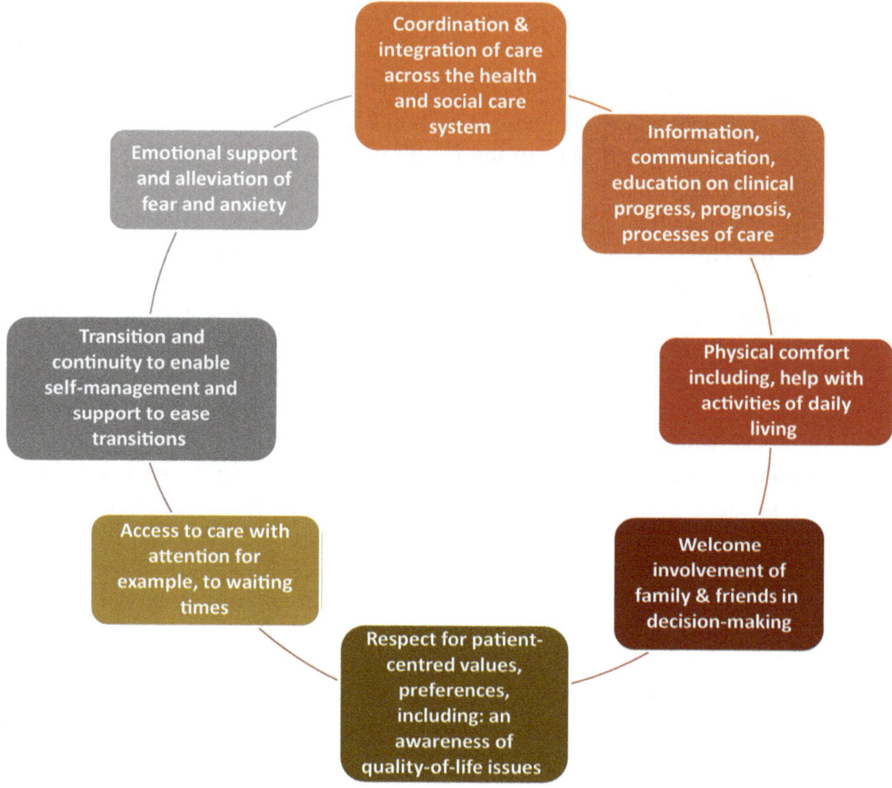


**Fig. 4.1** Interrelated principles of patient-centredness. (*Modified from the Department of Health NHS Patient Experience Framework NHS National Quality Board (NQB) 2011 Gateway reference number 17273*)

Additionally, attention to and integration of cultural and spiritual differences in care and care discussions may be a key patient-centred influencer in health outcomes [16].

## *Patient-Centred Environment*

Serious illness comes with significant baseline stress impacting health outcomes. These are fuelled by the condition itself, logistics such as travel, work absenteeism for patient/family, appointment scheduling and conflicts and health insurance challenges. Telehealth augmentation in most healthcare systems now confers the ability for home-based appointments when appropriate, offsetting a multifactorial burden on patients/family members. This also applies to integration of home-based monitoring apps and testing, e.g. home-based spirometry, oximetry and electrocardiogram [16–21].

The clinical environment can be a source of further stress or can support the patient/family in *stress reduction*. Noise, lengthy or complicated navigation of the system or buildings, crowds, unpleasant odours and lighting are environmental features that create/increase patient/family stress. Patient-centred environments are those that support logistical ease of navigation, streamline procedures and provide safe, welcoming environments with natural light and, wherever possible, physical comfort.

Colour, natural light, vegetal life, floral, herbal or woody natural fragrances and green spaces [22–26] not only make people feel happy but are repeatedly demonstrated to impact health outcomes [27–38] such as shorter hospitalisations and reduced need for postsurgical pain medications. Further improvements are seen in surgical outcomes, in-patient depression and cognition as well as hospital revenue and employee productivity [28–40]. The Center for Health Design, through the Pebbles Project, has generated data on extreme benefits in health outcomes and outputs (financial and volume), inspiring changes over the past couple decades in building construction. In parts of the USA, legislative specifications for new-build hospitals require square footage allocation for green space and natural light and a percentage of total budget for artwork preferably by local artists, as well as voluntary renovations of established healthcare facilities are redefining quality healthcare environment.

Despite many clinics and centres being housed in decades-old or even centuries-old buildings, making large changes a less likely prospect, considerate simple beautification and logistic modifications can support a patient-centred environment. Protocols for staff friendliness and helpfulness, and navigation support such as clear signposting, printed directions and available attendants can enhance the welcome of the environment.

Integrated approaches, incorporating mind-body methods (e.g. meditation, healthy diet, exercise, tai chi, yoga, singing) with conventional medical intervention, result in favourable health outcomes, contributing to a patient-centred environment and improved staff well-being. In reducing the stress response, vagus nerve activity and conditioning takes place, making it easier over time to induce a relaxation response and parasympathetic activation, which relaxes myocardium and slows heart rate, resulting in enhanced immune, cardiopulmonary, brain and even gastrointestinal responses [41–43]. Chronic stress shortens chromosomal telomeres associated with malignancy, autoimmunity and fibrosis, while integrative interventions halt and appear to increase telomere length [44–47]. Stress-relieving education provided in the clinical environment, through on-site programmes, or apprising patients of integrated opportunities for stress reduction, is a robust patient-centred strategy [41–43].

## *Patient-Centred Checklist: Assessment, Treatment and Counselling*

Checklists provide clinician support with an organised framework to improve patient comfort, safety and health outcomes while reducing patient suffering through comprehensive assessment and quality assurance measures [48–51]. The content of checklists is dependent on clinic focus and scope. A historical section of a checklist may include important diagnostic or symptom queries that might spark additional screening, assessment or interventions (e.g. as for depression or screening for sleep apnoea) or medical management considerations, (e.g. perceptions of worsening cough, medication-related nausea or diarrhoea, or extent of physical activity, or how much time is spent sitting in wheelchair prompting prevention queries regarding skin breakdown), A medication section reminds the clinician that prednisone may require stomach or bone protection depending on dose and potential duration of treatment. The prevention section of a checklist may include a review of vaccination status identifying a need for and update or further testing, e.g. annual hepatitis B or tuberculosis if on immunosuppression. Many examples of checklists are available and can be devised to fit unique patient population needs and revised over time to improve quality care.

## *Shared Decision-Making (SDM)*

Shared decision-making (SDM) offers clinicians an opportunity for power sharing within the consultation to empower the patient or their nominated informal caregiver to become the expert in their care. SDM is often eased by the use of decision aids albeit these require additional time and clinician training and an appreciation of health literacy. Attitudinal shift, an interdisciplinary team approach, patient activation, consideration of incentivisation or remuneration for healthcare providers through alignment with performance indicators and access to decision-making tools may help transition to a SDM approach [52]. Regulatory bodies offer repositories [53, 54] of decision aids to support SDM, with SDM guidelines expected in 2021 from the UK National Institute of Clinical and Healthcare Excellence (NICE) and the FDA patient-focused drug development (PFDD) unit. SDM training to achieve the 2024 targets of the NHS Long Term Plan personalised care programme is accessible through the virtual Personalised Care Institute [55].

## *Family-Centred Care*

Health conditions impact the entire family and/or those closely affiliated with the patient in an informal caring or supportive role. Caregiver research, of which the most studied in pulmonary diseases is lung cancer, is an emerging field initiated in dementia and cancer populations. Supporting the health and well-being of the caregiver directly impacts health outcomes of the patient. Family members instinctively recognise that their care influences health outcomes [6, 7, 56–60] and their responsibilities extend beyond assisting with activities of daily life (ADLs), nutritional support, medications, finances and interacting with healthcare system logistics while often living with anticipatory grief [61–66].

Caregivers across 26 health conditions were interviewed, with 92% impacted emotionally by the patient's illness owing to worry, thinking about future and patient's death (35%), frustrations (27%), anger (15%) and guilt (14%) [67]. Sleep loss occurred in 67% with 32% being worry-related and 38% to helping their loved one with personal hygiene or medication; others reported continually waking to check their loved one was still alive. Decline in caregiver health and depression were each reported at 92%. Caregiving was reported as taking a toll on daily activities (91%), family relationships (69%), work and study (52%) and finances (51%) [67].

These expressions of distress translate to detrimental health outcomes for caregivers and patients, when controlled for age, comorbidities, marital status and health condition of patient [68–77]. Iterative studies identify higher caregiver strain as leading to increased depression, stress and mortality. Mortality was increased at 63% generally and 84% at the highest levels of strain with 134% increase for cardiovascular events in caregivers over a mere 30-month period. Studies demonstrate increased caregiver depression as proportional to caregiver strain as well as increasing cardiovascular mortality [68, 69, 72–74, 78].

Identifiable predictors of caregivers at risk are baseline depressive symptoms, the perception of being overwhelmed, scoring high on the Zarit scale (a measure of caregiver strain) and scoring low on Bakis scale which assesses caregiver-perceived positive aspects of caring for a loved one. However, the introduction of targeted interventions led to significantly decreased strain, depression and adverse outcomes [78, 79]. Interventions included stress-reduction concepts as described above; education of stakeholders on anticipatory stress, strain, depression, health outcomes, resources and using protocols of assessment; empathetic communication with detailed attention to caregivers regarding time for self-care; purposeful engagement in pleasurable activities; and attention to nutrition and exercise.

Interventions to ameliorate the impact of caregiving strain are incremental and iterative in nature:

- *Screening* for depression, level of strain, and perception of being overwhelmed [79–83, 86, 87]. Simple questions expressing interest in the caregiver such as "...tell me how are *you* managing?" or noticing how the caregiver appears or behaves can provide insight. We advocate screening caregivers and patients routinely for depression and anxiety, additionally with the caregiver completing measures of strain/burden, e.g. Zarit and Bakis questionnaires.
- *Education* on screening results, health impact of caregiving strain and importance of strategies to antidote caregiver stress [84, 85]. Clear communication of the patient's health status, prognosis and shared decision-making in addressing changes that arise reduce stress for both the patient and family [86].
- *Healthcare structure and delivery* burden reduction, e.g. proactive support for respectful, whole-hearted assistance in manoeuvring logistics related to healthcare [84].
- *Advocacy* for healthcare policy that recognises the financial and physical demands of caring for a loved one, such that practical frameworks are instituted to support them, e.g. community home care, neighbourhood networking training and reimbursement strategies to provide logistical support to families [87, 88].

Planning for alone, family and/or social time each and collectively each has strong value in offsetting the effects of caregiver strain. The breadth of interventions can be programmatic/system-derived or self-created (e.g. playing musical instrument, painting or a bedtime decompression ritual) or self-elected (e.g. joining an exercise class or a support group).

## *Patient Advocacy Organisations*

Non-governmental patient organisations play an important role in engaging both patients and family members in education, research and advocacy - and often times in providing professional education. Patient organisations often raise awareness and engage patients regarding key disease transitions and areas of greatest concern to patients. A world café event, exemplifying the key influence of patient organisations, co-designed with patients and caregivers, identified that discussions on palliative care associated with fibrotic lung diseases should be included at the point of diagnosis. The Irish Lung Fibrosis Association (ILFA) recognised that approaches like world café events have potential to influence government policy to resolve persistent inadequacies in service provision. In the UK, the British Lung Foundation [89] has set out a 5-year plan to provide better care for people with lung disease. The BLF Taskforce for Lung Health includes 35 patients and healthcare professionals. Members work alongside partners in the pharmaceutical, diagnostics, device and digital industries, to improve lung health through promoting early detection, care and support with particular focus on access to care in the last year of life.

Patient organisations and support groups provide bonds and shared information on living that are beyond the abilities of a healthcare team. Patients and family members should be apprised of these opportunities that can be an important part of patient sustenance.

## *Health-Related Quality of Life (HRQoL)*

Patient-centredness in healthcare has a major influence on HRQoL (Fig. 4.2). The term health-related quality of life (HRQoL) focuses on aspects of health, which broadly encompasses psychosocial functioning alongside physical well-being, influenced by levels of impairment associated with the health condition. The term quality of life (QoL) is somewhat broader, taking into account non-health-related aspects.

Physical function, a measure of disability reflecting the degree of impairment due to symptom burden and other physical factors, is a main driver of other HRQoL components, such as mental health, fatigue, participation and work productivity [90]. HRQoL reflects the extent of ease or difficulty with which one is able to interface with their world [91] and to live a full and engaging life with loved ones and/or within the work environment.

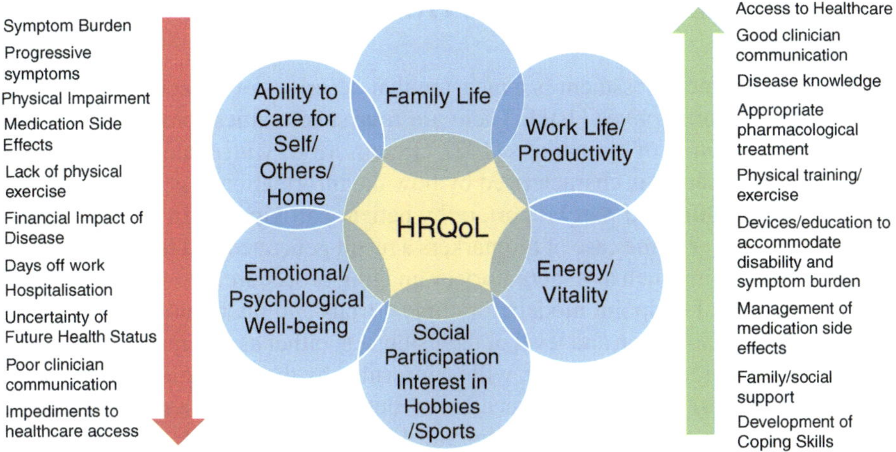


**Fig. 4.2** Core areas of HRQoL with factors that augment or diminish HRQoL. (*Courtesy of LA Saketkoo, with permission, rights reserved*)

The patient's self-assessment of HRQoL has been recognised as an important and independent prognostic factor of survival in advanced cancer and other conditions [15, 16]. HRQoL performs independently of common severity parameters used to predict survival such as tumour size, vascular events or organ damage scores. Higher HRQoL is expectedly associated with improved survival and lower HRQoL with higher mortality [92–96]. However, measurement of HRQoL may not simply be descriptive of health status, but rather facilitate actionable investigation and life-prolonging intervention. Across a spectrum of oncological diseases including lung cancer, evidence points towards the harmful effects of symptom distress on HRQoL but also on survival [92–96]. While the importance of HRQoL is recognised, the 'routine' use of PROMs in the field of lung cancer, for example, has not been widespread [97].

Implementing interventions to relieve symptom distress and increase HRQoL has been shown to extend survival. Defining modifiable elements of HRQoL and physical function portends large gains in the clinical care of respiratory and multi-organ system diseases, for example, post lung transplantation [98], and for aspects of mental health [99]. Clinicians lack the personal experience of patients' HRQoL and have been observed to consistently overestimate or underestimate patients' HRQoL scores [90]. Failure to capture the patient's perspective may result in sub-optimal or misdirected care.

Environmental factors [91, 100], including adaptive devices or aids, medications, cognitive training, anticipatory guidance and community support, are easily recognisable approaches to treat and diminish the impact of disability. Such interventions offer relief from restricting symptomatology potentially increasing patient participation in major life areas.

The subsequent chapters in this book explore HRQoL in greater depth, related to disease-specific contexts, palliative assessment and symptom management.

## Clinical Outcome Assessments: Overview

A clinical outcome assessment is a measure that describes or reflects how a patient feels, functions or survives [101]. There are four subclassifications of COAs with the potential addition of biomarkers [102], circumscribed with examples in Fig. 4.3. Each subclassification is characterised by how the information is generated, i.e. the patient, clinician or third-party report, or by patient participation in a performance-related measure, or in the case of biomarkers a result generated and reported through third-party handling such as a laboratory or imaging procedure. COAs are an important component of endpoint models for clinical trials and interventional and observational studies. Selection and level of inclusion, e.g. either as a primary, co-primary, secondary or exploratory endpoint, will be informed by the population and the intervention of interest [103]. Occurrence-based outcomes such as survival, all-cause mortality or time to clinical worsening are likely to be selected as primary endpoints, in clinical trials and observational studies [101].

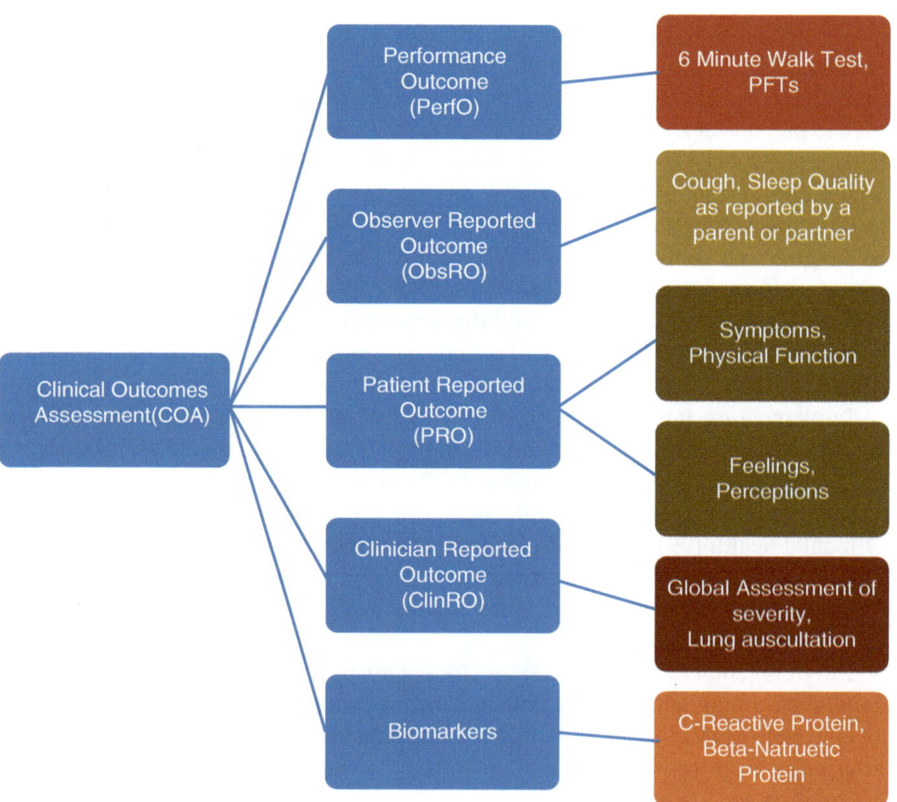


**Fig. 4.3** Framework of clinical outcomes assessments. (*Courtesy of AM Russell, with permission, rights reserved*)

A PRO is defined as a report that comes from the patient about their perceived status of their health condition without amendment, influence or interpretation by a clinician or anyone else [104]. Other patient-reported measures (PRMS) include the PREM, PEM and PAM.

Performance outcomes (PerfOs) are entirely dependent upon patient cooperation, motivation, confidence and capacity to perform procedure. An example of a PerfO is FVC, which may evoke anxiety related to thoughts of survival and associations of unpleasant after-effects such as headache or exhaustion for patients [105, 106]. These concerns justify cautious interpretation of results, consideration of the frequency with which the test is truly needed, their utility in clinical trial design and how to standardise performance experience.

Clinician-reported outcomes (ClinROs) are based on the clinicians' observation and interpretation of a physical finding, an examination, a global assessment of a patient's disease-specific or generic health status or an evaluation of the presence or absence of clinician-identified radiographic features. Observer-reported outcomes (ObsRO) are observations by someone other than the patient or clinician, such as a parent or caregiver, and do not include medical judgment or interpretation. ObsRO complements or replaces a patient's own report when the patient is unable to self-report. ObsRO is often employed in learning disability, complex mental ill health (e.g. dementia) and paediatrics [101] but can also inform adult screening, such as for obstructive sleep apnoea, when querying family members about breathing cessation during sleep, or querying change of exercise capacity in lung disease by family members' report of decelerating walking speed to accommodate the patient.

Biomarkers, debatably considered ClinROs, are objective measures evaluated as potential indicators of abnormal biological or pathogenic processes, or pharmacologic responses to an intervention. Examples include serological markers such as CRP for inflammation, BNP for myocardial strain or radiological assessment for change in tumour size or extent of UIP on HRCT.

## *COA Selection: Strategies and Measures*

The Patient-Reported Outcomes and Quality of Life Instruments Database (PROQOLID™) Mapi Research Trust created in 2002 holds ≥2300 clinical outcome assessments (COAs) that measure QoL, health status and symptoms across all therapeutic areas.[1] Selecting the most appropriate measure can be an overwhelming prospect. Careful consideration of what is to be measured, i.e. the 'concept of interest' (COI) is key to appropriate selection. Examination of a COA's content validity, reliability, ability to accurately discriminate and, if warranted, ability to demonstrate change over

[1] The PROQOLID™ database is supplied with new instruments through recommended sources such as FDA, the EMA and the research community. PROQOLID™ is accessible at https://eprovide.mapi-trust.org/.

time should also guide selection. Another essential consideration is feasibility, e.g. the degree to which the assessment is costly, safe, accessible and interpretable.

An example might be a COA measuring gait speed (e.g. 6MWT) as the primary endpoint in a drug study for pulmonary hypertension (PH) related to systemic sclerosis. There is strong argument that a COA such as time to clinical worsening (TTCW) (e.g. hospitalisation due to PH, drastic reduction in haemodynamics, new or increased need for oxygen supplementation) will more accurately reflect changes related to the actual COI, as the gait speed in this population tends to have multiple confounders such as musculoskeletal impairments and myopathy that would also factor into the outcome that resulted.

## *Operationalising Patient-Centredness*

Tools or instruments that measure and trend a patient's health experience can be of meaningful use to patients and a strong source of support to the clinician in three overarching areas:

(a) For *detection-intervention* to disclose areas requiring medical or other intervention in regard to patient health or environment, e.g. depression screening, severity scores, clinician checklists
(b) For appreciation of trends in *symptom-tracking* and other patient measures over time in conjunction with traditional markers and historical patient events, e.g. hospitalisation, exacerbations, antibiotic/steroid use
(c) To assist *patient-clinician discussion* whereby a patient might have the opportunity to comment first on why they believe a score has changed and the clinician then has opportunity to offer additional perspective and contributions from a clinical perspective [107]

Tracking symptom, functional or HRQoL scores enables patients and clinicians to identify trends that might lead up to recurrent complications, and provides an opportunity for patients and clinicians to recognise signals to inform anticipatory guidance. Thus tracking can be of meaningful use in alerting to signs and symptom changes that predict poor outcomes, e.g. hospitalisation, emergency visit, etc., and in developing strategies to prevent or ameliorate future complications through earlier intervention [16, 108–110].

Often, it is easy to overlook the propensity for psychological, emotional, physical and intellectual exhaustion for the dedicated clinician [111]. Patient-centred scores can provide the framework to help offset the intellectual and emotional investment of initiating and carrying difficult discussions such as those regarding important or milestone health changes e.g. transitioning to hospice care or lung transplantation assessment. Further, patient preference tools can guide the clinician in respectfully supporting the patient in expressing their treatment preferences:

- Providing important data on acceptability and capacity for compliance
- Ensuring the impact of treatment is not in fact worse than the disease itself

- Ensuring adequate preparation of the patient
- Enabling proactive and appropriate management of side effects
- Facilitating informed choice regarding therapy

A combination of the above utilities allows discussion for the clinician to explore patient and caregiver values, beliefs and expectations. It establishes a deep respect for patients and caregivers as care team partners and for their contributions as carrying valuable insights into cause and possible remedies of a developing clinical health challenge.

## Developing Patient-Reported Measures (PRMs)

Development and selection of PRMs requires critical rigour and appraisal. The FDA guidelines [104] provide a template for instrument development albeit not prescriptive in methodological detail. Additional resources [90] offer more detailed guidance on potential methodological approaches to PRM development. Adherence to and clear, transparent documentation of adherence to robust patient-centred methodology [112] are an essential component of measure development. A comprehensive literature review along with consultation with key stakeholders initiates determination of whether existing measures satisfy the assessment needs in question [113].

Population and circumstantial considerations for which the PRM is being developed influence subsequent utility (e.g. sensitivity to change, or content validity), for example, clinical trial populations may have less impaired physiological parameters than those on a palliative care pathway.

Qualitative approaches, such as interviews and focus groups, inform the content and language of a conceptual framework that give rise to question items or other instrument content. The term *mixed methods* refers to the utilisation of diverse methods of data acquisition or confirmation that usually converges to a final product/instrument. These may be mixed qualitative methods such as focus groups for content followed by stakeholder working groups and survey approaches to develop perhaps a narrative-based decision-making tool or by using combined qualitative and quantitative methods. An example might be a PRM developed with content and language obtained from focus groups, followed by concept ranking by stakeholders or statistical modelling of responses after question-item development. After appropriate field testing with stakeholders, psychometric analyses ensure systematic item reduction using classical test theory, confirmatory *factor analysis* or *item response theory such as Rasch analysis as a model of logistic regression*. Repeatability and responsiveness testing are conducted prior to longitudinal validity assessments [90, 113].

PRMs can also uniquely created by individual patients listing concepts most important to them (e.g. activity performance, symptom, healthcare experience) with a pre-determined response scale (e.g. VAS, Likert, etc.) for each item. Patients rate their current perception of each item on the response scale. These scores are tracked over time. Several widely utilised measures exist including the Patient-Specific Functional Scale (PSFS) [114] and the MACTAR [115].

## *Selecting Patient-Reported Measures (PRMs)*

In clinical practice and research, the choice of PRM is informed by an a priori hypothesis of how an intervention may impact patients, as informed by the best available evidence [116]. Outcome, motivation and experience measures are selected for the domains desired to be measured, in relation to the population and/or therapeutic area of interest. Familiarity, personal preference or historical reasons [117] are pitfalls in optimal PRM selection and surpassed by robust understanding, comparison and scrutiny for the best possible PRM for the circumstances. Practical issues, such as validated translations, copyrights and access to instruments, influence their selection [118].

PRMs may be symptom-specific or condition-specific. Condition-specific PRMs are generally expected to capture relevant details of the specific condition [119]. However, disease-specific PRMs often lack generalisability for comparisons across health conditions, thus supporting the value and complementary approach of using both a condition-specific and a generic PRM.

Several frameworks guide the selection of PROMs which also have utility in PREMs, PEMs and PAMs referred to collectively as PRMs. FDA guidelines determine the criteria that must be met to support labelling claims [104]; the Consensus-Based Standards for the Selection of Health Measurement Instruments (COSMIN) checklist assesses the psychometric properties of measures to determine methodological quality (Fig. 4.4: 120). These include a checklist for reliability, responsiveness and validity. Reliability connotes consistently reproducible measurements repeated over time in a defined population under stable conditions. Responsiveness refers to a PRM's ability to detect change over time in the domain(s) of interest [120].

The first level of validity are *content* and *face* validities representing patient-centred concepts generated through qualitative or mixed-methods approaches, i.e. the degree to which the content is truthful and makes sense. *Criterion validity* reflects the extent to which the PRM scores adequately compare against the 'gold standard' of measurement, e.g. a breathlesness measure (PRM) that repeatedly reflects change in pulmonary hypertension when compared with right heart catheterisation haemodynamic (gold standard), while *construct validity* assesses the degree to which the PRM correlates with scores of other 'non-gold-standard' instruments commonly used to measure the domain. *Cross-cultural validity* measures differences between relevant groups and/or is aligned with robust translation or cultural adaptation protocols [120]. All versions developed (including language adaptations) must be of good quality [121] with processes of modifications reported transparently.

The Consensus-Based Standards for the Health Measurement Instruments Outcome Measures in Effectiveness Trials (COMET) offer guidelines for selecting or administering and integrating PRMs into an endpoint model [122]. This checklist includes the following:

- Define the purpose and goals for collecting PRMs.
- In clinical research, ensure the endpoints are complementary to the concept of the study.
- Determine the resources that are available and what resources might be needed.
- Identify key barriers and consider appropriate solutions.

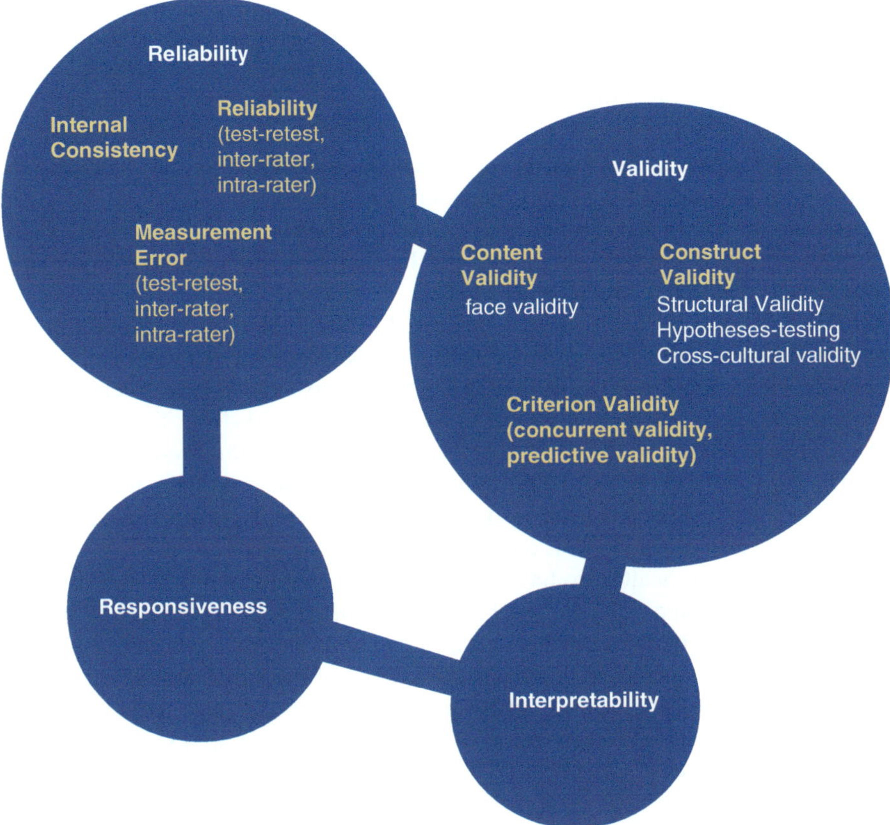


**Fig. 4.4** Interrelated core components for the development and evaluation of outcome measures. (*Adapted from the COSMIN Taxonomy Measurement of Properties*)

- Consider the heterogeneity of the groups of patients to be assessed and applicability of the selected PRMs.
- Determine how frequently patients should complete the PRM.
- Determine a consistent approach to administering PRMs.
- Consider if the scoring system is clear, available, easy to use and interpret and able to define a meaningful change.
- Determine how the analysis will be done and how the results will be presented.

## *Training in Administering Patient-Reported Measures*

Familiarity with PRMs is increasing for patients and clinicians [123–126]. Clarity and shared responsibility give rise to more meaningful interactions during PRM completion [127] or in context of an established trusting relationship [128]. The practice of precision medicine enables healthcare, treatments, practices or products to be specifically tailored to patient subgroups. PRM success is reliant upon meaningful selection and represents what is important to patients in their lived experiences. Patients rely on clinicians for clarity on the intent and interpretation of PRM scoring on both individual and population levels. PRM success requires a commitment to appropriate administration and sufficient thought and time for completion. Training programmes in oncology, paediatrics and lung transplantation [129] and generically through NHS Digital [130] have promoted global learning on PRM implementation. Guidelines also developed by ISOQOL further support clinicians, patients and researchers in PRM use [131].

PRM self-reflection can support patients to raise important discussion points with the clinician. PRM-driven self-reflection in palliative care enables patient stories to be told in their own words [107, 132] and clearly supports identification of or confers 'permission' to raise what matters to the patient [133–135]. Treatments may be selected according to PRMs of HRQoL in accordance with physiologic disease severity data that is relevant to the individual. If treatment options are similar in overall survival (OS) or progression-free survival (PFS) outcome measures, patients could base decisions on HRQoL outcome measures/data sets.

Digitalisation of healthcare has enabled the electronic administration of PRMs with cumulative mapping to Hospital Episode Statistics (HES) [136]. Data storage protocols are adapted from pre-existing biobanking and demographic registries. However, digital engagement is fraught with levels of inequity and potential disenfranchisement. Patients' level of activation/engagement, digital literacy, internet access, health status and personal preferences are considerations impacting the capacity for digital engagement.

## Types of Patient-Reported Measures

### *Patient Motivation/Engagement Measures*

PAMs or PEMs assess a person's inclination and ability to manage their own health and help to identify patients that are disengaged or overwhelmed and needing support [137, 138], as well as changing needs for support, e.g. improved awareness but still struggling or sufficiently active and engaged. Supportive interventions are adjusted according to the activation/engagement level, with the potential to improve health behaviour, health outcomes and experiences of care and reduce unplanned or emergency care.

Clinician presumptions overestimating patients' self-management capacity often deter a patient's admission to difficulties with health engagement. For example, the patient with caregiver responsibilities or with undisclosed learning disabilities may have suboptimal self-management, while increased support or education could increase patient activation. Conversely, hypervigilance regarding one's health can be identified with reassurance or confirmation to ameliorate anxiety regarding adequacy of their engagement.

The patient activation measure (PAM), a short 13-item scale comprising cognitive and behavioural components of patients' attitude towards their health, characterises patients' incremental preparedness and capacity to contribute to their health management [139]. The patient engagement measure (PEM) conceptualises conjoint cognitive (thinking), emotional (feeling) and conative (impetus to act) enactment in relation to one's health. The Patient Health Engagement Scale contains five ordinal items [140]. The Caregiving Health Engagement scale (CHE-s) is one instrument designed to identify specific areas for psychosocial support for caregivers [141]. PEMs can be concept specific such as the four-item Morisky Medication Adherence Scale (MMAS-4) [142] addressing barriers to medication-taking to support positive adherence behaviours.

## *Patient-Reported Experience Measures (PREMs)*

Patient-reported experience of healthcare services is an essential determinant and vital source of information for quality improvement [143]. PREMs provide standardised comparative information to monitor and measure service performance at local national and international levels [144]. PREMs provide value to clinicians through improved operations; to administrators through quality assurance and performance ratings; to health economists through evaluation of contracts and pay-for-performance schemes; to managers through performance assessment; to governments and the public for accountability purposes; and most importantly to patients for making informed decisions about their care. Used in conjunction with PROMs, PEMs and PAMs, they inform individual personalised health and care plans.

Patient experience can be assessed by generic or condition-specific PREMs. Conditon-specific PREMS for respiratory conditions are limited. The Commissioning for Quality in Rheumatoid Arthritis (CQRA) developed a PREM for RA [145] whose reliable and validated eight-domain RA-PREM maps to the eight domains of the NHS Patient Experience Framework (NPEF). The COPD patient-reported experience measure (PREM-C9) [146] addresses mild to severe disease, but does not map succinctly to the eight domains of the NPEF; and to date no large-scale validation studies are reported.

Hybrid measures such as the Consultation and Relational Empathy (CARE) patient-centred measure capture patient experience of clinician empathy. Its design is close in concept to the PREM model enabling an evaluation of the therapeutic relationship in the palliative care consultation [147].

Patient-reported experience data is a component in the healthcare quality frameworks of the US (US) Agency for Healthcare Research and Quality (AHRQ) and the Organisation for Economic Co-operation and Development (OECD), and in most countries of the developed world. Despite the ratification of a European patient charter [148], inequities in respiratory care persist across Europe [149]. Integrating translated and validated PREMS offers one approach to highlight such inequities, standardising and improving care.

## *Patient-Reported Outcome Measures (PROMs)*

PROMs capture the patients' own assessment of their health, symptom burden or health-related quality of life (HRQoL) and may be generic or condition-specific [150]. They are useful in clinical trials of treatment with palliative intent, often as a primary endpoint to quantify symptom relief, care or rehabilitation. Scales produce a score or grade which quantifies subjective qualitative and experiential information [121, 130] shifting focus from the 'quantity' of life gained to the 'quality' dimension, or the quantification of quality. For people living longer with long-term conditions and multi-morbidities, the 'quality' dimension is increasingly important as an outcome.

Perhaps due to overwhelming choice, lack of awareness or difficulties in access, there has been significant variance in the selection of validated PROMs in practice. For example, the European Society of Thoracic Surgeons reported 88% of all surgeons do not incorporate standardised PROMs into their clinical practice [151]. In cystic fibrosis a systematic review of PROs identified 27 PROMs in use predominantly disease-specific, across a variety of settings to assess the impact of physical, psychological, social or demographic variables on HRQoL [152]. It is reported that to alleviate distress some clinicians avoid using PROMs while others omit or adapt item content ineviatably impacting scores and interpretation [153] and others may administer PROMs but disconnect the information from the patient, overlooking opportunities to address important patient-centered issues.

In clinical practice the use of PROMs is now mandated in specific 'eligible' surgical procedures by regulatory bodies albeit the patient reserves the right to opt out. Service accreditation to collect and administer PROMs or to contract with an accredited PROMs supplier [154] ensures consistency in approach. PROM data generated in clinical practice and clinical trials informs not only individual but population-based treatment recommendations and health policy [129]. Further, PROM data contributes to the evidence patients and clinicians need to engage in informed shared decision-making [123, 155–157].

## *Generic Health Status Measures (GHSMs) with Utility Attributes*

*Generic health status measures* (GHSMs) are HRQoL scales also with utility in healthy populations. The Sickness Impact Profile (SIP) [158] is designed to assess the health impact of new treatments or services on individuals or populations by querying 136 behavioural items indicating health. The SIP was developed after querying 1000 respondents on sickness behaviour. The 36-Item Short Form Health

Survey (SF-36) [159, 160], though now the SF-6D more commonly assesses health economics, evaluates general health status with a strong emphasis on physical, social and emotional functioning but has received criticism for its population-specific questions on activities lacking global relevance [161]. Despite varying reference frames and response scales which may impact ease of utility, the SF-36 remains a widely used PROM.

The European Quality of Life Five Dimensions (EQ-5D™) developed by the EuroQoL Group is a generic measure of health used for clinical and economic evaluation [162]. The EQ-5D™ assesses five dimensions: mobility, the ability to self-care, usual activities, pain/discomfort and depression and includes a visual analogue scale (VAS) to capture health status. The National Institute for Health and Care Excellence (NICE) in the UK recommends the EQ-5D for health technology assessment [163], and it can be used with a condition-specific measure if an estimate of effectiveness of interventions is required in a specific disease [164].

In economic evaluations, utility values can be used to calculate quality-adjusted life-years (QALYs) or quality-adjusted time without symptoms or toxicity (Q-TWiST). Combining years of life, years of health condition with changing HRQoL, QALY/Q-TWiST approaches quantify the impact of specific health states in terms of years. The Q-TWiST applied to censored survival data is the approach favoured in clinical trials [90]. The purpose of both is to define health states and calculate cost utilities enabling comparisons of the impact of treatment across different health conditions [163].

## *Patient Preference*

Preference-based or 'utility measures' assign values across a wide spectrum of health conditions and situations. They are not considered HRQoL 'measures' but rather provide a HRQoL state against which a utility value or patient decisions can be associated. The metrics generated can inform economic decisions on treatment and supportive interventions to improve health status. At a population-based level as with GHSMs above, they can be a component of calculating quality-adjusted life-years (QALYs).

The trade-off between symptom palliation, treatment benefit, efficacy and safety can be measured as either a comparative advantage in how patients survive, feel or function or a comparative reduction in treatment-related side effects. Selection of the most appropriate instruments to measure these enables both clinical and economic appraisal.

The Standard Gamble (SG) technique asks the patient to make decisions regarding their hypothetical willingness to make sacrifices in order to gain relief from their illness, essentially offsetting risk against optimal health [165]. This approach may assist in supporting a patient to make choices about treatment offsetting side effects. For example, in IPF, anti-fibrotic medications pirfenidone and nintedanib slow disease progression to varying degrees without being curative, but both are associated with significant side effects, such as severe gastrointestinal symptoms or fatigue, impacting HRQoL. The decision to accept treatment is likely influenced by the outcome not being curative.

Time Trade-Off (TTO) is conceptually aligned to the QALY approach [90]. Unlike the SG it does not involve uncertainty and therefore is a preference-orientated approach; however the approach used is complex whereby a patient-centred paradigm strives for ease and simplicity.

## A Selection of PRMs for Respiratory Conditions

Here, brief summaries of a selection of PROMs to support palliative interventions in the respiratory field are discussed to illustrate real-world challenges of PRM selection [121]. The modified Medical Research Council (mMRC) Dyspnoea Scale widely used in COPD is integrated into COPD healthcare reviews as a key NICE Quality and Outcomes Framework indicator in the UK [166]. The mMRC measures perceived respiratory difficulty and is predictive of mortality in COPD and IPF [167–170].

The Functional Assessment of Chronic Illness Therapy-Fatigue Scale (FACIT-FS), a 13-item psychometrically robust, content-validated instrument, assesses fatigue/tiredness impact on daily activities and functioning across several chronic diseases [171–174]. Complementary quantitative and qualitative validation studies examine the utility of the FACIT-FS in respiratory diseases.

The St George's Respiratory Questionnaire (SGRQ) is a HRQoL condition-specific measure robustly developed for use in COPD measuring symptoms, activities (limited by the symptoms) and impacts (social and psychologic effect of the respiratory disease) [175]. Widely used and adapted for other respiratory diseases, it is a psychometrically strong measure of HRQoL in patients with IPF [176]. The SGRQ is able to distinguish between patients who experience a change in clinical status or those who remain stable over time [177] and an independent predictor of mortality in IPF [178].

A modified version of the SGRQ, the SGRQ-I, was developed for use in IPF, through Rasch modelling of a clinical trial data set which reduced the original 50 items to 34 IPF-relevant items [179, 180]. However, for unknown reasons, the SGRQ-I has not been widely adopted which warrants further exploration.

Over time several HRQoL and health status instruments have emerged for use in interstitial lung disease ILDs. The King's brief ILD (KBILD) questionnaire is a 15-item health status measure covering some aspects of HRQoL, anxiety, breathlessness and activities and physical symptom domains [181].

Two generations of KBILD questionnaires co-exist, KBILD-I, developed using confirmatory factor analysis (CFA), and KBILD-R developed using Rasch analysis an IRT approach [182]. The KBILD-I and KBILD-R share seven common items. The advantages and contextual differences for use are yet to be reported.

The ATAQ-IPF v.1 (86 items) and v.2 (74 items), developed with a US population in 2010, are questionnaires with a 4-point Likert scale (1, 'strongly disagree'; 2, 'disagree somewhat'; 3, 'agree somewhat'; and 4, 'strongly agree', with higher scores connoting greater impairment). Comprehensive measures due to their content length were perceived, perhaps unjustifiably, to be clinically unwieldy: v.1 has 14 domains with v.2 retaining 13 domains following the removal of 'spirituality'. The domains (v.1/v.2) contain respective items – cough (7/6), shortness of breath (7/7), planning (6/5), sleep (6/6), mortality (6/6), energy (6/5), mental and emotional well-being (7/7), spirituality (6/0), social activities (6/5), finances (6/6), independence (6/5), sexuality (5/5), relationships (6/6) and therapies (6/6).

The ATAQ-IPF v.1 and v.2 were used in clinical research settings. Collated responses (USA, 74; UK, 65) were subjected to further item reduction using Rasch analysis. The ATAQ-IPF-cA yielded 43 items across 10 domains [183]. The ATAQ having undergone further revisions was relaunched in 2020 as the L-IPF [184] containing 35 items within 2 modules (symptoms and impacts). The L-IPF requires longitudinal validation.

The IPF-PROM was developed using a mixed-methods approach, incorporating qualitative and consensus methodologies and embedding patient-centredness throughout. Six hundred fifty-seven patients, caregivers and HCPs consented and participated in the IPF-PROM development study from 2013 to 2018. The 12-item questionnaire assesses the psychological and physical experience of breathlessness, psychological well-being, energy level and global quality of life. The IPF-PROM is acceptable to patients and clinicians and meets the thresholds for reliability, validity, repeatability, sensitivity and responsiveness in an IPF population. Further longitudinal work is ongoing to establish qualitative and quantitative longitudinal validity and reliability in different IPF populations under licensed conditions.

An emotion thermometer (ET) reliant on the VAS has been developed and validated to evaluate distress in cancer. It is composed of five visual analogue scales which are demonstrated to have a positive predictive value in the domains distress, anxiety, depression, anger and need for help. It is a quick screening tool taking less than a minute to complete [185]. It has potential utility in other disease contexts.

## PRM Endpoints

Contemporary recommendations, developed by rigorous consensus methods, propose a minimum set of outcome measures, a 'core set', to be incorporated into future trials in ILD across seven domains: breathlessness, cough, health-related quality of life, imaging, lung physiology and function and mortality [105]. Collecting serial PRM data in observational and interventional studies and clinical trials is essential to determine tolerability, efficacy of medical interventions and overall impact of disease severity on HRQoL.

Further qualitative approaches that explore the acceptability of HRQoL and symptom measures to different patient populations preserve authentic patient-centred research.

The choice of PROMS has been hampered by a lack of standardised and validated instruments; yet the FDA increasingly requires patient experience data at the time of medicinal product approval to evaluate treatment effects [104]. Defining the concept and selecting the most appropriate endpoints that complement each other critically informs trial designs that generate meaningful data.

Primary endpoints include prespecified decline in pulmonary function, progression-free survival and hospitalisation-free survival (all-cause hospitalisation or death) in clinical trials in respiratory disease in addition to self-reported PROMs [186].

Secondary endpoints assess supportive concepts integral to determining treatment responsiveness. In the event that a disease-specific PROM is not available, a generic PROM is appropriate. Clinical trials being rich in correlative endpoints are a valuable testing ground for exploratory endpoints whether they are PRMs or biomarkers [105]. PRM endpoints assist either as an independent measure or along with other measures as a composite, being mindful that the weakest measure majorly influences its utility. The application of standardised operating procedures to guide the administration of PROMs ensures a consistent approach.

## Conclusion

Patient-centred methodology administered using patient-centred approaches has a great deal to contribute to clinical research and clinical practice in the respiratory field including support for the well-being of patients, family and clinicians. The scientific community holds a particular responsibility to rationalise its approach to PRM utilisation and the data generated.

Qualitative approaches lead to a better understanding of disease and treatment experiences and what matters to patients [187, 188], and thematic, framework, interpretative phenomenological and discourse analysis offer valuable insights into the lived experiences in life-limiting conditions such as lung fibrosis [65, 188–193].

High-quality patient-centred measures and strategies emerge from qualitative research with elicitation of concepts for item development from patients, family members, clinical experts and the literature. Patient involvement in the process at every stage ensures qualitative fit, influencing acceptability and overall utility of PRMs and the possibility they bring as an aid to shared/informed decision-making and their intrinsic value in the consultation.

Future research is needed on how the completion and feedback of PROMs shape and influence the process of building relationships with patients [194]. Patient-centred outcomes research (PCOR) is a growing specialty field receiving global investment and interest from multidisciplinary collaborations at the

American Thoracic and European Respiratory Societies. These global collective efforts can make a significant contribution to identifying future patient-centred research opportunities in chronic respiratory conditions from diagnosis to end of life care.

The question now lies in careful contextual and population-based examination of the instruments that exist, to identify true unmet needs in PRM assessments and as a community consolidate resources to address these gaps. Without efforts to identify standardised core sets, wide ranges of instruments create difficulties in comparing populations and treatment effects. With patients at the centre of clinical care and research, the collaborative clinical academic communities may accelerate optimal development, selections and uses of measures. Further, exploration of effective methods for PRM selection and time points of administration could bolster patient care and successful clinical trial design.

In regard to clinical care, research and policy-making, 'nothing about us, without us' strengthens the patient voice and participation [5], but the benefit reverberates to all stakeholders: clinicians, researchers, grantors and policy-makers, as the path of highest efficiency and greatest yield. Beyond being a popular but vague *buzzword,* the more *patient-centredness* can be held to high metric standards, the more likely the promise of healthcare excellence is in reach.

## References

1. Appleby J, Devlin N. Measuring success in the NHS. In: Using patient-assessed health outcomes to manage the performance of health care providers. London: King's Fund/Dr Foster; 2004.
2. Michie S, Miles J, Weinman J. Patient-centredness in chronic illness: what is it and does it matter? Patient Educ Couns. 2003;51(3):197–206.
3. Mead N, Bower P. Patient-centredness: a conceptual framework and review of the empirical literature. Soc Sci Med. 2000;51(7):1087–110.
4. Saha S, Beach MC, Cooper LA. Patient centeredness, cultural competence and healthcare quality. J Natl Med Assoc. 2008;100(11):1275–85.
5. Chu LF, Utengen A, Kadry B, et al. 'Nothing about us without us' – patient partnership in medical conferences. BMJ. 2016;354:i3883.
6. Collins SP, Levy PD, Holl JL, Butler J, Khan Y, Israel TL, Fonarow GC, Alikhaani J, Sarno E, Cook A, Yancy CW. Incorporating patient and caregiver experiences into cardio-vascular clinical trial design. JAMA Cardiol. 2017;2(11):1263–9. https://doi.org/10.1001/jamacardio.2017.3606.
7. Gierisch JM, Hughes JM, Williams JW Jr, Gordon AM, Goldstein KM. Qualitative exploration of engaging patients as advisors in a program of evidence synthesis: cobuilding the science to enhance impact. Med Care. 2019;57 Suppl 10 Suppl 3(10 Suppl 3):S246–52. https://doi.org/10.1097/MLR.0000000000001174. PMID: 31517795; PMCID: PMC6750153.
8. Balint E. The possibilities of patient-centred medicine. J R Coll Gen Pract. 1969;17:269–76.
9. Engel GI. The need for a new medical model: a challenge for biomedicine. Science. 1977;196:129–36.
10. Kitson A, Marshall A, Bassett K, Zeitz K. What are the core elements of patient-centred care? A narrative review and synthesis of the literature from health policy, medicine and nursing. J Adv Nurs. 2013;69(1):4–15.

11. Epstein RM, Stree RL Jr. Patient-centered communication in cancer care: promoting healing and reducing suffering. Bethesda: National Cancer Institute, NIH; 2007. Contract No.: 07-6225.
12. Wuyts WA, Peccatori FA, Russell AM. Patient-centred management in idiopathic pulmonary fibrosis: similar themes in three communication models. Eur Respir Rev. 2014;23(132):231–8. https://doi.org/10.1183/09059180.00001614.
13. Health Foundation. Health foundation person-centred care made simple. London: Health Foundation; 2015.
14. U.S. Department of Health and Human Services Food and Drug Administration (FDA). https://www.fda.gov/industry/prescription-drug-user-fee-amendments/voice-patient-series-reports-fdas-patient-focused-drug-development-initiative. Last accessed 26 Mar 2021.
15. The Picker Institute Principles of Person Centered Care. https://www.picker.org/about-us/picker-principles-of-person-centred-care/. Last accessed 28 Mar 2021.
16. Russell AM, Adamali H, Molyneaux PL, Lukey PT, Marshall RP, Renzoni EA, Wells AU, Maher TM. Daily home spirometry: an effective tool for detecting progression in idiopathic pulmonary fibrosis. Am J Respir Crit Care Med. 2016;194(8):989–97.
17. Johannson KA, Vittinghoff E, Morisset J, Lee JS, Balmes JR, Collard HR. Home monitoring improves endpoint efficiency in idiopathic pulmonary fibrosis. Eur Respir J. 2017;50:1602406.
18. Alexanderson H, Munters LA, Dastmalchi M, Loell I, Heimbürger M, Opava CH, Lundberg IE. Resistive home exercise in patients with recent-onset polymyositis and dermatomyositis -- a randomized controlled single-blinded study with a 2-year followup. J Rheumatol. 2014;41(6):1124–32.
19. Bernardi E, Pomidori L, Cassutti F, Cogo A. Home-based, moderate-intensity exercise training using a metronome improves the breathing pattern and oxygen saturation during exercise in patients with COPD. J Cardiopulm Rehabil Prev. 2018;38(6):E16–8.
20. Tuckson RV, Edmunds M, Hodgkins ML. Telehealth. N Engl J Med. 2017;377(16):1585–92.
21. Coats HL. African American elders' psychological-social-spiritual cultural experiences across serious illness: an integrative literature review through a palliative care lens. Ann Palliat Med. 2017;6(3):253–69. https://doi.org/10.21037/apm.2017.03.09. Epub 2017 Apr 17. PMID: 28595425; PMCID: PMC6280962.
22. Vujcic M, Tomicevic-Dubljevic J, Grbic M, Lecic-Tosevski D, Vukovic O, Toskovic O. Nature based solution for improving mental health and well-being in urban areas. Environ Res. 2017;158:385–92. https://doi.org/10.1016/j.envres.2017.06.030. Epub 2017 Jul 5.
23. Han AR, Park SA, Ahn BE. Reduced stress and improved physical functional ability in elderly with mental health problems following a horticultural therapy program. Complement Ther Med. 2018;38:19–23. https://doi.org/10.1016/j.ctim.2018.03.011. Epub 2018 Mar 28.
24. Nicholas SO, Giang AT, Yap PLK. The effectiveness of horticultural therapy on older adults: a systematic review. J Am Med Dir Assoc. 2019;20(10):1351.e1–1351.e11. https://doi.org/10.1016/j.jamda.2019.06.021. Epub 2019 Aug 8.
25. Freeman M, Ayers C, Peterson C, Kansagara D. Aromatherapy and essential oils: a map of the evidence. Washington, DC: Department of Veterans Affairs (US); 2019.
26. Sánchez-Vidaña DI, Ngai SP, He W, Chow JK, Lau BW, Tsang HW. The effectiveness of aromatherapy for depressive symptoms: a systematic review. Evid Based Complement Alternat Med. 2017:5869315. https://doi.org/10.1155/2017/5869315. Epub 2017 Jan 4. PMID: 28133489; PMCID: PMC5241490.
27. Ulrich RS. Effects of interior design on wellness: theory and recent scientific research. J Health Care Inter Des. 1991;3:97–109.
28. Ulrich RS. View through a window may influence recovery from surgery. Science. 1984;224(4647):420–1. https://doi.org/10.1126/science.6143402.
29. Schweitzer M, Gilpin L, Frampton S. Healing spaces: elements of environmental design that make an impact on health. J Altern Complement Med. 2004;10(Suppl 1):S71–83. https://doi.org/10.1089/1075553042245953.
30. Reiling J, Hughes RG, Murphy MR. The impact of facility design on patient safety. In: Hughes RG, editor. Patient safety and quality: an evidence-based handbook for nurses. Rockville: Agency for Healthcare Research and Quality (US); 2008. Chapter 28.

31. Designing for quality: hospitals look to the built environment to provide better patient care and outcomes. Qual Lett Healthc Lead. 2003;15(4):2–13, 1.
32. Healing environments: progress toward "evidence-based design". Russ Coiles Health Trends. 2001;13(11):8–12.
33. Brambilla A, Rebecchi A, Capolongo S. Evidence based hospital design. A literature review of the recent publications about the EBD impact of built environment on hospital occupants' and organizational outcomes. Ann Ig. 2019;31(2):165–80. https://doi.org/10.7416/ai.2019.2269.
34. Engineer A, Ida A, Sternberg EM. Healing spaces: designing physical environments to optimize health, wellbeing, and performance. Int J Environ Res Public Health. 2020;17(4):1155. https://doi.org/10.3390/ijerph17041155. PMID: 32059563; PMCID: PMC7068320.
35. Geimer-Flanders J. Creating a healing environment: rationale and research overview. Cleve Clin J Med. 2009;76 Suppl 2:S66–9. https://doi.org/10.3949/ccjm.76.s2.13.
36. Benedetti F, Colombo C, Barbini B, Campori E, Smeraldi E. Morning sunlight reduces length of hospitalization in bipolar depression. J Affect Disord. 2001;62(3):221–3. https://doi.org/10.1016/s0165-0327(00)00149-x.
37. Beauchemin KM, Hays P. Dying in the dark: sunshine, gender and outcomes in myocardial infarction. J R Soc Med. 1998;91(7):352–4. https://doi.org/10.1177/014107689809100703. PMID: 9771492; PMCID: PMC1296806.
38. Beauchemin KM, Hays P. Sunny hospital rooms expedite recovery from severe and refractory depressions. J Affect Disord. 1996;40(1–2):49–51. https://doi.org/10.1016/0165-0327(96)00040-7.
39. Eagle A. Interiors: distinctive design. Creating the [patient centered] room. Health Facil Manage. 2007;20(6):40–4.
40. Berry LL, Parker D, Coile RC Jr, Hamilton DK, O'Neill DD, Sadler BL. The business case for better buildings. Front Health Serv Manage. 2004;21(1):3–24.
41. Thayer JF, Loerbroks A, Sternberg EM. Inflammation and cardiorespiratory control: the role of the vagus nerve. Respir Physiol Neurobiol. 2011;178(3):387–94. https://doi.org/10.1016/j.resp.2011.05.016. Epub 2011 May 27.
42. Knowles LM, Skeath P, Jia M, Najafi B, Thayer J, Sternberg EM. New and future directions in integrative medicine research methods with a focus on aging populations: a review. Gerontology. 2016;62(4):467–76. https://doi.org/10.1159/000441494. Epub 2015 Nov 7.
43. Sternberg EM. Neural regulation of innate immunity: a coordinated nonspecific host response to pathogens. Nat Rev Immunol. 2006;6(4):318–28. https://doi.org/10.1038/nri1810. PMID: 16557263; PMCID: PMC1783839.
44. Duckworth A, Gibbons MA, Allen RJ, Almond H, Beaumont RN, Wood AR, Lunnon K, Lindsay MA, Wain LV, Tyrrell J, Scotton CJ. Telomere length and risk of idiopathic pulmonary fibrosis and chronic obstructive pulmonary disease: a mendelian randomisation study. Lancet Respir Med. 2021;9(3):285–94. https://doi.org/10.1016/S2213-2600(20)30364-7. Epub 2020 Nov 13.
45. Arsenis NC, You T, Ogawa EF, Tinsley GM, Zuo L. Physical activity and telomere length: impact of aging and potential mechanisms of action. Oncotarget. 2017;8(27):45008–19. https://doi.org/10.18632/oncotarget.16726. PMID: 28410238; PMCID: PMC5546536.
46. Ornish D, Lin J, Chan JM, Epel E, Kemp C, Weidner G, Marlin R, Frenda SJ, Magbanua MJM, Daubenmier J, Estay I, Hills NK, Chainani-Wu N, Carroll PR, Blackburn EH. Effect of comprehensive lifestyle changes on telomerase activity and telomere length in men with biopsy-proven low-risk prostate cancer: 5-year follow-up of a descriptive pilot study. Lancet Oncol. 2013;14(11):1112–20. https://doi.org/10.1016/S1470-2045(13)70366-8. Epub 2013 Sep 17.
47. Ornish D, Lin J, Daubenmier J, Weidner G, Epel E, Kemp C, Magbanua MJ, Marlin R, Yglecias L, Carroll PR, Blackburn EH. Increased telomerase activity and comprehensive lifestyle changes: a pilot study. Lancet Oncol. 2008;9(11):1048–57. https://doi.org/10.1016/S1470-2045(08)70234-1. Epub 2008 Sep 15. Erratum in: Lancet Oncol. 2008;9(12):1124.
48. Gasperino J. The Leapfrog initiative for intensive care unit physician staffing and its impact on intensive care unit performance: a narrative review. Health Policy. 2011;102(2–3):223–8. https://doi.org/10.1016/j.healthpol.2011.02.005. Epub 2011 Mar 24.

49. Tritou I, Vakaki M, Sfakiotaki R, Kalaitzaki K, Raissaki M. Pediatric thyroid ultrasound: a radiologist's checklist. Pediatr Radiol. 2020;50(4):563–74. https://doi.org/10.1007/s00247-019-04602-2. Epub 2020 Mar 12.
50. Williams PD, Williams AR, Kelly KP, Dobos C, Gieseking A, Connor R, Ridder L, Potter N, Del Favero D. A symptom checklist for children with cancer: the Therapy-Related Symptom Checklist-Children. Cancer Nurs. 2012;35(2):89–98. https://doi.org/10.1097/NCC.0b013e31821a51f6.
51. Gao MC, Martin PB, Motal J, Gingras LF, Chai C, Maikoff ME, Sarkisian AM, Rosenthal N, Eiss BM. A multidisciplinary discharge timeout checklist improves patient education and captures discharge process errors. Qual Manag Health Care. 2018;27(2):63–8. https://doi.org/10.1097/QMH.0000000000000168.
52. Health Foundation. The making good decisions in collaboration programme (MAGIC): evaluation. 2013. https://www.health.org.uk/publications/the-magic-programme-evaluation. Accessed 6 Apr 2021 at 10:00.
53. National Institute of Clinical Excellence. https://www.nice.org.uk/about/what-we-do/our-programmes/nice-guidance/nice-guidelines/shared-decision-making. Accessed 6 Apr 2021 at 10:00.
54. U.S. Department of Health and Human Services Food and Drug Administration. https://www.fda.gov/drugs/development-approval-process-drugs/fda-patient-focused-drug-development-guidance-series-enhancing-incorporation-patients-voice-medical. Accessed 6 Apr 2021 at 10:00.
55. Personalised Care Institute. https://www.personalisedcareinstitute.org.uk/. Accessed 6 Apr 2021 at 10:00.
56. Ho AHY, Car J, Ho MR, Tan-Ho G, Choo PY, Patinadan PV, Chong PH, Ong WY, Fan G, Tan YP, Neimeyer RA, Chochinov HM. A novel Family Dignity Intervention (FDI) for enhancing and informing holistic palliative care in Asia: study protocol for a randomized controlled trial. Trials. 2017;18(1):587. https://doi.org/10.1186/s13063-017-2325-5. PMID: 29202863; PMCID: PMC5715529.
57. Kornblith AB, Herr HW, Ofman US, Scher HI, Holland JC. Quality of life of patients with prostate cancer and their spouses. The value of a data base in clinical care. Cancer. 1994;73(11):2791–802. https://doi.org/10.1002/1097-0142(19940601)73:11<2791::aid-cncr2820731123>3.0.co;2-9.
58. Weitzenkamp DA, Gerhart KA, Charlifue SW, Whiteneck GG, Savic G. Spouses of spinal cord injury survivors: the added impact of caregiving. Arch Phys Med Rehabil. 1997;78(8):822–7. https://doi.org/10.1016/s0003-9993(97)90194-5.
59. Youngblood NM, Hines J. The influence of the family's perception of disability on rehabilitation outcomes. Rehabil Nurs. 1992;17(6):323–6. https://doi.org/10.1002/j.2048-7940.1992.tb01268.x.
60. Moor CC, van Manen MJG, van Hagen PM, Miedema JR, van den Toorn LM, Gür-Demirel Y, Berendse APC, van Laar JAM, Wijsenbeek MS. Needs, perceptions and education in sarcoidosis: a live interactive survey of patients and partners. Lung. 2018;196(5):569–75. https://doi.org/10.1007/s00408-018-0144-4. Epub 2018 Aug 7. PMID: 30088094; PMCID: PMC6153596.
61. Sandford D, Reynolds P. The psychological distress that idiopathic pulmonary fibrosis patients and caregivers experience. The invisible injury that adds complexity to management and treatment. Respirology. 2019;24:89. https://doi.org/10.1111/resp.13699_254.
62. Tan JY, Molassiotis A, et al. Emotional distress and quality of life among informal caregivers of lung cancer patients: an exploratory study. Eur J Cancer Care. 2018;27:e12691.
63. Strang S, et al. Family caregivers' heavy and overloaded burden in advanced chronic obstructive pulmonary disease. J Palliat Med. 2018;21:1768–72.
64. Verma S, et al. Caregiver's burden in pulmonary arterial hypertension: a clinical review. J Exerc Rehabil. 2016;12:386.

65. Russell AM, Ripamonti E, Vancheri C. Qualitative European survey of patients with idiopathic pulmonary fibrosis: patients' perspectives of the disease and treatment. BMC Pulm Med. 2016;16:1–7.
66. Adelman RD, et al. Caregiver burden: a clinical review. JAMA. 2014;311:1052–60.
67. Golics CJ, et al. Int J Gen Med. 2013;6:787–98. Published 2013 Sep 18. https://doi.org/10.2147/IJGM.S45156.
68. Schulz R, Beach SR, Friedman EM. Caregiving factors as predictors of care recipient mortality. Am J Geriatr Psychiatry. 2021;29(3):295–303. https://doi.org/10.1016/j.jagp.2020.06.025. Epub 2020 Jul 5. PMID: 32718853; PMCID: PMC7782207.
69. Vitaliano PP, Scanlan JM, Zhang J, Savage MV, Hirsch IB, Siegler IC. A path model of chronic stress, the metabolic syndrome, and coronary heart disease. Psychosom Med. 2002;64(3):418–35. https://doi.org/10.1097/00006842-200205000-00006.
70. Moon HE, Haley WE, Rote SM, Sears JS. Caregiver well-being and burden: variations by race/ethnicity and care recipient nativity status. Innov Aging. 2020;4(6):igaa045. https://doi.org/10.1093/geroni/igaa045. PMID: 33241124; PMCID: PMC7679974.
71. Perkins M, Howard VJ, Wadley VG, Crowe M, Safford MM, Haley WE, Howard G, Roth DL. Caregiving strain and all-cause mortality: evidence from the REGARDS study. J Gerontol B Psychol Sci Soc Sci. 2013;68:504–12.
72. Mausbach BT, Roepke SK, Ziegler MG, Milic M, von Känel R, Dimsdale JE, Mills PJ, Patterson TL, Allison MA, Ancoli-Israel S, Grant I. Association between chronic caregiving stress and impaired endothelial function in the elderly. J Am Coll Cardiol. 2010;55(23):2599–606. https://doi.org/10.1016/j.jacc.2009.11.093. PMID: 20513601; PMCID: PMC2892624.
73. Lee S, Colditz GA, Berkman LF, Kawachi I. Caregiving and risk of coronary heart disease in U.S. women: a prospective study. Am J Prev Med. 2003;24(2):113–9. https://doi.org/10.1016/s0749-3797(02)00582-2.
74. Lee S, Colditz G, Berkman L, Kawachi I. Caregiving to children and grandchildren and risk of coronary heart disease in women. Am J Public Health. 2003;93(11):1939–44. https://doi.org/10.2105/ajph.93.11.1939. PMID: 14600070; PMCID: PMC1448080.
75. Kitko L, McIlvennan CK, Bidwell JT, Dionne-Odom JN, Dunlay SM, Lewis LM, Meadows G, Sattler ELP, Schulz R, Strömberg A, American Heart Association Council on Cardiovascular and Stroke Nursing, Council on Quality of Care and Outcomes Research, Council on Clinical Cardiology; and Council on Lifestyle and Cardiometabolic Health. Family caregiving for individuals with heart failure: a scientific statement from the American Heart Association. Circulation. 2020;141(22):e864–78. https://doi.org/10.1161/CIR.0000000000000768. Epub 2020 Apr 30.
76. Schulz R, Beach SR, Czaja SJ, Martire LM, Monin JK. Family caregiving for older adults. Annu Rev Psychol. 2020;71:635–59. https://doi.org/10.1146/annurev-psych-010419-050754. PMID: 31905111; PMCID: PMC7291827.
77. Haley WE, Roth DL, Howard G, Safford MM. Caregiving strain and estimated risk for stroke and coronary heart disease among spouse caregivers: differential effects by race and sex. Stroke. 2010;41:331–6.
78. Schulz R, Beach SR. Caregiving as a risk factor for mortality: the Caregiver Health Effects Study. JAMA. 1999;282(23):2215–9. https://doi.org/10.1001/jama.282.23.2215.
79. Tsai CF, Hwang WS, Lee JJ, Wang WF, Huang LC, Huang LK, Lee WJ, Sung PS, Liu YC, Hsu CC, Fuh JL. Predictors of caregiver burden in aged caregivers of demented older patients. BMC Geriatr. 2021;21(1):59. https://doi.org/10.1186/s12877-021-02007-1. PMID: 33446114; PMCID: PMC7809883.
80. Kroenke K, Spitzer RL, Williams JB. The PHQ-9: validity of a brief depression severity measure. J Gen Intern Med. 2001;16(9):606–13.
81. Epstein-Lubow G, Gaudiano BA, Hinckley M, Salloway S, Miller IW. Evidence for the validity of the American Medical Association's Caregiver Self-Assessment Questionnaire as a screening measure for depression. J Am Geriatr Soc. 2010;58(2):387–8.

82. Zarit SH, Todd PA, Zarit JM. Subjective burden of husbands and wives as caregivers: a longitudinal study. Gerontologist. 1986;26:260–6.
83. Robinson BC. Validation of a caregiver strain index. J Gerontol. 1983;38:344–8.
84. Ptomey LT, Vidoni ED, Montenegro-Montenegro E, Thompson MA, Sherman JR, Gorczyca AM, Greene JL, Washburn RA, Donnelly JE. The feasibility of remotely delivered exercise session in adults with Alzheimer's disease and their caregivers. J Aging Phys Act. 2019;27(5):670–7. https://doi.org/10.1123/japa.2018-0298. PMID: 30747564; PMCID: PMC6891121.
85. Mausbach BT, Harmell AL, Moore RC, Chattillion EA. Influence of caregiver burden on the association between daily fluctuations in pleasant activities and mood: a daily diary analysis. Behav Res Ther. 2011;49(1):74–9. https://doi.org/10.1016/j.brat.2010.11.004. Epub 2010 Nov 22. PMID: 21130981; PMCID: PMC3025044.
86. Lindell KO, Nouraie M, Klesen MJ, Klein S, Gibson KF, Kass DJ, Rosenzweig MQ. Randomised clinical trial of an early palliative care intervention (SUPPORT) for patients with idiopathic pulmonary fibrosis (IPF) and their caregivers: protocol and key design considerations. BMJ Open Respir Res. 2018;5(1):e000272. https://doi.org/10.1136/bmjresp-2017-000272.
87. https://medium.com/@JoeBiden/the-biden-plan-for-mobilizing-american-talent-and-heart-to-create-a-21st-century-caregiving-and-af5ba2a2dfeb. Last accessed 29 Mar 2021.
88. Lee J, Cagle JG. Measures of financial burden for families dealing with serious illness: a systematic review and analysis. Palliat Med. 2021;35(2):280–94. https://doi.org/10.1177/0269216320973161. Epub 2020 Dec 4.
89. British Lung Foundation. https://www.blf.org.uk/taskforce. Accessed 06 04 21 10:00h.
90. Fayers PM, Machin D. Quality of life: the assessment, analysis and interpretation of patient-reported outcomes. 2nd ed. Chichester/Hoboken: John Wiley & Sons Ltd; 2007.
91. Saketkoo LA, Escorpizo R, Keen KJ, Fligelstone K, Distler O. International Classification of Functioning, Disability and Health core Set construction in systemic sclerosis and other rheumatic diseases: a EUSTAR initiative. Rheumatology. 2012;51:2170–6.
92. Liang JW, Cheung YK, Willey JZ, et al. Quality of life independently predicts long-term mortality but not vascular events: the Northern Manhattan Study. Qual Life Res. 2017;26:2219–28. https://doi.org/10.1007/s11136-017-1567-8.
93. Kanwal F, Gralnek IM, Hays RD, et al. Health-related quality of life predicts mortality in patients with advanced chronic liver disease. Clin Gastroenterol Hepatol. 2009;7:793–9. https://doi.org/10.1016/j.cgh.2009.03.013.
94. Irwin KE, Greer JA, Khatib J, Temel JS, Pirl WF. Early palliative care and metastatic non-small cell lung cancer: potential mechanisms of prolonged survival. Chron Respir Dis. 2013;10:35–47. https://doi.org/10.1177/1479972312471549.
95. Giese-Davis J, Collie K, Rancourt KMS, et al. Decrease in depression symptoms is associated with longer survival in patients with metastatic breast cancer: a secondary analysis. J Clin Oncol. 2011;29:413–20. https://doi.org/10.1200/JCO.2010.28.4455.
96. Bakitas M, Lyons KD, Hegel MT, et al. Effects of a palliative care intervention on clinical outcomes in patients with advanced cancer: the project ENABLE II randomized controlled trial. JAMA. 2009;302:741–9. https://doi.org/10.1001/jama.2009.1198.
97. Molassiotis AW, Uyterlinde PJ, Hollen L, Sarna P, Palmer M. Krishnasamy supportive care in lung cancer: milestones over the past 40 years. J Thorac Oncol. 2015;10(1):10–8.
98. Stącel T, Jaworska I, Zawadzki F, Wajda-Pokrontka M, Tatoj Z, Urlik M, et al. Assessment of quality of life among patients after lung transplantation: a single-center study. transplantation proceedings. Transplant Proc. 2020;52(7):2165–72. https://doi.org/10.1016/j.transproceed.2020.03.048.
99. Kolaitis NA, Singer JP. Defining success in lung transplantation: from survival to quality of life. Semin Respir Crit Care Med. 2018;39(2):255–68.
100. Alvarelhão J, Silva A, Martins A, Queirós A, Amaro A, Rocha N, Lains J. Comparing the content of instruments assessing environmental factors using the International Classification

of Functioning, Disability and Health. J Rehabil Med. 2012;44(1):1–6. https://doi.org/10.2340/16501977-0905.
101. United States Food and Drug Administration. Clinical Outcome Assessments (COA) qualification program resources. www.fda.gov . Last Accessed 29 Mar 2021.
102. Powers JH, Patrick DL, Walton MK, Marquis P, Cano S, Hobart J, et al. Clinician-reported outcome assessments of treatment benefit: report of the ISPOR clinical outcome assessment emerging good practices task force. Value Health J Int Soc Pharmacoecon Outcomes Res. 2017;20(1):2–14.
103. Saketkoo LA, Mittoo S, Huscher D, Khanna D, Dellaripa PF, Distler O, Flaherty KR, Frankel S, Oddis CV, Denton CP, Fischer A, Kowal-Bielecka OM, LeSage D, Merkel PA, Phillips K, Pittrow D, Swigris J, Antoniou K, Baughman RP, Castelino FV, Christmann RB, Christopher-Stine L, Collard HR, Cottin V, Danoff S, Highland KB, Hummers L, Shah AA, Kim DS, Lynch DA, Miller FW, Proudman SM, Richeldi L, Ryu JH, Sandorfi N, Sarver C, Wells AU, Strand V, Matteson EL, Brown KK, Seibold JR, CTD-ILD Special Interest Group. Connective tissue disease related interstitial lung diseases and idiopathic pulmonary fibrosis: provisional core sets of domains and instruments for use in clinical trials. Thorax. 2014;69(5):428–36. https://doi.org/10.1136/thoraxjnl-2013-204202. Epub 2013 Dec 24. Erratum in: Thorax. 2014;69(9):834. CTD-ILD Special Interest Group [added]; multiple investigator names added. PMID: 24368713; PMCID: PMC3995282.
104. U.S. Department of Health and Human Services Food and Drug Administration (FDA). Guidance for industry patient-reported outcome measures: use in medical product development to support labeling claims. Maryland FDA 2009 http://www.fda.gov/downloads/Drugs/Guidances/UCM193282.pdf.
105. Saketkoo LA, Mittoo S, Frankel S, et al. Reconciling healthcare professional and patient perspectives in the development of disease activity and response criteria in connective tissue disease-related interstitial lung diseases. J Rheumatol. 2014;41(4):792–8.
106. Saketkoo LA, Mittoo S, Huscher D, et al. Connective tissue disease related interstitial lung diseases and idiopathic pulmonary fibrosis: provisional core sets of domains and instruments for use in clinical trials. Thorax. 2014;69(5):428–36.
107. Coulter A, Roberts S, Dixon A. Delivering better services for people with long term conditions: building the house of care. London: The King's Fund; 2013.
108. Moor CC, Mostard M, Grutters J, et al. Home monitoring in patients with IPF: a RCT. Am J Respir Crit Care Med. 2020;202(3):393–401.
109. Pletta KH, Kerr BR, Eickhoff JC, Allen GS, Jain SR, Moreno MA. Pediatric asthma action plans: national cross-sectional online survey of parents' perceptions. JMIR Pediatr Parent. 2020;3(2):e21863. https://doi.org/10.2196/21863. PMID: 33164900; PMCID: PMC7683255.
110. Kelly C, Grundy S, Lynes D, Evans DJ, Gudur S, Milan SJ, Spencer S. Self-management for bronchiectasis. Cochrane Database Syst Rev. 2018;2(2):CD012528. https://doi.org/10.1002/14651858.CD012528.pub2. PMID: 29411860; PMCID: PMC6491127.
111. National Academies of Sciences, Engineering, and Medicine. 2019. Taking action against clinician burnout: a systems approach to professional well-being. Washington, DC: The National Academies Press. https://doi.org/10.17226/25521.
112. Tong A, Sainsbury P, Craig J. Consolidated criteria for reporting qualitative research (COREQ): a 32-item checklist for interviews and focus groups. International J Qual Health Care. 2007;19(6):349–57.
113. Russell AM Development and testing of an Idiopathic Pulmonary Fibrosis (IPF) Patient Reported Outcome Measure (PROM) Doctoral Thesis; 2018. Imperial College London.
114. Stratford P, Gill C, Westaway M, Binkley J. Assessing disability and change on individual patients: a report of a patient specific measure. Physiother Can. 1995;47:258–63.
115. Tugwell P, Bombardier C, Buchanan WW, et al. The MACTAR patients preference disability questionnaire: an individualized functional priority approach for assessing improvement in physical disability in clinical trials in rheumatoid arthritis. J Rheumatol. 1987;14:446–51.

116. Calvert M, Blazeby J, Altman DG, Revicki DA, Moher D, Brundage MD. Reporting of patient-reported outcomes in randomized trials: the CONSORT PRO extension. JAMA. 2013;309(8):814–22.
117. Russell A-M, Sprangers MA, Wibberley S, Snell N, Rose DM, Swigris JJ. The need for patient-centred clinical research in idiopathic pulmonary fibrosis. BMC Med. 2015;13(1):240.
118. Emery MP, Perrier LL, Acquadro C. Patient-reported outcome and quality of life instruments database (PROQOLID): frequently asked questions. Health Qual Life Outcomes. 2005;3:12.
119. Devlin N, Appleby J. Getting the most out of PROMs: putting health outcomes at the heart of NHS decision-making (The King's Fund). 2010. https://www.kingsfund.org.uk/sites/files/kf/Getting-the-most-out-of-PROMs-Nancy-Devlin-John-Appleby-Kings-Fund-March-2010.pdf.
120. Mokkink LB, Terwee CB, Patrick DL, Alonso J, Stratford PW, Knol DL, et al. The COSMIN study reached international consensus on taxonomy, terminology, and definitions of measurement properties for health-related patient-reported outcomes. J Clin Epidemiol. 2010;63(7):737–45.
121. McKenna SP. Measuring patient-reported outcomes: moving beyond misplaced common sense to hard science. BMC Med. 2011;9:86.
122. Prinsen CAC, Vohra S, Rose MR, King-Jones S, Ishaque S, Bhaloo Z, et al. Core Outcome Measures in Effectiveness Trials (COMET) initiative: protocol for an international Delphi study to achieve consensus on how to select outcome measurement instruments for outcomes included in a 'core outcome set'. Trials. 2014;15(1):247.
123. Greenhalgh J, Abhyankar P, McCluskey S, Takeuchi E, Velikova G. How do doctors refer to patient-reported outcome measures (PROMS) in oncology consultations? Qual Life Res. 2013;22(5):939–50.
124. National Health Service England. National Patient Reported Outcome Measures (PROMs) programme consultation report. Leeds Insight and Feedback Team NHSE; 2017.
125. Boyce MB, Browne JP, Greenhalgh J. The experiences of professionals with using information from patient-reported outcome measures to improve the quality of healthcare: a systematic review of qualitative research. BMJ Qual Saf. 2014;23(6):508–18.
126. Nelson EC, Eftimovska E, Lind C, Hager A, Wasson JH, Lindblad S. Patient reported outcome measures in practice. BMJ (Online). 2015;350:g7818.
127. Krawczyk M, Sawatzky R. Relational use of an electronic quality of life and practice support system in hospital palliative consult care: a pilot study. Palliat Support Care. 2018;17:208–13.
128. Gamlen E, Arber A. First assessments by specialist cancer nurses in the community: an ethnography. Eur J Oncol Nurs. 2013;17(6):797–801.
129. Santana MJ, Haverman L, Absolom K, Takeuchi E, Feeny D, Grootenhuis M, et al. Training clinicians in how to use patient-reported outcome measures in routine clinical practice. Qual Life Res. 2015;24(7):1707–18.
130. Health and Social Care Information Centre (HSCIC). Patient Reported Outcome Measures (PROMs) in England: a guide to PROMs methodology. London: NHS digital [Health and Social Care Information Centre]; 2017.
131. International Society for Quality of Life Research. User's guide to implementing patient-reported outcomes assessment in clinical practice. 2011. http://www.isoqol.org/UserFiles/file/UsersGuide.pdf.
132. Annells M, Koch T. The real stuff': implications for nursing of assessing and measuring a terminally ill person's quality of life. J Clin Nurs. 2001;10(6):806–12.
133. Santana MJ, Feeny D. Framework to assess the effects of using patient-reported outcome measures in chronic care management. Qual Life Res. 2014;23(5):1505–13.
134. Feldman-Stewart D, Brundage M. A conceptual framework for patient-provider communication: a tool in the PRO research tool box. Qual Life Res. 2009;18:109–14.
135. Neale J, Strang J. Philosophical ruminations on measurement: methodological orientations of patient reported outcome measures (PROMS). J Ment Health. 2015;24(3):123–5.
136. Department of Health. Digital strategy: leading the culture change in health and care; 2012.
137. NHSE Independent evaluation of the feasibility of using the Patient Activation Measure in the NHS in England: NHSE 03964: 20/11/2015.
138. NHSE PAM implementation quick guide NHSE 07888: 04/04/2018.

139. Hibbard JH, Greene J, Shi Y, Mittler J, Scanlon D. Taking the long view: how well do patient activation scores predict outcomes four years later? Med Care Res Rev. 2015;72(3):324–37. https://doi.org/10.1177/1077558715573871.
140. Graffigna G, Barello S, Bonanomi A, Lozza E. Measuring patient engagement: development and psychometric properties of the Patient Health Engagement (PHE) Scale. Front Psychol. 2015;6:274. https://doi.org/10.3389/fpsyg.2015.00274.
141. Barello S, Castiglioni C, Bonanomi A, Graffigna G. The Caregiving Health Engagement Scale (CHE-s): development and initial validation of a new questionnaire for measuring family caregiver engagement in healthcare. BMC Public Health. 2019;19(1):1562. https://doi.org/10.1186/s12889-019-7743-8. PMID: 31771546; PMCID: PMC6880352.
142. Morisky DE, Green LW, Levine DM. Concurrent and predictive validity of a self-reported measure of medication adherence. Med Care. 1986;24:67–74. https://doi.org/10.1097/00005650-198601000-00007.
143. Raleigh V, Graham C, Thompson J, Sizmur S, Jabbal J, Coulter A. Patients' experience of using hospital services: an analysis of trends in inpatient surveys in NHS acute trusts in England, 2005–13 The King's fund London 2015.
144. De Rosis S, Cerasuolo D, Nuti S. Using patient-reported measures to drive change in healthcare: the experience of the digital, continuous and systematic PREMs observatory in Italy. BMC Health Serv Res. 2020;20:315. https://doi.org/10.1186/s12913-020-05099-4.
145. Bosworth A, Cox M, O'Brien A, Jones P, Sargeant I, Elliott A, Bukhari M. Development and Validation of a Patient Reported Experience Measure (PREM) for patients with Rheumatoid Arthritis (RA) and other rheumatic conditions. Curr Rheumatol Rev. 2015;11:1–7.
146. Hodson M, Roberts CM, Andrew S, et al. Development and first validation of a patient-reported experience measure in chronic obstructive pulmonary disease (PREM-C9). Thorax. 2019;74:600–3.
147. Mercer SW, McConnachie A, Maxwell M, Heaney DH, Watt GCM. Relevance and performance of the Consultation and Relational Empathy (CARE) measure in general practice. Fam Pract. 2005;22(3):328–34.
148. IPF World. European IPF Patient Charter. www.ipfcharter.org/the-charter/ Date last updated: 2015. Date last accessed: 06 04 21.
149. Bonella F, Wijsenbeek M, MolinaMolina M, Duck A, Mele R, Geissler K, Wuyts W. European IPF Patient Charter: unmet needs and a call to action for healthcare policymakers. Eur Respir J. 2016;47(2):597–606. https://doi.org/10.1183/13993003.01204-2015.
150. Higgins JPT, Green S. Cochrane handbook for systematic reviews of interventions: the Cochrane collaboration; 2011.
151. Pompili C, Novoa N, Balduyck B. Clinical evaluation of quality of life: a survey among members of European Society of Thoracic Surgeons (ESTS). Interact Cardiovasc Thorac Surg. 2015;21(4):415–9.
152. Ratnayake I, Ahern S, Ruseckaite R. A systematic review of patient-reported outcome measures (PROMs) in cystic fibrosis. BMJ Open. 2020;10:e033867. https://doi.org/10.1136/bmjopen-2019-033867.
153. Hughes R, Aspinal F, Addington-Hall JM, Dunckley M, Faull C, Higginson I. It just didn't work: the realities of quality assessment in the English health care context. Int J Nurs Stud. 2004;41(7):705–12.
154. NHS England National PROMs Programme Guidance. 2017. https://www.england.nhs.uk/ourwork/insight/proms/. Accessed 06 04 21.
155. Ahmed S, Berzon RA, Revicki DA, Lenderking WR, Moinpour CM, Basch E, et al. The use of patient-reported outcomes (PRO) within comparative effectiveness research: implications for clinical practice and health care policy. Med Care. 2012;50(12):1060–70.
156. Detmar SB, Muller MJ, Schornagel JH, Wever LD, Aaronson NK. Health-related quality-of-life assessments and patient-physician communication: a randomized controlled trial. JAMA. 2002;288(23):3027–34.
157. Valderas JM, Kotzeva A, Espallargues M, Guyatt G, Ferrans CE, Halyard MY, et al. The impact of measuring patient-reported outcomes in clinical practice: a systematic review of the literature. Qual Life Res. 2008;17(2):179–93.

158. Bergner M, Bobbitt RA, Carter WB, Gilson BS. The Sickness Impact Profile: development and final revision of a health status measure. Med Care. 1981;19(8):787–805.
159. Ware J Jr, Kosinski M, Keller SD. A 12-Item Short-Form Health Survey: construction of scales and preliminary tests of reliability and validity. Med Care. 1996;34(3):220–33.
160. Martinez TY, Pereira CAC, dos Santos ML, Ciconelli RM, Guimarães SM, Martinez JAB. Evaluation of the short-form 36-item questionnaire to measure health-related quality of life in patients with idiopathic pulmonary fibrosis. Chest. 2000;117(6):1627–32.
161. Ware JES, Sherbourne CD. The MOS 36-item Short-Form Health Survey (SF-36): I. Conceptual framework and item selection. Med Care. 1992;30:473–83.
162. van Reenen M, Janssen B. EQ-5D-5L User Guide: basic information on how to use the EQ-5D-5L instrument. The Netherlands: EuroQol Research Foundation; 2015.
163. National Institute of Clinical Excellence. Guide to the methods of technology appraisal. Process and methods London: 2013 Contract No.: PMG9.
164. Herdman M, Gudex C, Lloyd A, Janssen MF, Kind P, Parkin D, et al. Development and preliminary testing of the new five-level version of EQ-5D (EQ-5D-5L). Qual Life Res. 2011;20(10):1727–36.
165. Stiggelbout AM, de Vogel-Voogt E. Health state utilities: a framework for studying the gap between the imagined and the real. Value Health. 2008;11(1):76–87.
166. Excellence NIfHaC. Indicators for the NICE menu for the QOF: COPD NM104. London: NICE; 2015.
167. Manali ED, Stathopoulos GT, Kollintza A, Kalomenidis I, Emili JM, Sotiropoulou C, et al. The Medical Research Council chronic dyspnea score predicts the survival of patients with idiopathic pulmonary fibrosis. Respir Med. 2008;102(4):586–92.
168. Mura M, Porretta MA, Bargagli E, Sergiacomi G, Zompatori M, Sverzellati N, et al. Predicting survival in newly diagnosed idiopathic pulmonary fibrosis: a 3-year prospective study. Eur Respir J. 2012;40(1):101–9.
169. Jones PW, Adamek L, Nadeau G, Banik N. Comparisons of health status scores with MRC grades in COPD: implications for the GOLD 2011 classification. Eur Respir J. 2013;42(3):647–54.
170. Rajala K, Lehto JT, Sutinen E, Kautiainen H, Myllärniemi M, Saarto T. mMRC dyspnoea scale indicates impaired quality of life and increased pain in patients with idiopathic pulmonary fibrosis. ERJ Open Research. 2017;3(4):00084-2017.
171. Cella D, Lai JS, Chang CH, Peterman A, Slavin M. Fatigue in cancer patients compared with fatigue in the general United States population. Cancer. 2002;15:528–38. https://doi.org/10.1002/cncr.10245.
172. Acaster S, Dickerhoof R, DeBusk K, Bernard K, Strauss W, Allen LF. Qualitative and quantitative validation of the FACIT-fatigue scale in iron deficiency anemia. Health Qual Life Outcomes. 2015;13:60. https://doi.org/10.1186/s12955-015-0257-x.
173. Cella D, Wilson H, Shalhoub H, et al. Content validity and psychometric evaluation of functional assessment of chronic illness therapy-fatigue in patients with psoriatic arthritis. J Patient Rep Outcomes. 2019;3:30. https://doi.org/10.1186/s41687-019-0115-4.
174. Eek D, Ivanescu C, Corredoira L, Meyers O, Cella D. Content validity and psychometric evaluation of the functional assessment of chronic illness therapy-fatigue scale in patients with chronic lymphocytic leukemia. J Patient Rep Outcomes. 2021;5(1):27. https://doi.org/10.1186/s41687-021-00294-1.
175. Jones PW, Quirk FH, Baveystock CM. The St George's respiratory questionnaire. Respir Med. 85;(Suppl B):25–31.
176. Swigris JJ, Esser D, Conoscenti CS, Brown KK. The psychometric properties of the St George's Respiratory Questionnaire (SGRQ) in patients with idiopathic pulmonary fibrosis: a literature review. Health Qual Life Outcomes. 2014;12(1):124.
177. Richeldi L, du Bois RM, Raghu G, Azuma A, Brown KK, Costabel U, et al. Efficacy and safety of nintedanib in idiopathic pulmonary fibrosis. N Engl J Med. 2014;370(22):2071–82.

178. Furukawa T, Taniguchi H, Ando M, Kondoh Y, Kataoka K, Nishiyama O, et al. The St. George's Respiratory Questionnaire as a prognostic factor in IPF. Respir Res. 2017;18(1):18.
179. Yorke J, Jones PW, Swigris JJ. Development and validity testing of an IPF-specific version of the St George's Respiratory Questionnaire. Thorax. 2010;65(10):921–6.
180. Andrich D. Rasch models for measurement: SAGE Publications. Thousand Oaks: SAGE Publications, Inc; 1988.
181. Patel AS, Siegert RJ, Brignall K, Gordon P, Steer S, Desai SR, et al. The development and validation of the King's Brief Interstitial Lung Disease (K-BILD) health status questionnaire. Thorax. 2012;67(9):804–10.
182. Patel AS, Siegert RJ, Bajwah S, Brignall K, Gosker HR, Moxham J, et al. Rasch analysis and impact factor methods both yield valid and comparable measures of health status in interstitial lung disease. J Clin Epidemiol. 2015;68(9):1019–27.
183. Yorke J, Spencer LG, Duck A, Ratcliffe S, Kwong GN, Longshaw MS, et al. Cross-Atlantic modification and validation of the A Tool to Assess Quality of Life in Idiopathic Pulmonary Fibrosis (ATAQ-IPF-cA). BMJ Open Respir Res. 2014;1(1):e000024.
184. Swigris JJ, Andrae DA, Churney T, Johnson N, Scholand MB, White ES, Matsui A, Raimundo K, Evans CJ. Development and initial validation analyses of the living with idiopathic pulmonary fibrosis questionnaire. Am J Respir Crit Care Med. 2020;202(12):1689–97. https://doi.org/10.1164/rccm.202002-0415OC.
185. Mitchell AJ, Kaar S, Coggan C, Herdman J. Acceptability of common screening methods used to detect distress and related mood disorders-preferences of cancer specialists and non-specialists. Psychooncology. 2008;17:226–36.
186. Finkelstein DM, Schoenfeld DA. Combining mortality and longitudinal measures in clinical trials. Stat Med. 1999;18(11):1341–54.
187. Overgaard D, Kaldan G, Marsaa K, Nielsen TL, Shaker SB, Egerod I. The lived experience with idiopathic pulmonary fibrosis: a qualitative study. Eur Respir J. 2016;47(5):1472–80.
188. Belkin A, Albright K, Swigris JJ. A qualitative study of informal caregivers' perspectives on the effects of idiopathic pulmonary fibrosis. BMJ Open Respir Res. 2014;1:e000007.
189. Schoenheit G, Becattelli I, Cohen AH. Living with idiopathic pulmonary fibrosis: an in-depth qualitative survey of European patients. Chron Respir Dis. 2011;8(4):225–31.
190. Giot C, Maronati M, Becattelli I, Schoenheit G. Idiopathic pulmonary fibrosis: an EU patient perspective survey; 2013.
191. Duck A, Spencer LG, Bailey S, Leonard C, Ormes J, Caress AL. Perceptions, experiences and needs of patients with idiopathic pulmonary fibrosis. J Adv Nurs. 2015;71:1055–65.
192. Bajwah S, Koffman J, Higginson IJ, Ross JR, Wells AU, Birring SS, et al. 'I wish I knew more ...' the end-of-life planning and information needs for end-stage fibrotic interstitial lung disease: views of patients, carers and health professionals. BMJ Support Palliat Care. 2013;3(1):84–90.
193. Sampson C, Gill BH, Harrison NK, Nelson AM, Byrne A. The care needs of patients with idiopathic pulmonary fibrosis and their carers (CaNoPy): results of a qualitative study. BMC Pulm Med. 2015;15:155.
194. Greenhalgh J, Gooding K, Gibbons E, et al. How do patient reported outcome measures (PROMs) support clinician-patient communication and patient care? A realist synthesis. J Patient Rep Outcomes. 2018;2:42. https://doi.org/10.1186/s41687-018-0061-6.

# Chapter 5
# Quality of Life in Chronic Lung Disease

**Matthew Koslow and Jeffrey Swigris**

## Introduction

Despite tremendous advances in understanding the pathophysiology of chronic lung diseases and the environmental and genetic influences on their development, therapeutic options to reverse many of these diseases are limited. Thus, chronic lung diseases can cause great suffering, but healthcare providers can ease the burden of disease for patients and their caregivers. For many chronic lung diseases, medicinal therapies can slow or halt progression, and these, in combination with other pharmacological or non-drug interventions and a thoughtful, empathic approach to care, aim to relieve the burdens of disease, reduce physical impairment, preserve independence, and maintain quality of life (QOL) – to keep patients living as well as possible for as long as possible.

### *What Is QOL, and Why Is It So Important?*

QOL is an abstract construct, reasonably understood and recognized as important by all people. QOL is loosely defined as overall enjoyment or satisfaction with one's station in life. The World Health Organization defines health as "a state of complete physical, mental and social well-being not merely the absence of disease…" and further defines QOL as an individual's perception of their position in life in the context of the culture and value systems in which they live (and in relation to their goals, expectations, standards, and concerns). The most comprehensive assessment

M. Koslow (✉) · J. Swigris
Interstitial Lung Disease Program, Department of Medicine, National Jewish Health, Denver, CO, USA
e-mail: koslowm@njhealth.org; SwigrisJ@NJHealth.org


K. O. Lindell, S. K. Danoff (eds.), *Palliative Care in Lung Disease*, Respiratory Medicine, https://doi.org/10.1007/978-3-030-81788-6_5

of QOL would integrate a person's perceptions about their life for each of 16 life dimensions: material comforts, physical health and personal safety, relationships with family, having and raising children, relationship with a spouse/partner, having close friends, helping and encouraging others, participating in activities relating to local/national government and/or public affairs, learning, understanding oneself, independence, work, expressing oneself, socializing, reading/listening to music/entertainment, and participation in active recreation. Obviously, not all dimensions are applicable to all people, and how much value is placed on any one of them will vary from person to person – these make QOL a very personal construct.

For many patients with chronic disease, QOL is valued as much or more than how long they live. However, the medical community has traditionally defined health and well-being from a perspective of deficit, focusing on physical morbidity and mortality. In order to effectively intervene and improve QOL for patients with any chronic condition, we have needed to develop greater understanding of how diseases impact QOL. For any chronic lung disease, QOL correlates only weakly to moderately strong with clinical measures of disease severity, like pulmonary function or imaging studies; thus, knowing results for them leaves much to know about a person's (or cohort's) QOL – it must be measured directly.

## *What Is Health-Related Quality of Life?*

Health-related quality of life (HRQL) is an individual's satisfaction or happiness with domains of life as they affect or are affected by "health." The assessment of HRQL is an attempt to determine how the variables within the construct of health (e.g., a disease and things associated with it, like the physical symptoms it causes; its impact on emotional well-being; and its treatment and longitudinal management) affect dimensions of life determined to be important to people in general (diseased or well) or those dimensions most important to patients with a specific disease (condition-specific HRQL) [1].

When making decisions about health (e.g., to have a procedure, take a medicine, enroll in hospice), patients will consciously or subconsciously integrate QOL as they attempt to forecast how a choice will impact their lives. To make such a judgment, patients must have access to reliable information about the potential benefits and harms of candidate choices.

## Case Discussion

A 65-year-old man (martial arts instructor, married, father of two, lifelong nonsmoker) developed fatigue and breathlessness over several months. He was initially diagnosed with mild sleep apnea and mild pulmonary hypertension, but after 24 months and consultations with three different physicians, he was ultimately diagnosed with pulmonary fibrosis. He searched the internet, receiving numerous hits for "idiopathic pulmonary fibrosis" and became depressed when he read about its poor prognosis. He asked: "Will I need oxygen? How fast will this progress? What should I do with my martial arts studio? What will life look like for me in 1, 2, 3 years?"

The approach to his management should include an assessment (formal or informal) of his current QOL, consideration of the dimensions of life most important to him, discussions of therapeutic options, and a plan for promoting and maintaining QOL no matter the stage or severity of his disease.

## Measuring QOL or HRQL

QOL or HRQL is formally assessed through the administration of questionnaires (tools or instruments) that contain one or more questions (items). For multidimensional questionnaires, the items tap (ask about) different dimensions (domains), and the dimensions may or may not be apparent to the respondent. Questionnaires may be completed in paper and pencil format or electronically (on a tablet or computer, on- or offline), depending on how it was developed.

Questionnaires are generic or disease/condition specific, and there are literally thousands of them to choose from. Many questionnaires are in the public domain; others are proprietary. MAPI Research Trust (mapi-trust.org) is a trustworthy, respected, nonprofit organization that oversees licensing and distribution of several thousand questionnaires.

Generic questionnaires have been used to determine allocation of healthcare resources and allow comparison of outcomes across disease states or, for many questionnaires with normative response data, comparison of patients with a condition to people in the general population. The World Health Organization's 100-item questionnaire (WHOQOL-100) is an example of a generic QOL questionnaire [2].

By focusing on the domains of interest (and including items generated through discussions or interviews with patients with the condition of interest), *disease-specific questionnaires* are typically more sensitive to change than generic questionnaires in the population of interest. The St. George's Respiratory Questionnaire (SGRQ) is an example of a condition-specific questionnaire: it was developed for assessment of patients with airflow limitation, asthma, or COPD [3].

## Which Questionnaire Is Best?

There is probably no such thing as a "best" questionnaire for assessing QOL or HRQL in patients with chronic lung disease. There are many questionnaires available with acceptable measurement properties in patients with chronic lung disease. However, which one(s) to use depends on the purpose for which it is employed. For example, "Are assessments being done for clinical care or in the context of a research study?", "What is already known about QOL in the population of interest?", "How the condition affects QOL?", "Is that information applicable?", "What does the clinician or researcher want to learn/study?", "How granular does she/he want the data to be (e.g., Would a summary score suffice, or are scores for particular domains of interest desired?)?", "If there is an intervention and what aspects of the condition is the intervention expected to affect?", "Are there data to support the questionnaire's performance in the population under study (e.g., Does it measure what it purports to measure? Is it responsive/sensitive to change over time?)?", and on and on.

Equally important are the content of the candidate questionnaires (do they measure things that align with the objectives of the particular study?), their overall psychometric soundness, and the strength of the foundation of data that show they can capture information of interest under similar circumstances.

We believe it is most useful to administer a generic questionnaire and a condition- or symptom-specific questionnaire when QOL or HRQL is an outcome of interest in a research study.

## Main Drivers of Impairment

Currently, there are no cures – other than lung transplantation – for chronic lung diseases. For many chronic lung diseases, therapies may not affect or alleviate symptoms; thus, patients are forced to live with suboptimal physical health. Dyspnea, cough, and fatigue are symptoms common to all chronic lung diseases, including all forms of interstitial (including cystic) lung disease, chronic obstructive pulmonary disease, and suppurative lung conditions; and for many, symptoms are strong drivers of QOL impairment.

*Dyspnea*, the sensation of breathlessness, is derived from the Greek *dys,* meaning "painful," and *pneuma,* meaning "breath." It is experienced to some degree by nearly every patient with chronic lung disease. Dyspnea results in avoidance of activities that provoke breathlessness, which induces downstream effects including physical deconditioning, fatigue, impaired emotional well-being, and social isolation [4].

Among patients with chronic lung disease, the source of dyspnea may be multifactorial. The identification and treatment of modifiable sources (e.g., heart failure, coronary artery disease, pulmonary hypertension, deconditioning, obesity, muscular weakness, and sleep disorders) may improve dyspnea – and QOL by extension [5]. Because chronic lung diseases are incurable, often progressive, and in most cases not reliably reversible to significant degrees, we believe conducting an exhaustive search for modifiable sources is warranted for all patients.

***Cough*** In some patients with chronic lung disease, cough is the most bothersome symptom. In these and other patients with chronic lung disease, cough may occur in episodes or "spells" that leave patients breathless and anxious [6]. Patients with chronic lung disease report frustration in their inability to control cough; its frequency and severity often leave them physically exhausted, and cough may interfere with sleep or social activities (e.g., going to the movies, a play, a friend's house for dinner). Cough also leaves many patients embarrassed and stigmatized. It's no surprise cough is a driver of QOL impairment in patients with chronic lung disease. As with dyspnea, an exhaustive search for contributors to chronic cough is warranted [7]. In many of our patients with ILD, cough is a sign of peripheral oxygen desaturation, but whether cough in these situations is a direct result of hypoxemia or (we believe more likely) tachypnea and rapid inspiratory flow or rapid chest wall expansion in the setting of a hypersensitive cough response is unknown [8].

***Fatigue*** Fatigue is incredibly common in patients with chronic lung disease. Like dyspnea and cough, fatigue can lead to decreased physical activity and less social participation and increased dependence on caregivers. Although not as widely recognized as a symptom of chronic lung disease as dyspnea and cough, fatigue is debilitating for many patients with chronic lung disease. Patients describe not having the energy to do the things they need or want to do – things they view as giving their life purpose or enjoyment, things that add quality to their lives [9]. As with dyspnea and cough, any of several factors may contribute to fatigue in patients with chronic lung disease, including sleep disorders, drug side effects, and mood disturbance.

***Anxiety and depression*** Patients with any chronic physical disease are susceptible to developing anxiety or depression, which are very common in patients with chronic lung disease [10]. For example, in some studies, nearly 50% of patients with fibrotic ILD have clinically meaningful depression and symptoms of anxiety [11], and their caregivers are at risk to develop these symptoms, too [12]. Debilitating and distressing physical symptoms, uncertain futures and the real possibility of shortened survival, and worry over how families will get on if they die are just a few of the ways chronic lung disease affects patients' emotional well-being. Screening for depression and anxiety at every visit is important in the longitudinal care of patients with chronic lung disease [13].

***Sleep quality*** Sleep is a state of restoration, and poor sleep quality has important daytime consequences. Sleep is frequently disturbed among patients with ILD (or other chronic lung diseases), resulting in insomnia, daytime fatigue and sleepiness, mood disturbances, and QOL impairment [14–16].

***Lack of knowledge and lack of control*** Many patients with chronic lung disease feel powerless over it; they lack control over symptoms; their unpredictable disease courses create worry and unease; working harder does not necessarily equate with improvements in many clinical disease severity variables like pulmonary physiology (i.e., patients cannot exercise their way out of emphysema or pulmonary fibrosis); the only knowledge many patients have about their disease is what they read after typing the name of their condition into a search engine – and the information they see may be partly or entirely wrong and not applicable to or misinterpreted by them. All of these can detract from patients' QOL.

## Improving QOL in Patients with Chronic Lung Disease

Despite the profound burden of symptoms and uncertainty associated with many chronic lung diseases, there is much that can be done to improve how patients feel and function – and by extension, their QOL. Nonmedicinal interventions can play an essential role.

### *Pulmonary Rehabilitation*

Pulmonary rehabilitation – the backbone of which is exercise training – improves QOL in patients with chronic lung disease. Although pulmonary rehabilitation was designed for (and leads to inarguable improvements in QOL among) patients with COPD, a number of studies have demonstrated that pulmonary rehabilitation benefits patients with other chronic lung diseases [17]. Dowman and colleagues conducted the largest trial of exercise training in patients with interstitial lung disease [18]. The treatment group attended twice-weekly supervised, outpatient exercise sessions, each of which included 30 minutes of aerobic exercise and upper and lower limb resistance training while using supplemental oxygen to maintain SpO2 $\geq$ 88%. Subjects demonstrated clinically meaningful improvements in 6MWD, dyspnea, and HRQL. Patients who were most impaired at baseline and those who increased exercise intensity per protocol benefited most. Durability of improvements correlated with baseline physiology prompting the investigators to argue for referral of patients early in the course of their disease.

Despite the compelling evidence supporting the benefits of pulmonary rehabilitation for chronic lung diseases, access remains a major obstacle for many patients. An estimated 50% of those referred to pulmonary rehabilitation will never attend, and 33% do not complete the program [19]. Home-based pulmonary rehabilitation has been proposed as an alternative model to improve access and adherence. Holland and her colleagues randomized 166 subjects to a home-based program or a traditional outpatient program to test their hypothesis that the home-based model would overcome many patient-related barriers to attendance such as travel, inconvenient session times, and disruption to patients' daily routines. Indeed, the home-based group had short-term gains in both 6MWD and HRQL that were equal or greater than the traditional center-based program, and a greater proportion completed the program [20]. Several investigators have demonstrated similar feasibility and success with home-based rehabilitation for COPD [21–23], asthma [24], lung cancer [25], bronchiectasis [26], fibrotic ILD [27], IPF [28], neuromuscular disease [29], and pulmonary hypertension [30] and even in children and adolescents with chronic lung disease [31]. Dr. Anne Holland and her team have developed a state-of-the-art home-based rehabilitation model called "HomeBase" which is an excellent online resource (homebaserehab.net) that provides guidance to health professionals on developing a home-based pulmonary rehabilitation program for their patients [32].

## *Oxygen*

As with pulmonary rehabilitation, much of what we know about oxygen supplementation is derived from studies of COPD patients. Long-term oxygen therapy is one of the few interventions that improves survival of COPD patients [33, 34]. Oxygen supplementation is considered standard of care for resting severe hypoxemia (SpO2 at or below <88%) [35], and, in addition to the survival benefit, it may improve pulmonary hemodynamics [36], sleep quality [37], neuropsychological scores (cognition) [38], and mood [39]. Supplemental oxygen may also improve renal blood flow, reducing salt and water retention [40], and reduce secondary polycythemia [41]. The benefits of oxygen supplementation for COPD patients with severe *resting* hypoxemia have been extrapolated to other chronic lung conditions such as ILD, pulmonary hypertension, cystic fibrosis, and neuromuscular disorders [42]. However, whether it improves QOL in patients who have chronic lung disease and resting hypoxemia is likely but has not been rigorously studied. Data for ambulatory oxygen supplementation are somewhat conflicting.

Ambulatory oxygen therapy (AOT) is the use of supplemental oxygen during exercise or with activities of daily life. Several studies indicate that supplemental oxygen improves exercise endurance and maximal work rate and reduces breathlessness [43, 44]. By using supplemental oxygen, patients who normally desaturate during activity are able to exercise at higher intensity, for longer, and thus gain more from exercise training [45]. The effect of AOT on activities of daily living and its impact on QOL is less straightforward.

The long-term oxygen therapy (LTOT) trial was conducted to test whether long-term treatment with supplemental oxygen improved survival among COPD patients with moderate resting desaturation (SpO2 89–93%) and was expanded to include those with isolated moderate exercise-induced desaturation. Investigators found that supplemental oxygen did not reduce mortality or the risk of hospitalization, nor were their meaningful benefits on QOL, depression, anxiety, or functional status [46]. There were several limitations to LTOT, including that SpO2 was not monitored to ensure that normoxia was maintained among subjects randomized to oxygen.

Exercise hypoxemia is more severe in patients with fibrotic ILD than in patients with COPD, independent of resting SpO2 and baseline pulmonary physiology [47]; thus, data derived from patients with COPD may not apply to patients with other chronic lung disease (e.g., fibrotic ILD). In the AmbOx trial [48], Visca and co-investigators conducted the first randomized controlled trial on the impact of ambulatory oxygen on HRQL measures among fibrotic ILD patients with isolated exertional hypoxemia (Spo 88% or less during 6MWT). Ambulatory oxygen was associated with clinically significant improvements in breathlessness, walking ability, and overall HRQL. Twenty-one subjects participated in qualitative interviews before and after oxygen use: although most reported initial "apprehension" prior to using AOT, in most (15/21), views changed because "they could do more," and most (16/21) continued with oxygen therapy after the study trial.

However, as expected, not all subjects interviewed had a positive experience. Patients and caregivers reported physical and psychological obstacles. Graney and colleagues describe the potential for positive or negative effects when oxygen enters the lives of patients and their caregivers; supplemental oxygen often alters the dynamics of the home and may affect relationships and social interactions [49].

Providers who prescribe supplemental oxygen to patients may help patients transition by offering "information, realistic hope and a plan" [50]. The need for oxygen, which often coincides with disease progression, is a time "when their [patients' and caregivers'] QOL is most threatened, and they are forced to adapt to a new normal" [50]. Providers need to recognize these moments, reassess the needs, and provide essential information that creates the opportunity for oxygen to improve QOL. This may include examples of patients with similar conditions that have adapted to using oxygen, which allows them to continue doing the things they love.

## *Sleep Quality*

Emerging research indicates that improving sleep quality may translate into better HRQL for patients with chronic lung diseases. Effective treatment of OSA among patients with IPF is associated with improvements in daily living activities per the Functional Outcomes of Sleep Questionnaire [51]. In a 2015 study, patients with IPF and moderate to severe OSA were classified according to compliance with continuous positive airway pressure (CPAP) treatment for OSA. Those with good compliance (CPAP use for at least 4 hours per night and 70% of nights per week) demonstrated a statistically significant improvement in all QOL and sleep quality [52].

One challenge facing clinicians, who care for patients with chronic lung disease, is to recognize and diagnose sleep disorders at an early stage, so successful treatment can be initiated. It is also critical to realize that patients with chronic lung disease may have sleep-disordered breathing despite the absence of typical risk factors like elevated BMI [14, 15].

Given the high prevalence of sleep-disordered breathing (SDB) among patients with chronic lung disease; the possible presence of SDB despite the absence of common risk factors; the tangled associations among SDB, mood disturbance/anxiety, dyspnea, and fatigue; and the reasonable expectation that treating sleep disorders could improve outcomes most meaningful to patients, we believe it is appropriate to screen all patients with chronic lung disease for SDB.

### *Social Support*

We encourage all our patients with chronic lung disease to consider involvement in support networks. There are reputable, trustworthy organizations that offer information, educational resources and social support for patients with various chronic lung conditions (e.g., the American Lung Association, the British Lung Foundation, the Pulmonary Fibrosis Foundation, the LAM Foundation, the Cystic Fibrosis Foundation) along with their caregivers. Patients and caregivers who take advantage of these offerings gain knowledge about their disease and, by interacting with others going through the same struggles, realize they are not alone in their battle against chronic lung disease.

### *Talking to Patients*

We practitioners who care for patients with chronic lung disease can play a large role in helping to improve or maintain patients' QOL. The way we talk to patients and their caregivers – the words we use, the tone of our voice, our physical demeanor – can have profound effects on patients' well-being. Being realistic without taking away hope, delivering truth without being dogmatic, and using language that lets patients know we are their partners (and will walk with them through the entirety of their disease course, no matter where it takes them) are key attributes that we can use as we care for patients with any chronic lung disease.

## Back to Our Case

He was clearly and understandably anxious about having chronic lung disease, but in detailed discussions, we determined he did not have generalized anxiety or clinical depression. Much of his outlook was shaped by the misinformation he gathered by doing his own internet search. We partnered with him and shared science-derived, fact-based information. His mild physiological impairment and very gradual decline over the last 3 years suggested the probability of him dying within the next 3 years was not great. However, we told him that we would be here to keep a watchful eye on his disease status and symptoms via quarterly clinic visits (and more frequently if the need arose). We talked to him about the importance of adhering to CPAP therapy for his OSA, participating in a formal pulmonary rehabilitation program and then carrying on with a home-based exercise regimen, using supplemental oxygen with the goal of maintaining normoxia, considering participation in his local support group, using the Pulmonary Fibrosis Foundation website as an informational hub, and considering us as partners to him and his caregiver wife as they navigate his disease journey.

**Table 5.1** A quality of life checklist for the provider, patient, and caregiver

| | |
|---|---|
| Listen | Listen with empathy and understand the current challenges facing patient and caregiver |
| Interests | Encourage activities which bring meaning to patients' lives |
| Friends | Explore available support groups |
| Education | Examine knowledge regarding their disease (treatments and prognosis) and correct misunderstandings, manage expectations, and empower |
| Exercise | Encourage pulmonary rehabilitation and other forms of exercise |
| Oxygen | Evaluate the need for supplemental oxygen at rest, exertion, and sleep. Provide solutions to ambulatory oxygen limitations (e.g., appropriate POC) |
| Sleep | Screen for sleep-disordered breathing |

## Conclusions

Patients with chronic lung disease are at risk for substantially impaired QOL. Threats to their QOL include intrusive, activity-limiting symptoms; mood disturbance and anxiety; having to live with the real possibility of shortened survival; a lack of knowledge about their disease; misinformation they may be exposed to; and feelings of isolation and a lack of support. There are several interventions and opportunities for practitioners to intervene and help boost, bolster, and maintain QOL in these patients. Table 5.1 offers a suggestion of key points to consider during the clinical encounter discussion.

## References

1. Ware JE Jr. The status of health assessment 1994. Annu Rev Public Health. 1995;16:327–54.
2. The World Health Organization Quality of Life Assessment (WHOQOL): development and general psychometric properties. Soc Sci Med. 1998;46(12):1569–85.
3. Meguro M, Barley EA, Spencer S, Jones PW. Development and validation of an improved, COPD-specific version of the St. George Respiratory Questionnaire. Chest. 2007;132(2):456–63.
4. Nishiyama O, Taniguchi H, Kondoh Y, et al. A simple assessment of dyspnoea as a prognostic indicator in idiopathic pulmonary fibrosis. Eur Respir J. 2010;36(5):1067–72.
5. Garibaldi BT, Danoff SK. Symptom-based management of the idiopathic interstitial pneumonia. Respirology. 2016;21(8):1357–65.
6. Smyrnios NA, Irwin RS, Curley FJ, French CL. From a prospective study of chronic cough: diagnostic and therapeutic aspects in older adults. Arch Intern Med. 1998;158(11):1222–8.
7. Irwin RS, Baumann MH, Bolser DC, et al. Diagnosis and management of cough executive summary: ACCP evidence-based clinical practice guidelines. Chest. 2006;129(1 Suppl):1S–23S.
8. Hope-Gill BD, Hilldrup S, Davies C, Newton RP, Harrison NK. A study of the cough reflex in idiopathic pulmonary fibrosis. Am J Respir Crit Care Med. 2003;168(8):995–1002.
9. Swigris JJ, Stewart AL, Gould MK, Wilson SR. Patients' perspectives on how idiopathic pulmonary fibrosis affects the quality of their lives. Health Qual Life Outcomes. 2005;3:61.
10. Holland AE, Fiore JF Jr, Bell EC, et al. Dyspnoea and comorbidity contribute to anxiety and depression in interstitial lung disease. Respirology. 2014;19(8):1215–21.

11. Behr J, Kreuter M, Hoeper MM, et al. Management of patients with idiopathic pulmonary fibrosis in clinical practice: the INSIGHTS-IPF registry. Eur Respir J. 2015;46(1):186–96.
12. Jacome C, Figueiredo D, Gabriel R, Cruz J, Marques A. Predicting anxiety and depression among family carers of people with Chronic Obstructive Pulmonary Disease. Int Psychogeriatr. 2014;26(7):1191–9.
13. Ryerson CJ, Arean PA, Berkeley J, et al. Depression is a common and chronic comorbidity in patients with interstitial lung disease. Respirology. 2012;17(3):525–32.
14. Krishnan V, McCormack MC, Mathai SC, et al. Sleep quality and health-related quality of life in idiopathic pulmonary fibrosis. Chest. 2008;134(4):693–8.
15. Mermigkis C, Stagaki E, Amfilochiou A, et al. Sleep quality and associated daytime consequences in patients with idiopathic pulmonary fibrosis. Med Princ Pract. 2009;18(1):10–5.
16. Cho JG, Teoh A, Roberts M, Wheatley J. The prevalence of poor sleep quality and its associated factors in patients with interstitial lung disease: a cross-sectional analysis. ERJ Open Res. 2019;5(3):00062-2019.
17. Spruit MA, Singh SJ, Garvey C, et al. An official American Thoracic Society/European Respiratory Society statement: key concepts and advances in pulmonary rehabilitation. Am J Respir Crit Care Med. 2013;188(8):e13–64.
18. Dowman LM, McDonald CF, Hill CJ, et al. The evidence of benefits of exercise training in interstitial lung disease: a randomised controlled trial. Thorax. 2017;72(7):610–9.
19. Keating A, Lee A, Holland AE. What prevents people with chronic obstructive pulmonary disease from attending pulmonary rehabilitation? A systematic review. Chron Respir Dis. 2011;8(2):89–99.
20. Holland AE, Mahal A, Hill CJ, et al. Home-based rehabilitation for COPD using minimal resources: a randomised, controlled equivalence trial. Thorax. 2017;72(1):57–65.
21. Horton EJ, Mitchell KE, Johnson-Warrington V, et al. Comparison of a structured home-based rehabilitation programme with conventional supervised pulmonary rehabilitation: a randomised non-inferiority trial. Thorax. 2018;73(1):29–36.
22. Benzo R, Vickers K, Novotny PJ, et al. Health coaching and chronic obstructive pulmonary disease rehospitalization. A randomized study. Am J Respir Crit Care Med. 2016;194(6):672–80.
23. Benzo RP, Kramer KM, Hoult JP, Anderson PM, Begue IM, Seifert SJ. Development and feasibility of a home pulmonary rehabilitation program with health coaching. Respir Care. 2018;63(2):131–40.
24. Grosbois JM, Coquart J, Fry S, et al. Long-term effect of home-based pulmonary rehabilitation in severe asthma. Respir Med. 2019;157:36–41.
25. Edbrooke L, Denehy L, Granger CL, Kapp S, Aranda S. Home-based rehabilitation in inoperable non-small cell lung cancer-the patient experience. Support Care Cancer. 2020;28(1):99–112.
26. Jose A, Holland AE, Oliveira CS, et al. Does home-based pulmonary rehabilitation improve functional capacity, peripheral muscle strength and quality of life in patients with bronchiectasis compared to standard care? Braz J Phys Ther. 2017;21(6):473–80.
27. Wallaert B, Duthoit L, Drumez E, et al. Long-term evaluation of home-based pulmonary rehabilitation in patients with fibrotic idiopathic interstitial pneumonias. ERJ Open Res. 2019;5(2):00045-2019.
28. Ozalevli S, Karaali HK, Ilgin D, Ucan ES. Effect of home-based pulmonary rehabilitation in patients with idiopathic pulmonary fibrosis. Multidiscip Respir Med. 2010;5(1):31–7.
29. Kagaya H, Takahashi H, Sugawara K, Kasai C, Kiyokawa N, Shioya T. Effective home-based pulmonary rehabilitation in patients with restrictive lung diseases. Tohoku J Exp Med. 2009;218(3):215–9.
30. Inagaki T, Terada J, Tanabe N, et al. Home-based pulmonary rehabilitation in patients with inoperable or residual chronic thromboembolic pulmonary hypertension: a preliminary study. Respir Investig. 2014;52(6):357–64.
31. Nunez IR, Araos DZ, Delgado CM. Effects of home-based respiratory muscle training in children and adolescents with chronic lung disease. J Bras Pneumol. 2014;40(6):626–33.
32. Holland A. HomeBase pulmonary rehab. https://homebaserehab.net.

33. Continuous or nocturnal oxygen therapy in hypoxemic chronic obstructive lung disease: a clinical trial. Nocturnal Oxygen Therapy Trial Group. Ann Intern Med. 1980;93(3):391–8.
34. Long term domiciliary oxygen therapy in chronic hypoxic cor pulmonale complicating chronic bronchitis and emphysema. Report of the Medical Research Council Working Party. Lancet. 1981;1(8222):681–6.
35. Rodriguez-Roisin R, Rabe KF, Vestbo J, et al. Global Initiative for Chronic Obstructive Lung Disease (GOLD) 20th anniversary: a brief history of time. Eur Respir J. 2017;50(1):1700671.
36. Timms RM, Khaja FU, Williams GW. Hemodynamic response to oxygen therapy in chronic obstructive pulmonary disease. Ann Intern Med. 1985;102(1):29–36.
37. Calverley PM, Brezinova V, Douglas NJ, Catterall JR, Flenley DC. The effect of oxygenation on sleep quality in chronic bronchitis and emphysema. Am Rev Respir Dis. 1982;126(2):206–10.
38. Heaton RK, Grant I, McSweeny AJ, Adams KM, Petty TL. Psychologic effects of continuous and nocturnal oxygen therapy in hypoxemic chronic obstructive pulmonary disease. Arch Intern Med. 1983;143(10):1941–7.
39. Borak J, Sliwinski P, Tobiasz M, Gorecka D, Zielinski J. Psychological status of COPD patients before and after one year of long-term oxygen therapy. Monaldi Arch Chest Dis. 1996;51(1):7–11.
40. Bratel T, Ljungman S, Runold M, Stenvinkel P. Renal function in hypoxaemic chronic obstructive pulmonary disease: effects of long-term oxygen treatment. Respir Med. 2003;97(4):308–16.
41. Chambellan A, Chailleux E, Similowski T, Group AO. Prognostic value of the hematocrit in patients with severe COPD receiving long-term oxygen therapy. Chest. 2005;128(3):1201–8.
42. Hardinge M, Annandale J, Bourne S, et al. British Thoracic Society guidelines for home oxygen use in adults. Thorax. 2015;70 Suppl 1:i1–43.
43. Bradley JM, Lasserson T, Elborn S, Macmahon J, O'Neill B. A systematic review of randomized controlled trials examining the short-term benefit of ambulatory oxygen in COPD. Chest. 2007;131(1):278–85.
44. Bradley JM, O'Neill B. Short-term ambulatory oxygen for chronic obstructive pulmonary disease. Cochrane Database Syst Rev. 2005;(4):CD004356.
45. Dyer F, Callaghan J, Cheema K, Bott J. Ambulatory oxygen improves the effectiveness of pulmonary rehabilitation in selected patients with chronic obstructive pulmonary disease. Chron Respir Dis. 2012;9(2):83–91.
46. Long-Term Oxygen Treatment Trial Research G, Albert RK, Au DH, et al. A randomized trial of long-term oxygen for COPD with moderate desaturation. N Engl J Med. 2016;375(17):1617–27.
47. Du Plessis JP, Fernandes S, Jamal R, et al. Exertional hypoxemia is more severe in fibrotic interstitial lung disease than in COPD. Respirology. 2018;23(4):392–8.
48. Visca D, Mori L, Tsipouri V, et al. Effect of ambulatory oxygen on quality of life for patients with fibrotic lung disease (AmbOx): a prospective, open-label, mixed-method, crossover randomised controlled trial. Lancet Respir Med. 2018;6(10):759–70.
49. Graney BA, Wamboldt FS, Baird S, et al. Informal caregivers experience of supplemental oxygen in pulmonary fibrosis. Health Qual Life Outcomes. 2017;15(1):133.
50. Swigris JJ. Transitions and touchpoints in idiopathic pulmonary fibrosis. BMJ Open Respir Res. 2018;5(1):e000317.
51. Weaver TE, Laizner AM, Evans LK, et al. An instrument to measure functional status outcomes for disorders of excessive sleepiness. Sleep. 1997;20(10):835–43.
52. Mermigkis C, Mermigkis D, Varouchakis G, Schiza S. CPAP treatment in patients with idiopathic pulmonary fibrosis and obstructive sleep apnea--therapeutic difficulties and dilemmas. Sleep Breath. 2012;16(1):1–3.

# Chapter 6
# Breathlessness

**Irene J. Higginson, Charles C. Reilly, and Matthew Maddocks**

## Introduction

Breathlessness is one of the most common, burdensome and neglected symptoms affecting patients in palliative and end of life care, in particular those with advanced or progressive lung disease [1, 2], and represents a major clinical management challenge [1, 3–5]. It has a devastating impact on patients' lives, severely impacting their well-being and quality of life and their family, friends and caregivers [6–8], causing additional anxiety and social isolation for the patient and their family and carers [9–11]. Breathlessness results in high health, social and informal care costs and is one of the most frequent causes of emergency hospital admission and attendance [9–14]. In people with advanced disease and breathlessness, the informal care costs, e.g. time spent helping with daily tasks and loss of earnings, can increase the overall societal costs (i.e. when added to formal care costs) by >250% [15].

In the advanced stages of lung disease, including at the end of life, breathlessness often increases in severity, becomes debilitating and frightening and often results in emergency department visits and hospitalisation [10, 11, 16–18]. People with such breathlessness often have multiple symptoms, which also increase as their diseases progress [9, 19]. Our research [20] has estimated that worldwide over 75 million

I. J. Higginson (✉) · M. Maddocks
Cicely Saunders Institute of Palliative Care, Policy and Rehabilitation, King's College London, London, UK
e-mail: irene.higginson@kcl.ac.uk; matthew.maddocks@kcl.ac.uk

C. C. Reilly
Cicely Saunders Institute of Palliative Care, Policy and Rehabilitation, King's College London, London, UK

Department of Physiotherapy, King's College Hospital NHS Foundation Trust, London, UK
e-mail: charles.reilly@nhs.net



K. O. Lindell, S. K. Danoff (eds.), *Palliative Care in Lung Disease*, Respiratory Medicine, https://doi.org/10.1007/978-3-030-81788-6_6

people experience breathlessness each year, including more than 90% of the 65 million people with severe lung disease, over 50% of the 10 million with incurable cancer and 50% of the 23 million with heart failure.

## What Do We Mean By Breathlessness?

Breathlessness, also called dyspnoea or dyspnea, is widely accepted as a subjective experience of breathing discomfort that consists of qualitatively distinct sensations that vary in intensity [6]. The experience of breathlessness derives from interactions among multiple physiological, psychological, social and environmental factors and may induce secondary physiological and behavioural responses. Importantly, as this definition makes it clear with the use of subjective experience, breathlessness can only be perceived by the person experiencing it [6].

As Table 6.1 illustrates, although terminology and classification are evolving, palliative care most often focuses on patients whose breathlessness persists despite optimal treatment of their underlying disease. This is referred to as chronic breathlessness or refractory breathlessness [3, 21–24]. The concept of episodic breathlessness has developed, with acute episodes of intense breathlessness, often overlaying chronic or refractory breathlessness (see Fig. 6.1 and Table 6.1) [25–30]. These episodes are often acutely distressing and frightening, leading to emergency hospital attendance [25, 27].

## What Is the Mechanism of Breathlessness in Advanced Diseases?

Breathing is essential for life. It is normal to increase the work of breathing and become breathless during increased physical activity, when more oxygen is required and more carbon dioxide needs to be eliminated. In health, the lungs have a great capacity to meet these metabolic demands, by increasing both the rate and depth of breathing; this increased work of breathing is what we perceive and subjectively experience as breathlessness. In health, breathlessness recovery is rapid, therefore often not distressing.

In patients affected by lung diseases such as COPD and ILD and those with cancer, the lung capacity is reduced, increasing the demand in the respiratory muscle pump, resulting in symptomatic breathlessness during daily activities or at rest, which is very distressing for the individual. The experience of breathlessness is temporally and qualitatively different to other symptoms. It steadily increases over time (chronic or refractory breathlessness) with exacerbations (acute or episodic breathlessness) limiting mobility and everyday function [31–34]. At its most severe,

**Table 6.1** What's in a name: emerging and common definitions of chronic, refractory and episodic breathlessness?

| Term | Citation | Definition | Strengths | Limitations |
|---|---|---|---|---|
| ATS breathlessness definition of dyspnoea or breathlessness | American Thoracic Society statement [6] | A subjective experience of breathing discomfort that consists of qualitatively distinct sensations that vary in intensity | Based on international consensus<br>Widely used and accepted | Does not reflect the breathlessness experienced in more severe disease, which continues despite treatment of the underlying condition |
| Intractable breathlessness | Booth et al. (2008) [42] | Breathlessness that persists despite treatment of the disease | Clear that breathlessness is difficult to manage | Suggests breathlessness cannot be alleviated |
| Refractory breathlessness | Booth et al. (2009) [116]<br>Horton and Rocker (2010) [117] | Breathlessness that persists despite optimal treatment of the underlying condition | Common term in published literature<br>102 matches on PubMed in 2018, 6 in the title<br>Includes chronic and episodic breathlessness [118] | 'Refractory' may suggest complete resistance to treatment which is not always the case<br>Term is used in varying ways in the literature |
| Chronic breathlessness | Bowden et al. (2011) [119] | Episodes of breathlessness lasting more than 3 months | Common term in published literature<br>76 matches on PubMed in 2018, 5 in the title | Can be defined more narrowly as breathlessness for more than 4–8 weeks, or 'long term'<br>May miss episodes of breathlessness |
| Chronic refractory breathlessness | Currow et al. (2013) [120–122] | Chronic breathlessness which is refractory to treatments for the underlying condition | Emerging term<br>34 matches on PubMed<br>Explicitly states both 'chronic' and 'refractory' | As for refractory breathlessness may suggest complete resistance to treatment |
| Episodic breathlessness | Simon et al. (2013) [25, 27] | Severe worsening of breathlessness intensity or unpleasantness beyond usual fluctuations in the patient's perception [28–30] | Is characterised as one form of refractory breathlessness<br>Highlights the importance of unpleasant episodes that often drive hospital use [118] | Is a newly emerging term with varying definitions<br>29 matches on PubMed<br>Is sometimes called 'acute' or 'breakthrough' breathlessness |

(continued)

**Table 6.1** (continued)

| Term | Citation | Definition | Strengths | Limitations |
|---|---|---|---|---|
| Chronic breathlessness syndrome | Johnson et al. (2017) [123] | Breathlessness that persists despite optimal treatment of the underlying pathophysiology and results in disability for the patient | Recent consensus Inclusion of impact of breathlessness related 'experience' and 'disability' Clinical syndrome may lead to increased awareness of its importance for clinicians and others | New term. Does not reflect the World Health Organisation's new definition of disability in the International Classification of Functioning, Disability and Health (ICF 2001) |

Triggered, normal breathless level
Late onset, quick recovery
(e.g, heavy exertion, getting very excited)
Triggered, predictable (typical for exertional breathlessness)
Always triggered – certain level of trigger causes predictable severity of breathlessness
"still able to breathe."
Triggered, unpredictable
Triggered but unpredictable, not related to level of trigger
"it's unpredictable."
Non-triggered: attack-like
Non-triggered (unpredictable), out-of-the-blue, no warning – quick onset, often severe
"it hits you."
Non-triggered or triggered: wave-like (COPD specific)
Gradually onset, mostly severe, "don't panic"
"You can't stop it."

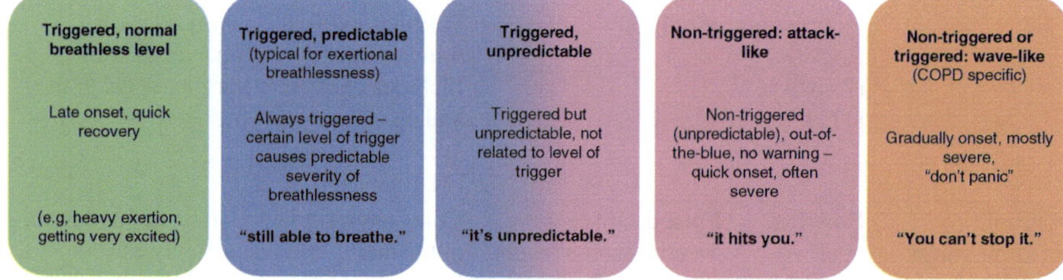

**Fig. 6.1** Emergent phenotypes of breathlessness according to the nature of episodes experienced, which may have different mechanisms. Episodic breathlessness is found in COPD, IPF and cancer patients [25, 26]

breathlessness is interpreted as an immediate threat to life and often results in hospitalisation [35].

Breathlessness, as in all definitions above (see Table 6.1), is a distressing, multidimensional sensation resulting from complex interactions between physiological, environmental, cultural and social factors, with a considerable emotional component. This requires mechanisms for arousal, detection and triggering of appropriate motor responses to correct actual or threatened disturbances to homeostasis, likely involving common corticolimbic pathways [36, 37]. There are no sensory afferents solely responsible for the sensation of breathlessness [7, 38, 39]. Instead, the three interrelated axes are involved. It is important in palliative care treatment, education and research to consider these three axes together, in contrast with earlier 'silo' or single-discipline approaches.

## *Lung-Brain*

The sensation of breathlessness is closely related to the sensation of respiratory effort, suggesting common neurophysiological origins [35]. Respiratory effort is increased when the load on the respiratory muscles increases, the capacity of the respiratory muscles decreases or there is a combination of both factors. When there is load-capacity imbalance, neural drive to the respiratory muscles (neural respiratory drive, NRD) from the medullary respiratory centre increases to maintain gas exchange. The conscious awareness of the level of NRD is important to the perception of breathlessness (see Fig. 6.1) [32, 34, 40].

Breathlessness therefore involves cortical integration of sensory information from awareness of NRD (reflecting the load on respiratory muscles), and afferent feedback from the respiratory system (sensory and/or chemical) [36, 37]. When there is increased work of breathing and lung capacity is reduced (e.g. patients with chronic respiratory disease), a mismatch can occur between increasing NRD and the ability of the respiratory muscles to increase the level of ventilation [40, 41]. Increasing requirements for oxygen (because the lungs do not work well, or the muscles need more oxygen) increases the load on the respiratory system, which in turn increases NRD. This alters afferent feedback and changes in the sensorimotor cortex (intensity) and limbic pathways (unpleasantness/distress) [42] modulating breathlessness and its distinct sensations [35, 40].

This mismatch between increasing NRD and the underlying response occurs irrespective of the underlying cause (obstructive lung diseases, e.g. COPD, or restrictive lung diseases, e.g. ILD) [41]. Recent research using functional neuroimaging has identified a relatively consistent set of brain areas and networks that are associated with breathlessness. However, the brain is not a passive signal transducer; a person's expectations and mood are major contributors to the function of the brain networks that generate perceptions of breathlessness, highlighting the importance of the brain-lung axis [43]. These findings also suggest that other symptoms which commonly occur when people have breathlessness, such as lack of sleep or pain, anxiety and depression, will all contribute to lower mood and lead to lower threshold or amplification of an individual's perception (experience) of breathlessness. Therefore, a holistic approach to management should also address these symptoms.

## *Behavioural-Functional*

Breathlessness produces a 'spiral of disability' whereby physical inactivity causes deconditioning, reduced functional capacity and increased NRD and breathlessness at progressively lower workloads [35, 44–48]. Deconditioning also leads to muscle wasting weakness, especially of the quadricep muscles (thighs) [49]. Skeletal muscle aerobic function is reduced, leading to lactic acidosis induced by exercise at relatively low workloads [50]. This increases NRD due to $CO_2$ generated by bicarbonate buffering and hydrogen ion stimulation thereby increasing breathlessness.

### *Psychosocial*

Emotion affects the anticipation, perception of and response to afferent information [7]. Panic and anxiety are common responses to breathlessness, modulated by context, culture and prior experiences [51]. Respiratory afferent information may be translated into neural code and transmitted to a subcortical gating area. This allows sensations to reach consciousness via distinct areas of sensorimotor and affective cortex [52]. In chronic respiratory disease, there is evidence of relative 'desensitisation' to respiratory afferent information [34].

Neuroimaging studies suggest plasticity in pathways traditionally associated with the perception of noxious stimuli, including breathlessness [53–56]. This potentially allows treatment of breathlessness-related distress without a reduction in NRD or the associated sensorimotor activation.

## Assessment and Management of Breathlessness in Palliative Care for People with Lung Disease: A Holistic and Interdisciplinary Approach

These three axes to the generation of breathlessness have critical implications for assessment and management. They demonstrate how firstly assessment must be based on the individuality of the patient's experience of breathlessness. Management of breathlessness must go well beyond the lungs; it needs to consider muscle strength, managing functioning, thinking as well as affecting the brain response, by, for example, the flow of air across the face. A perfect treatment would affect all three axes; see Fig. 6.2. This is something that needs careful explanation to patients and families, as there is often a focus on only the lungs, and patients can move into a 'disability' cycle of doing less. Breathlessness leads to physical inactivity, causing muscle deconditioning, which itself drives breathlessness, further physical inactivity and so on. The management of breathlessness, therefore, must be holistic and use multidisciplinary approaches. Booth proposed a model of treatment based on breathing (efficient breathing), thinking (avoiding negative thoughts) and functioning (prevention of deconditioning) which addresses most aspects of the axes outlined above. These approaches are often combined in holistic breathlessness-triggered services; see below. Figure 6.3 outlines a flowchart of the steps in management.

The exertional nature of breathlessness, and the fact that breathlessness is a normal part of life, also means that reduction of breathlessness, control of breathing and relief of its distress and negative impact on quality of life are usually the therapeutic goal, rather than complete elimination of breathlessness.

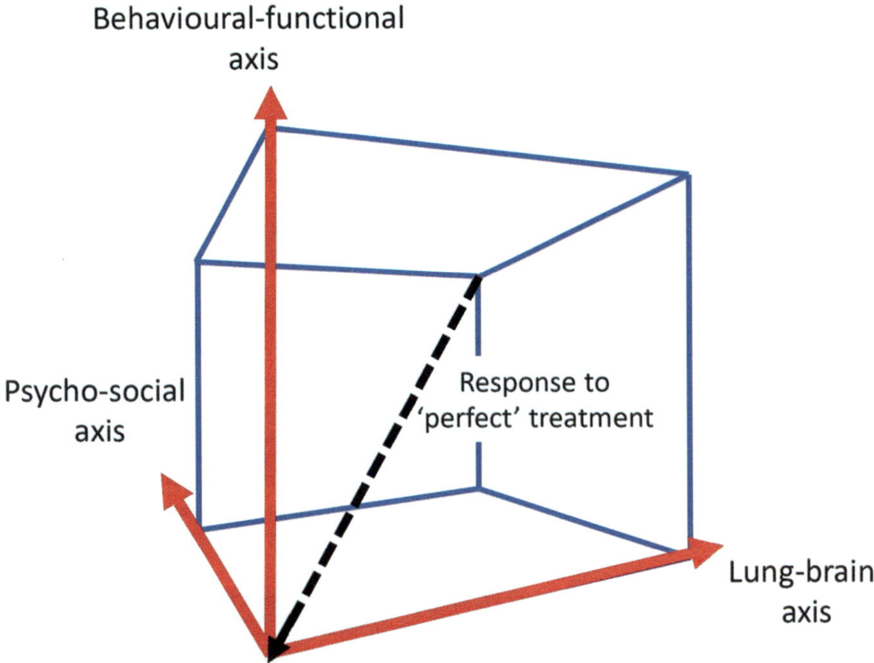


**Fig. 6.2** Hypothesised baseline and post-treatment responses of breathlessness in palliative care. On each axis, movement towards the origin indicates improvement. The hypothesised response to a holistic intervention is shown, improving on all three axes. The exertional nature of breathlessness means that reduction rather than elimination of the symptom is the therapeutic goal. Patients with episodic breathlessness (Fig. 6.1) may be particularly aided by treatments which affect the psychosocial axis, because of the short duration of the breathlessness

## Assessment of Breathlessness

The nature of breathlessness outlined above establishes why breathlessness assessment should focus on assessing breathlessness as what the patient says it is.

There is a plethora of assessment tools available to measure breathlessness. The modified Medical Research Council Breathlessness Scale is widely used in the assessment of breathlessness. It is a useful measure to categorise populations, correlates with quality of life [57] and may be helpful in explaining the nature of the population to respiratory or other clinicians. However, it is unlikely to be sensitive to change over time in palliative care patients, who mostly have an mMRC score of 3 (stops for breath after walking ~100 yards (91 metres) or after few minutes on the level) or 4 (too breathless to leave the house, or breathless when dressing or undressing), the two worst categories [20, 58].

Systematic reviews have appraised the different measures. Bausewein and co-workers [58] assessed measures with regard to validity, reliability, appropriateness and responsiveness to change in advanced disease. The tools were then examined for their usefulness in measuring important components of breathlessness in

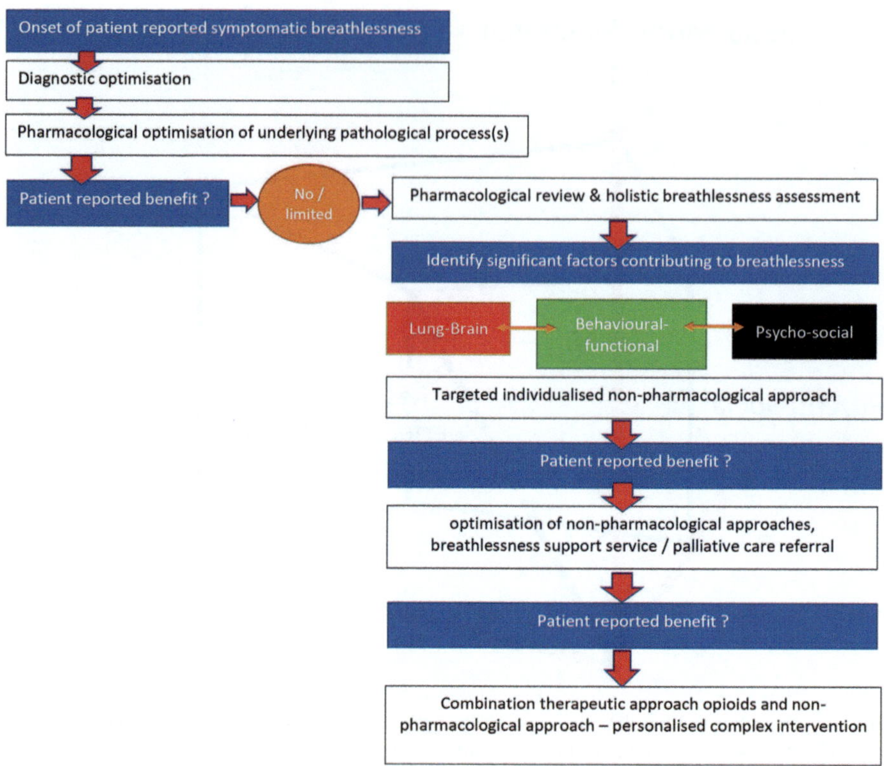


**Fig. 6.3** Proposed steps in the management of breathlessness. (Copyright: Reilly, Higginson, Maddocks developed for this chapter)

advanced disease. This review recommended applying a combination of measures to assess breathlessness, using a single item, such as numerical rating scale (NRS), and then one of the better validated multidimensional measures (such as the Chronic Respiratory Questionnaire). In research, other methods (such as qualitative techniques) could be useful to gauge psychosocial and carer distress for the assessment of breathlessness in advanced disease [58]. A systematic review by Dorman and co-workers [59] appraised measures with particular emphasis on construct validity and responsiveness for use in palliative care. They concluded that NRS and some breathlessness-specific measures were first-line choices. The National Cancer Research Institute Palliative Care Breathlessness Subgroup consensus statement (2009) recommended that breathlessness severity should be assessed in research using a single-item measure, but that researchers should also consider including a measure of fatigue, mastery, emotional state and sleep [7]. The American Thoracic Society classified assessment measures according to the domains of sensory-perceptual experience, affective distress and symptom/disease impact or burden [6]. People living with advanced disease and breathlessness report concerns across six domains of 'total breathlessness', and it is worthwhile considering whether these aspects should be considered in assessment of breathlessness: (1) physical including function, (2) emotional concerns, (3) social impact, (4) spiritual distress, (5) impact of control in relation to an episode of breathlessness and within the wider context and (6) context (episodic and/or chronic) [60].

This patient group will often report multiple symptoms with breathlessness co-existing alongside pain, depression, anxiety and fatigue [9]. In the clinic setting, time does not allow for a detailed assessment of each symptom; therefore composite measures, e.g. the Palliative care Outcome Scale (POS) or Edmonton Symptom Assessment Scale (ESAS), are clinically valuable [61].

Many of the breathlessness-specific measures developed for research, rather than clinical practice, provide valuable information on the perception of breathlessness, its impact on day-to-day life and factors which exacerbate the symptom, but are not sensitive enough to detect small but significant changes that may occur in the symptom in a patient with advanced disease. In addition, a minimally clinically important difference has been described for only some of these tools, and for others this information is not available.

Unidimensional measures, like the NRS, or clinical measures like the POS are more suitable for repeated measures than disease-specific tools as they take only a short time to complete and have been shown to be sensitive to change. Lovell and co-workers found that the NRS assessing worst breathlessness (defined as 'How bad has your breathlessness felt at its worst over the past 24 hours?') captured change in a randomised trial across multiple domains when compared with qualitative interviews with patients [62]. Interestingly changes in the single NRS was slightly more closely aligned to changes in the qualitative comments than was the well validated Chronic Respiratory Questionnaire, but the study was small, and the domains of the Chronic Respiratory Questionnaire may provide useful information for planning clinical interventions and understanding the impacts of breathlessness. The NRS worst breathlessness may be an appropriate measure in practice and research in this population. Care should be taken in using the NRS, different wordings have been used over time, and sometimes no wording was specified [62]. The validation of Lovell and co-workers relates only to the wording used in their study. Additional characteristics of breathlessness that can be assessed clinically include its time course [19], triggers and nature (episodic or continuous) [26, 27]. These features may be particularly helpful in palliative care to determine symptom prognosis and which management strategies to pursue. Studying individual trajectories of patients with COPD or lung cancer, Bausewein and co-workers [19] found four distinct patterns: fluctuation, increasing, stable and decreasing breathlessness. Similarly, Simon and co-workers [26] explored experiences of episodic breathlessness, characterised by time-limited 'severe worsening of breathlessness intensity or unpleasantness beyond usual fluctuations in the patient's perception' [27], and found clearly distinguishable triggers. A standardised classification system will help aid clinical assessment, define trial populations, compare findings of studies accurately and help determine which sub-groups of patients respond to which treatments.

The impact of breathlessness on daily living can also be explored. Questions about breathlessness in the context of daily living and brief physical tests can highlight patients who could benefit from additional symptom management. The 6-minute walk [63] and incremental/endurance shuttle walk [64, 65] are commonly used to assess functional exercise capacity. Nonetheless, issues with the time and space required to perform these tests prevent widespread implementation in palliative care. For example, the 6-minute walk requires a 30 m flat course and both require a repeat walk following adequate rest. These also suffer from floor effects when the patient cannot ambulate 10 metres and/or needs frequent rests. A range of simpler and shorter tests are available within gerontology literature, including gait speed, sit-to-stand tests, the Short Physical Performance Battery and the Stair Power Climb Test. The psychometric properties of these in COPD are currently strongest for the 4-metre gait speed [66, 67] and five sit-to-stand tests [68]. The former requires patients to walk at their normal walking speed with or without walking aids along a flat, unobstructed 4 m course. The latter uses standardised instructions and measures the time taken for the patient to stand up and sit down five times from a chair, without the use of the upper limbs, as quickly as possible.

The intricacies of breathlessness make it difficult to identify physiological parameters that relate strongly with its sensation. In advanced disease, traditional lung function measurements, such as $FEV_1$, are poorly related with patient-reported breathlessness and its impact. Effort-dependent testing manoeuvres are often difficult for breathless patients to perform. An emerging physiological correlate to breathlessness is neural respiratory drive (NRD) (see above for model of breathlessness), which reflects the balance between the load *on* and the capacity *of* the respiratory muscle pump. NRD can be quantified from the electromyogram (EMG) of the crural diaphragm (EMGdi) using a multipair oesophageal electrode catheter and/or from parasternal intercostal muscles, recorded from surface electrodes (sEMGpara). Both EMGdi and sEMGpara provide real-time breath-by-breath measures of NRD that reflect disease severity and provide a physiological correlate to breathlessness in advanced chronic respiratory disease [31, 34, 69, 70].

In research, functional neuroimaging has identified areas of the brain, in particular the insula, cingulate and sensory cortices, the amygdala and the periaqueductal grey matter, which are involved in the generation of breathlessness. It has identified that the brain is not merely a passive signal transducer and that expectations and mood influence perception [43, 55].

In clinical practice our current first-line recommendations for assessment of breathlessness in the clinical settings are a 0–10 NRS of worst breathlessness [62], plus a comprehensive palliative care assessment measure, such as the POS or ESAS, and, ideally, if the patient is well enough, some simple functional assessments, such as the five sit-to-stand tests or the 1-minute sit-to-stand test. If further information on breathlessness is needed, then the Chronic Respiratory Questionnaire and/or information on episodes of breathlessness, their impact and average breathlessness may be helpful (see Table 6.2).

**Table 6.2** Suggested assessment of patients needing palliative care and with breathlessness in the clinical setting, with measures that are likely to detect change over time

**First-line measures**
**0–10 numerical rating scale (NRS) of worst breathlessness**

How bad your breathlessness felt at its worst over the past 24 hours?

| | 0 | 1 | 2 | 3 | 4 | 5 | 6 | 7 | 8 | 9 | 10 |
|---|---|---|---|---|---|---|---|---|---|---|---|
| Not breathless at all | | | | | | ☐ | NRSWorF04 | | | | The worst possible breathlessness |

**Palliative care Outcome Scale (POS) (or Edmonton Symptom Assessment System)**
See www.pos-pal.org for latest version available free and instructions for use, analysis and interpretation.

Q1. What have been your main problems or concerns over the past 3 days?

1. ______
2. ______
3. ______

Q2. Below is a list symptoms, which you may or may not have experienced. For each symptom, please tick one box that best descrobes how it has affected you over the past 3 days.

| | *Not at all* | *Slightly* | *Moderately* | *Severely* | *Overwhelmingly* |
|---|---|---|---|---|---|
| Pain | 0 ☐ | 1 ☐ | 2 ☐ | 3 ☐ | 4 ☐ |
| Shortness of breath | 0 ☐ | 1 ☐ | 2 ☐ | 3 ☐ | 4 ☐ |
| Weakness or lack of energy | 0 ☐ | 1 ☐ | 2 ☐ | 3 ☐ | 4 ☐ |
| Nausea (feeling like you are going to be sick) | 0 ☐ | 1 ☐ | 2 ☐ | 3 ☐ | 4 ☐ |
| Vomiting (being sick) | 0 ☐ | 1 ☐ | 2 ☐ | 3 ☐ | 4 ☐ |
| Poor appetite | 0 ☐ | 1 ☐ | 2 ☐ | 3 ☐ | 4 ☐ |
| Constipation | 0 ☐ | 1 ☐ | 2 ☐ | 3 ☐ | 4 ☐ |
| Sore or dry mouth | 0 ☐ | 1 ☐ | 2 ☐ | 3 ☐ | 4 ☐ |
| Drowsiness | 0 ☐ | 1 ☐ | 2 ☐ | 3 ☐ | 4 ☐ |
| Poor mobility | 0 ☐ | 1 ☐ | 2 ☐ | 3 ☐ | 4 ☐ |

Please list any other symptoms not mentioned above, and tick one box to show how they have affected you over the past 3 days.

| | | | | | |
|---|---|---|---|---|---|
| 1. ______ | 0 ☐ | 1 ☐ | 2 ☐ | 3 ☐ | 4 ☐ |
| 2. ______ | 0 ☐ | 1 ☐ | 2 ☐ | 3 ☐ | 4 ☐ |
| 3. ______ | 0 ☐ | 1 ☐ | 2 ☐ | 3 ☐ | 4 ☐ |

(continued)

**Table 6.2** (continued)

Over the past 3 days:

| | *Not at all* | *Occasionally* | *Sometimes* | *Most of the time* | *Always* |
|---|---|---|---|---|---|
| Q3. Have you been feeling anxious or worried about your illness or treatment? | 0 ☐ | 1 ☐ | 2 ☐ | 3 ☐ | 4 ☐ |
| Q4. Have any of your family or friends been anxious or worried about you? | 0 ☐ | 1 ☐ | 2 ☐ | 3 ☐ | 4 ☐ |
| Q5. Have you been feeling depressed? | 0 ☐ | 1 ☐ | 2 ☐ | 3 ☐ | 4 ☐ |

| | *Always* | *Most of the time* | *Sometimes* | *Occasionally* | *Not at all* |
|---|---|---|---|---|---|
| Q6. Have you felt at peace? | 0 ☐ | 1 ☐ | 2 ☐ | 3 ☐ | 4 ☐ |
| Q7. Have you been able to share how you are feeling with your family or friends as much as you wanted? | 0 ☐ | 1 ☐ | 2 ☐ | 3 ☐ | 4 ☐ |
| Q8. Have you had as much information as you wanted? | 0 ☐ | 1 ☐ | 2 ☐ | 3 ☐ | 4 ☐ |

| | *Problems addressed/ No problems* | *Problems mostly addressed* | *Problems partly addressed* | *Problems hardly addressed* | *Problems not addressed* |
|---|---|---|---|---|---|
| Q9. Have any practical problems resulting from your illness been addressed? (such as financial or personal) | 0 ☐ | 1 ☐ | 2 ☐ | 3 ☐ | 4 ☐ |

**Five sit-to-stand tests**

Time taken for the patient to stand up and sit down five times from a chair, without the use of the upper limbs, as quickly as possible

**Second-line measures and scales that might be added where appropriate, to assess specific aspects:**

0–10 NRS 'average breathlessness' over the past 24 hours
Number and nature of episodes of breathlessness
Chronic Respiratory Questionnaire
Quality of life measures
Short Physical Performance Battery

## Non-pharmacological Treatments and Interventions

There are multiple non-pharmacological interventions that offer first-line treatment options for the management of breathlessness and complement pharmacological treatments where breathlessness persists. The evidence base for these treatments is strongest in non-cancer respiratory diseases, especially in COPD, and in practice many are used in combination [71].

Breathing retraining techniques help to address altered breathing patterns, including increased respiratory rate, apical breathing and excessive accessory muscle use, which reduce the efficiency of ventilation and increase work of breathing [72]. Common techniques include pursed-lip breathing, diaphragmatic breathing and breathing control or timed breathing. Each patient's breathing pattern, underlying condition(s) and pathophysiology should be considered to select use [73]. Systematic review evidence in COPD finds breathing retraining techniques can improve function [72]. The impact on breathlessness is difficult to discern, as these techniques aim to encourage physical activity and exertion, which itself can lead breathlessness intensity.

Mobility aids are an evidence-based inexpensive intervention to improve breathlessness and function. Studies in COPD find that use of a rollator (wheeled walker) improves walking performance [74–76], especially in patients with severe and debilitating breathlessness [77]. They offer support and stability and help increase ventilatory capacity and reduced metabolic cost [78, 79].

The use of a hand-held fan to direct airflow towards the face is a simple intervention that patients can use to self-manage their breathlessness. The fan is an inexpensive, easy to obtain, portable and non-stigmatising piece of equipment [80]. An alternative is cooling the face with wipes or a spray of sterile cooled water. Plausible routes to reduce breathlessness include cooling nasal receptors and moderating afferent signals to the respiratory centre [81]. In qualitative studies most patients reported some or substantial benefit from use of a fan, to relieve their breathlessness severity and reduce recovery time after physical exertion. Trial evidence is mixed [82] though most studies show a favourable direction of effect. Some patients dislike the cooling sensation [80] of a fan but a brief therapeutic trial is worthwhile.

Education and self-management help patients and family/carers to stay independent despite their breathlessness. The advice that breathlessness itself is not dangerous and breathlessness on exertion will settle with rest can be powerful. Advice on positions to aid recovery or during an episode of breathlessness can also be valuable [83]. Common examples include a 'forward-lean' position [84], relaxed sitting and high side lying [71] as shown in the extract from the leaflet from the King's Breathlessness Support Service (Fig. 6.4).

Advice on activity pacing aims to help patients to moderate their behavioural response to breathlessness, avoiding extremes of rest or activity and 'boom or bust' situations where patients push themselves too much, and then face a prolonged period of recovery. Energy conservation, with careful planning and enforced pacing during activities, can help performance without compromising the time that everyday tasks take [85, 86].

Individually tailored exercise should be considered as it can help to counter the 'disability spiral' by improving by exposing patients to being breathless while staying in control, which itself can reduce the anxiety related to breathlessness [87]. Exercises that target the legs and mobility are most helpful. By improving the patients' physical capacity, the ventilatory demand for activities becomes lower, and so the exertion is reduced, thereby reducing breathlessness. Pulmonary rehabilitation, which combines exercise training and education, has a very strong effect on breathlessness and

**1.High side lying**

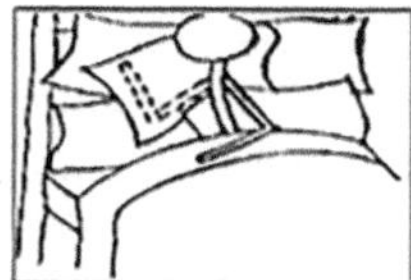

- Make sure your head and chest are supported
- Bend your top leg over
- Put your lower arm under the pillows.

**2.Forward lean sitting**

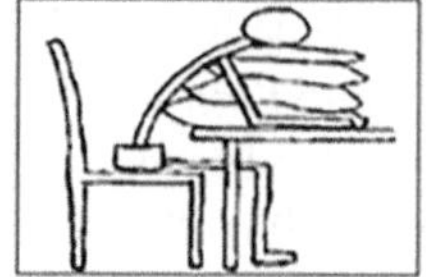

- Pile several pillows on a table
- Relax your head ont them
- Relax your arms on the table Do not try this position if tou have neck problems or are uncomfortable with things near your face.

**3. Relaxed sitting position**

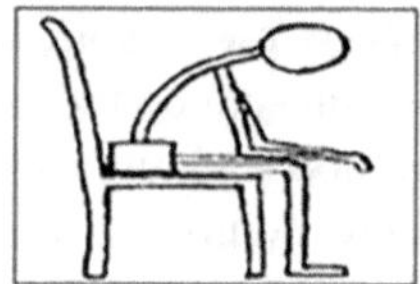

- Sit on a chair
- Rest your elbows on your thighs
- Relax your hands and wrists.

**4.Relaxed standing**

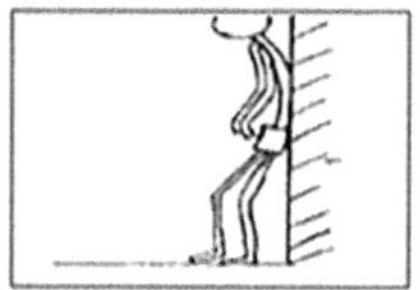

- Lean against a wall
- Relax your shoulders, arms and neck.

**5. Forward lean standing**

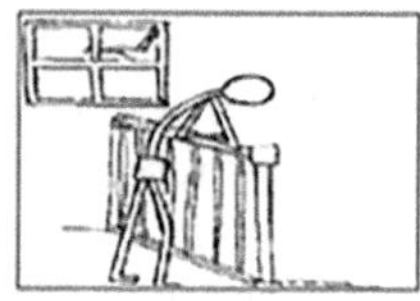

- Lean against a banister, fence or wall but keep a comfortable distance.
- Relax your hands, wrists and neck.

**Fig. 6.4** Positions to ease breathlessness. For full leaflet see https://www.kcl.ac.uk/cicelysaunders/attachments/breathlessness-final/positions-to-ease-breathlessness.pdf

function, and should not be overlooked as a resource if patients are well enough to take part [88]. Supervised training formats generally lead to most benefit [89], but unsupervised home training is effective if completed regularly. Some patients may prefer mind-body exercises (e.g. yoga and tai chi). More passive approaches, e.g. neuromuscular muscle stimulation [90] (to strengthen the thigh muscles) or partitioned training, may also suit patients where exertional breathlessness is severely limiting [91]. The low demand of these modalities on ventilation makes them suited to the severely breathless patient. Other non-pharmacological interventions include using music, visualisation, guided imagery, auditory distraction and acupressure or acupuncture.

## Pharmacological Treatments

The European Respiratory Society (ERS) and the American Thoracic Society (ATS) have both concluded that beyond oxygen and opioids, there is not a robust evidence base for other pharmacological agents in the management of breathlessness currently [6, 92]. The ATS further recommends funding for large-scale multi-institutional investigations into drugs for breathlessness [6].

Relevant systematic reviews of effectiveness and clinical trials are available for opioids, oxygen and benzodiazepines [24, 42, 93–97]. Opioids by mouth and injection can reduce breathlessness; their effects are modest, and the optimal dosing, titration and potential issues arising from long-term use (e.g. safety, tolerance, dependence, misuse) remain to be determined. There is recent controversy as to the degree of benefit from opioids [24, 98]. There are some concerns regarding adverse cardiac and respiratory effects of long-term use of opioids, especially in older people with COPD [99–101], although the studies are population-based and are limited by confounding [102, 103].

Further, not all patients may be suitable for or want to take opioids, especially those living with non-malignant disease [93, 104, 105], and many clinicians are reluctant to prescribe them. In one Dutch study, only 2% of people with advanced COPD were prescribed strong opioids [16]. Evidence does currently not support the use of nebulised opioids or transmucosal fentanyl [24].

Oxygen has a clear and accepted role in hypoxic patients. However, in mildly or non-hypoxaemic breathless patients, the benefit derived from oxygen is similar to medical air, and there are limitations to its use (e.g. safety, cost) [97, 106]. There are no randomised trials of oxygen in interstitial lung disease.

The evidence from Cochrane reviews does not support a role for benzodiazepines, except as second- or third-line treatment if opioids fail, as there is no overall evidence of benefit and some evidence of possible harms [95, 107].

Antidepressants are another option to explore, particularly given their low risk of respiratory depression and dependence, though data are limited and current evidence does not support their use outside of research trials. A double-blind randomised trial of 223 participants with chronic breathlessness and a modified Medical Research Council Breathlessness Scale ≥2 compared sertraline 25–100 mg (titrated upwards over 9 days) with placebo over 4 weeks. There was no difference between study arms on the primary outcome, which was the proportion who had an improvement in intensity of current breathlessness >15% from baseline on a 100 mm visual analogue scale. Following the results from a feasibility trial and case studies into mirtazapine for breathlessness [108–110], a randomised trial is currently underway. Other treatments are also in the trial stage.

## Holistic Breathlessness-Triggered Services

Understanding breathlessness as a multidimensional construct leads to development of multimodal interventions that include both non-pharmacological and pharmacological treatments. Progress has been made in randomised trials of specialist breathlessness support services, which integrate palliative, respiratory and rehabilitation care. These can reduce the distress of breathlessness, improve self-reported breathlessness mastery, lead to high levels of patient satisfaction and are cost neutral or potentially cost saving [20, 111, 112]. The breathlessness support service in our trial provided tailored pharmacological and non-pharmacological interventions over 6 weeks (Table 6.3). Patients had a clinic consultation with palliative care and respiratory medicine clinicians, followed by a home assessment with a physiotherapist and/or occupational therapist 2–3 weeks later. They were provided with a self-help

**Table 6.3** Breathlessness-triggered support service (BSS) and timing

| Time | Type of contact with clinic | Content of meeting |
|---|---|---|
| Week 1 | First outpatient clinic visit/ contact | *Before visit:* Patients were offered free transport or if required disabled parking for the clinic appointments<br>*At visit*<br>Welcome<br>Functional test, e.g. five sit-to-stand tests<br>Completion of Palliative care Outcome Scale by patient, to aid clinical assessment<br>*Contact with respiratory medicine physician*<br>Explore the symptom of breathlessness and its triggers<br>Establish underlying cause of breathlessness<br>Optimise disease-orientated management (check medications used correctly, appropriate treatments)<br>Review of previous investigations<br>Verbal and handwritten handover of notes from respiratory physician to palliative medicine to ensure patients do not have to repeat information<br>*Contact with palliative medicine physician*<br>Experience of breathlessness<br>Development of crises plan<br>Burden on patient and family<br>Symptom burden (other than breathlessness), with recommendations to patients and GP of any appropriate treatments<br>Psychosocial and spiritual issues<br>Introduction of non-pharmacological measures such as the hand-held fan, water spray<br>Review together and provide breathlessness pack to take away, with information leaflets on managing breathlessness, a 'poem' (a mantra (laminated) to put up in the house and to read and follow when in acute breathlessness developed by Jenny Taylor at St Christopher's Hospice), a chart of positions (laminated) to use when in acute breathlessness, fan/water spray<br>*Following visit*: After each clinic appointment, a letter was sent to the patient (to reinforce self-management) summarising the diagnosis, assessment results and plan for treatment, with a copy sent to the referring clinicians and the general practitioner. This and an e-mail were also sent to physiotherapy/occupational therapy to aid their visit. If required urgent contact/phone call with GP |

**Table 6.3** (continued)

| Time | Type of contact with clinic | Content of meeting |
|---|---|---|
| Week 2–3 | Home visit | Based on the patients' needs as assessed during clinic attendance and then home visit:<br>*Physiotherapy input*<br>Review of the positions of breathlessness<br>Provision of a walking aid<br>Breathing control techniques and anxiety-panic cycle<br>Management of exacerbations in COPD<br>Home programme of exercise (DVD, personalised sheet)<br>Cough minimisation techniques<br>Pacing and fatigue management<br>Sputum clearance techniques<br>Ambulatory oxygen assessments<br>Referral to pulmonary rehabilitation<br>*Occupational therapy input*<br>Assessment of activities of daily living (ADL) (mobility/transfers, self-care and domestic ADL)<br>Assessment for aids and minor adoptions and referral for provision of equipment<br>Wheelchair prescription<br>Education on planning, pacing and energy conservation techniques to patients and carers<br>Referral to other community services (local/out of area), as appropriate<br>Assess the need for social support and liaison with the BSS social worker, as appropriate<br>Liaison with the BSS team regarding interventions and feedback |
| Week 2–3 | Telephone call | *Carer assessment*<br>Carer assessment including understanding of disease and symptoms and information needs and coping strategies, if indicated at clinic assessment |
| Week 4–6 | Second outpatient clinic visit or equivalent contact and discharge | *Contact with palliative medicine*<br>Re-evaluation of breathlessness and other symptoms, repeat measures including POS and sit to stand<br>Check use of fan, spray, pack, DVD, etc., further guidance given<br>Change of medications recommended if required, with contact with GP regarding future planned treatments if required<br>Referral to medical and/or palliative care services if appropriate<br>Discharge from service<br>Provided with information on drop-in patient/family information centre for further resources<br>*Following visit:* After clinic appointment a letter was sent to the patient (to reinforce self-management) summarising the progress made, further recommendations and plan for treatment, with a copy sent to the referring clinicians and the general practitioner |

home toolkit (Fig. 6.5). The primary outcome, CRQ mastery at 6 weeks, was significantly better compared to control (mean difference 0.58, 95% CI 0.01 to 1.15, $P = 0.048$). However, the other dyspnoea outcomes such as numerical ratings scales and other CRQ domains did not differ significantly.

A systematic review and meta-analysis of holistic breathlessness-triggered services combined evidence from 18 different services. Most used a short-term delivery format with four to six contacts over 4–6 weeks and were interdisciplinary and used palliative care staff for their symptom management expertise [113, 114]. The most commonly used non-pharmacological treatments included the hand-held fan, breathing retraining techniques, psychological support and relaxation techniques. In patient and family interviews ($n = 216$), those accessing services valued the tailored education, self-management interventions and the expert staff providing what they perceived as person-centred, dignified care [71]. Pooling study findings in meta-analyses showed the services led to reductions in distress due to breathlessness [$n = 324$; NRS mean difference (MD) −2.30, 95%CI −4.43 to −0.16, $P = 0.03$] and Hospital Anxiety and Depression Scale (HADS) depression scores ($n = 408$, MD −1.67, 95%CI −2.52 to −0.81, $P < 0.001$) compared with usual care. They also tended to improve Chronic Respiratory Questionnaire (CRQ) mastery ($n = 259$, MD 0.23, 95%CI −0.10 to 0.55, $P = 0.17$) and HADS anxiety scores ($n = 552$, MD −1.59, 95%CI −3.22 to 0.05, $P = 0.06$) [71]. An in-depth look at individual patient's data found outcomes of reduced mastery and distress were influenced by baseline scores (with the most distressed benefitting the most), but diagnosis or lung function did not change outcome [115].

## Future Directions for Research

Research into breathlessness has been relatively neglected in comparison with other common symptoms, such as pain. Sustained interdisciplinary research is needed. There are important therapeutic options to explore including:

- Phenotyping patients; classification by trajectory, trigger or nature; and understanding the psychophysiological mechanism underlying breathlessness, to help target interventions
- The economic impacts of holistic breathlessness services, and the potential role of these given as digital or remote health interventions, which may be especially important to avoid travel and risk of infection
- Understanding the longer-term effects of brief non-pharmacological interventions on breathlessness severity/patient mastery/function/quality of life/healthcare costs
- Determining the most appropriate outcomes including for patients and carers and on service use
- The cost-effectiveness of early interventions, including with breathlessness support services, to optimise patients' function, symptom burden and psychological distress as a consequence of the onset of chronic breathlessness

- Improving the pharmacologic treatments including opioid dosing, titration and long-term use, repurposing and new medicines, including the potential role of antidepressants
- Interventions to meet needs of carers and families, including within holistic breathlessness-triggered services or as digital or remote health interventions

## References

1. Maddocks M, Lovell N, Booth S, Man WD, Higginson IJ. Palliative care and management of troublesome symptoms for people with chronic obstructive pulmonary disease. Lancet (London, England). 2017;390(10098):988–1002.
2. Moens K, Higginson IJ, Harding R, Euro I. Are there differences in the prevalence of palliative care-related problems in people living with advanced cancer and eight non-cancer conditions? A systematic review. J Pain Symptom Manage. 2014;48(4):660–77.
3. Currow DC, Abernethy AP, Allcroft P, Banzett RB, Bausewein C, Booth S, Carrieri-Kohlman V, Davidson P, Disler R, Donesky D, et al. The need to research refractory breathlessness. Eur Respir J. 2016;47(1):342–3.
4. Ecenarro PS, Iguiniz MI, Tejada SP, Malanda NM, Imizcoz MA, Marlasca LA, Navarrete BA. Management of COPD in end-of-life care by Spanish pulmonologists. COPD. 2018;15(2):171–76.
5. Rocker GM, Simpson AC, Horton R. Palliative care in advanced lung disease: the challenge of integrating palliation into everyday care. Chest. 2015;148(3):801–9.
6. Parshall MB, Schwartzstein RM, Adams L, Banzett RB, Manning HL, Bourbeau J, Calverley PM, Gift AG, Harver A, Lareau SC, et al. An official American Thoracic Society statement: update on the mechanisms, assessment, and management of dyspnea. Am J Respir Crit Care Med. 2012;185(4):435–52.
7. Dorman S, Jolley C, Abernethy A, Currow D, Johnson M, Farquhar M, Griffiths G, Peel T, Moosavi S, Byrne A, et al. Researching breathlessness in palliative care: consensus statement of the National Cancer Research Institute Palliative Care Breathlessness Subgroup. Palliat Med. 2009;23(3):213–27.
8. Dudgeon DJ. Managing dyspnea and cough. Hematol Oncol Clin North Am. 2002;16(3):557–77, viii.
9. Bausewein C, Booth S, Gysels M, Kuhnbach R, Haberland B, Higginson IJ. Understanding breathlessness: cross-sectional comparison of symptom burden and palliative care needs in chronic obstructive pulmonary disease and cancer. J Palliat Med. 2010;13(9):1109–18.
10. Gysels MH, Higginson IJ. The lived experience of breathlessness and its implications for care: a qualitative comparison in cancer, COPD, heart failure and MND. BMC Palliat Care. 2011;10:15.
11. Malik FA, Gysels M, Higginson IJ. Living with breathlessness: a survey of caregivers of breathless patients with lung cancer or heart failure. Palliat Med. 2013;27(7):647–56.
12. Bone AE, Gao W, Gomes B, Sleeman KE, Maddocks M, Wright J, Yi D, Higginson IJ, Evans CJ, Elderly OP. Factors associated with transition from community settings to hospital as place of death for adults aged 75 and older: a population-based mortality follow-back survey. J Am Geriatr Soc. 2016;64(11):2210–7.
13. Currow DC, Johnson MJ. Chronic breathlessness: silent and deadly. Curr Opin Support Palliat Care. 2016;10(3):221–2.
14. Siegel M, Bigelow S. Palliative care symptom management in the emergency department: the ABC's of symptom management for the emergency physician. J Emerg Med. 2018;54(1):25–32.

15. Dzingina MD, McCrone P, Higginson IJ. Does the EQ-5D capture the concerns measured by the Palliative care Outcome Scale? Mapping the Palliative care Outcome Scale onto the EQ-5D using statistical methods. Palliat Med. 2017;31(8):716–25.
16. Janssen DJA, Spruit MA, Uszko-Lencer NH, Schols JMGA, Wouters EFM. Symptoms, comorbidities, and health care in advanced chronic obstructive pulmonary disease or chronic heart failure. J Palliat Med. 2011;14(6):735–43.
17. Janssen DJ, Wouters EF, Schols JM, Spruit MA. Self-perceived symptoms and care needs of patients with severe to very severe chronic obstructive pulmonary disease, congestive heart failure or chronic renal failure and its consequences for their closest relatives: the research protocol. BMC Palliat Care. 2008;7:5.
18. Janssen DJ, Spruit MA, Schols JM, Wouters EF. A call for high-quality advance care planning in outpatients with severe COPD or chronic heart failure. Chest. 2011;139(5):1081–8.
19. Bausewein C, Booth S, Gysels M, Kuhnbach R, Haberland B, Higginson IJ. Individual breathlessness trajectories do not match summary trajectories in advanced cancer and chronic obstructive pulmonary disease: results from a longitudinal study. Palliat Med. 2010;24(8):777–86.
20. Higginson IJ, Bausewein C, Reilly CC, Gao W, Gysels M, Dzingina M, McCrone P, Booth S, Jolley CJ, Moxham J. An integrated palliative and respiratory care service for patients with advanced disease and refractory breathlessness: a randomised controlled trial. Lancet Respir Med. 2014;2(12):979–87.
21. Currow DC, Dal Grande E, Ferreira D, Johnson MJ, McCaffrey N, Ekstrom M. Chronic breathlessness associated with poorer physical and mental health-related quality of life (SF-12) across all adult age groups. Thorax. 2017;72(12):1151–3.
22. Barbetta C, Currow DC, Johnson MJ. Non-opioid medications for the relief of chronic breathlessness: current evidence. Expert Rev Respir Med. 2017;11(4):333–41.
23. Dzingina MD, Reilly CC, Bausewein C, Jolley CJ, Moxham J, McCrone P, Higginson IJ, Yi D. Variations in the cost of formal and informal health care for patients with advanced chronic disease and refractory breathlessness: a cross-sectional secondary analysis. Palliat Med. 2017;31(4):369–77.
24. Barnes H, McDonald J, Smallwood N, Manser R. Opioids for the palliation of refractory breathlessness in adults with advanced disease and terminal illness. Cochrane Database Syst Rev. 2016;3:CD011008.
25. Simon ST, Higginson IJ, Benalia H, Gysels M, Murtagh FE, Spicer J, Bausewein C. Episodic and continuous breathlessness: a new categorization of breathlessness. J Pain Symptom Manage. 2013;45(6):1019–29.
26. Simon ST, Higginson IJ, Benalia H, Gysels M, Murtagh FE, Spicer J, Bausewein C. Episodes of breathlessness: types and patterns - a qualitative study exploring experiences of patients with advanced diseases. Palliat Med. 2013;27(6):524–32.
27. Simon ST, Bausewein C, Schildmann E, Higginson IJ, Magnussen H, Scheve C, Ramsenthaler C. Episodic breathlessness in patients with advanced disease: a systematic review. J Pain Symptom Manage. 2013;45(3):561–78.
28. Mercadante S. Episodic breathlessness in patients with advanced cancer: characteristics and management. Drugs. 2018, Feb 22, e-publication ahead of print.
29. Linde P, Hanke G, Voltz R, Simon ST. Unpredictable episodic breathlessness in patients with advanced chronic obstructive pulmonary disease and lung cancer: a qualitative study. Support Care Cancer. 2018;26(4):1097–104.
30. Mercadante S, Fusco F, Caruselli A, Cartoni C, Masedu F, Valenti M, Aielli F. Background and episodic breathlessness in advanced cancer patients followed at home. Curr Med Res Opin. 2017;33(1):155–60.
31. Murphy PB, Kumar A, Reilly C, Jolley C, Walterspacher S, Fedele F, Hopkinson NS, Man WD-C, Polkey MI, Moxham J, et al. Neural respiratory drive as a physiological biomarker to monitor change during acute exacerbations of COPD. Thorax. 2011;66(7):602–8.

32. Luo YM, Li RF, Jolley C, Wu HD, Steier J, Moxham J, Zhong NS. Neural respiratory drive in patients with COPD during exercise tests. Respiration. 2011;81(4):294–301.
33. Qin YY, Steier J, Jolley C, Moxham J, Zhong NS, Luo YM. Efficiency of neural drive during exercise in patients with COPD and healthy subjects. Chest. 2010;138(6):1309–15.
34. Jolley CJ, Luo YM, Steier J, Reilly C, Seymour J, Lunt A, Ward K, Rafferty GF, Polkey MI, Moxham J. Neural respiratory drive in healthy subjects and in COPD. Eur Respir J. 2009;33(2):289–97.
35. Jolley CJ, Moxham J. A physiological model of patient-reported breathlessness during daily activities in COPD. Eur Respir Rev. 2009;18(112):66–79.
36. Gracely RH, Undem BJ, Banzett RB. Cough, pain and dyspnoea: similarities and differences. Pulm Pharmacol Ther. 2007;20(4):433–7.
37. Banzett RB, Mulnier HE, Murphy K, Rosen SD, Wise RJ, Adams L. Breathlessness in humans activates insular cortex. Neuroreport. 2000;11(10):2117–20.
38. Edgecombe J, Wilcock A, Carr D, Clarke D, Corcoran R, Tattersfield AE. Re: dyspnea in the advanced cancer patient. J Pain Symptom Manage. 1999;18(5):313–5.
39. Feathers LS, Wilcock A, Manderson C, Weller R, Tattersfield AE. Measuring inspiratory muscle weakness in patients with cancer and breathlessness. J Pain Symptom Manage. 2003;25(4):305–6.
40. Jolley CJ, Luo YM, Steier J, Rafferty GF, Polkey MI, Moxham J. Neural respiratory drive and breathlessness in COPD. Eur Respir J. 2015;45(2):355–64.
41. Faisal A, Alghamdi BJ, Ciavaglia CE, Elbehairy AF, Webb KA, Ora J, Neder JA, O'Donnell DE. Common mechanisms of dyspnea in chronic interstitial and obstructive lung disorders. Am J Respir Crit Care Med. 2016;193(3):299–309.
42. Booth S, Moosavi SH, Higginson IJ. The etiology and management of intractable breathlessness in patients with advanced cancer: a systematic review of pharmacological therapy. Nat Clin Pract Oncol. 2008;5(2):90–100.
43. Marlow LL, Faull OK, Finnegan SL, Pattinson KTS. Breathlessness and the brain: the role of expectation. Curr Opin Support Palliat Care. 2019;13(3):200–10.
44. Seymour JM, Moore L, Jolley CJ, Ward K, Creasey J, Steier JS, Yung B, Man WD, Hart N, Polkey MI, et al. Outpatient pulmonary rehabilitation following acute exacerbations of COPD. Thorax. 2010;65(5):423–8.
45. Maddocks M, Jones M, Snell T, Connolly B, de Wolf-Linder S, Moxham J, Rafferty GF. Ankle dorsiflexor muscle size, composition and force with ageing and chronic obstructive pulmonary disease. Exp Physiol. 2014;99(8):1078–88.
46. Maddocks M, Shrikrishna D, Vitoriano S, Natanek SA, Tanner RJ, Hart N, Kemp PR, Moxham J, Polkey MI, Hopkinson NS. Skeletal muscle adiposity is associated with physical activity, exercise capacity and fibre shift in COPD. Eur Respir J. 2014;44:1188–98.
47. Maddocks M, Taylor V, Klezlova R, England R, Manderson C, Wilcock A. When will I get my breath back? Recovery time of exercise-induced breathlessness in patients with thoracic cancer. Lung Cancer. 2012;76(1):128–9.
48. Wilcock A, Maddocks M, Lewis M, England R, Manderson C. Symptoms limiting activity in cancer patients with breathlessness on exertion: ask about muscle fatigue. Thorax. 2008;63(1):91–2.
49. Bernard S, LeBlanc P, Whittom F, Carrier G, Jobin J, Belleau R, Maltais F. Peripheral muscle weakness in patients with chronic obstructive pulmonary disease. Am J Respir Crit Care Med. 1998;158(2):629–34.
50. Debigare R, Maltais F. Last word on point:counterpoint: the major limitation to exercise performance in COPD is 1) inadequate energy supply to the respiratory and locomotor muscles, 2) lower limb muscle dysfunction, 3) dynamic hyperinflation. J Appl Physiol (1985). 2008;105(2):764.
51. Hallas CN, Howard C, Theadom A, Wray J. Negative beliefs about breathlessness increases panic for patients with chronic respiratory disease. Psychol Health Med. 2012;17(4):467–77.

52. Davenport PW, Vovk A. Cortical and subcortical central neural pathways in respiratory sensations. Respir Physiol Neurobiol. 2009;167(1):72–86.
53. Herigstad M, Faull OK, Hayen A, Evans E, Hardinge FM, Wiech K, KTS P. Treating breathlessness via the brain: changes in brain activity over a course of pulmonary rehabilitation. Eur Respir J. 2017;50(3):1701029.
54. Hayen A, Wanigasekera V, Faull OK, Campbell SF, Garry PS, Raby SJM, Robertson J, Webster R, Wise RG, Herigstad M, et al. Opioid suppression of conditioned anticipatory brain responses to breathlessness. Neuroimage. 2017;150:383–94.
55. Faull OK, Hayen A, Pattinson KTS. Breathlessness and the body: neuroimaging clues for the inferential leap. Cortex. 2017;95:211–21.
56. Pattinson KT, Johnson MJ. Neuroimaging of central breathlessness mechanisms. Curr Opin Support Palliat Care. 2014;8(3):225–33.
57. Henoch I, Strang S, Lofdahl CG, Ekberg-Jansson A. Health-related quality of life in a nationwide cohort of patients with COPD related to other characteristics. Eur Clin Respir J. 2016;3:31459.
58. Bausewein C, Farquhar M, Booth S, Gysels M, Higginson IJ. Measurement of breathlessness in advanced disease: a systematic review. Respir Med. 2007;101(3):399–410.
59. Dorman S, Byrne A, Edwards A. Which measurement scales should we use to measure breathlessness in palliative care? A systematic review. Palliat Med. 2007;21(3):177–91.
60. Lovell N, Etkind SN, Bajwah S, Maddocks M, Higginson IJ. Control and context are central for people with advanced illness experiencing breathlessness: a systematic review and thematic synthesis. J Pain Symptom Manage. 2019;57(1):140–155.e142.
61. Higginson IJ, Simon ST, Benalia H, Downing J, Daveson BA, Harding R, Bausewein C. Which questions of two commonly used multidimensional palliative care patient reported outcome measures are most useful? Results from the European and African PRISMA survey. BMJ Support Palliat Care. 2012;2(1):36–42.
62. Lovell N, Etkind SN, Bajwah S, Maddocks M, Higginson IJ. To what extent do the NRS and CRQ capture change in patients' experience of breathlessness in advanced disease? Findings from a mixed-methods double-blind randomized feasibility trial. J Pain Symptom Manage. 2019;58(3):369–381 e367.
63. Brooks D, Solway S, Gibbons WJ. ATS statement on six-minute walk test. Am J Respir Crit Care Med. 2003;167(9):1287.
64. Singh SJ, Morgan MD, Scott S, Walters D, Hardman AE. Development of a shuttle walking test of disability in patients with chronic airways obstruction. Thorax. 1992;47(12):1019–24.
65. Revill SM, Morgan MDL, Singh SJ, Williams J, Hardman AE. The endurance shuttle walk: a new field test for the assessment of endurance capacity in chronic obstructive pulmonary disease. Thorax. 1999;54(3):213–22.
66. Kon SS, Canavan JL, Nolan CM, Clark AL, Jones SE, Cullinan P, Polkey MI, Man WD. The 4-metre gait speed in COPD: responsiveness and minimal clinically important difference. Eur Respir J. 2013;43:1298–305.
67. Kon SS, Patel MS, Canavan JL, Clark AL, Jones SE, Nolan CM, Cullinan P, Polkey MI, Man WD. Reliability and validity of 4-metre gait speed in COPD. Eur Respir J. 2013;42(2):333–40.
68. Jones SE, Kon SS, Canavan JL, Patel MS, Clark AL, Nolan CM, Polkey MI, Man WD. The five-repetition sit-to-stand test as a functional outcome measure in COPD. Thorax. 2013;68(11):1015–20.
69. Reilly CC, Ward K, Jolley CJ, Lunt AC, Steier J, Elston C, Polkey MI, Rafferty GF, Moxham J. Neural respiratory drive, pulmonary mechanics and breathlessness in patients with cystic fibrosis. Thorax. 2011;66(3):240–6.
70. Reilly CC, Jolley CJ, Elston C, Moxham J, Rafferty GF. Measurement of parasternal intercostal electromyogram during an infective exacerbation in patients with cystic fibrosis. Eur Respir J. 2012;40(4):977–81.
71. Brighton LJ, Miller S, Farquhar M, Booth S, Yi D, Gao W, Bajwah S, Man WD, Higginson IJ, Maddocks M. Holistic services for people with advanced disease and chronic breathlessness: a systematic review and meta-analysis. Thorax. 2019;74(3):270–81.

72. Holland AE, Hill CJ, Jones AY, McDonald CF. Breathing exercises for chronic obstructive pulmonary disease. Cochrane Database Syst Rev. 2012;10:Cd008250.
73. Bott J, Blumenthal S, Buxton M, Ellum S, Falconer C, Garrod R, Harvey A, Hughes T, Lincoln M, Mikelsons C, et al. Guidelines for the physiotherapy management of the adult, medical, spontaneously breathing patient. Thorax. 2009;64 Suppl 1:i1–51.
74. Solway S, Brooks D, Lau L, Goldstein R. The short-term effect of a rollator on functional exercise capacity among individuals with severe COPD. Chest. 2002;122(1):56–65.
75. Gupta R, Goldstein R, Brooks D. The acute effects of a rollator in individuals with COPD. J Cardiopulm Rehabil. 2006;26(2):107–11.
76. Vaes AW, Meijer K, Delbressine JM, Wiechert J, Willems P, Wouters EF, Franssen FM, Spruit MA. Efficacy of walking aids on self-paced outdoor walking in individuals with COPD: a randomized cross-over trial. Respirology. 2015;20(6):932–9.
77. Crisafulli E, Costi S, De Blasio F, Biscione G, Americi F, Penza S, Eutropio E, Pasqua F, Fabbri LM, Clini EM. Effects of a walking aid in COPD patients receiving oxygen therapy. Chest. 2007;131(4):1068–74.
78. Probst VS, Troosters T, Coosemans I, Spruit MA, Pitta Fde O, Decramer M, Gosselink R. Mechanisms of improvement in exercise capacity using a rollator in patients with COPD. Chest. 2004;126(4):1102–7.
79. Hill K, Dolmage TE, Woon LJ, Brooks D, Goldstein RS. Rollator use does not consistently change the metabolic cost of walking in people with chronic obstructive pulmonary disease. Arch Phys Med Rehabil. 2012;93(6):1077–80.
80. Luckett T, Phillips J, Johnson MJ, Farquhar M, Swan F, Assen T, Bhattarai P, Booth S. Contributions of a hand-held fan to self-management of chronic breathlessness. Eur Respir J. 2017;50(2):1700262.
81. Spathis A, Booth S, Moffat C, Hurst R, Ryan R, Chin C, Burkin J. The Breathing, Thinking, Functioning clinical model: a proposal to facilitate evidence-based breathlessness management in chronic respiratory disease. NPJ Prim Care Respir Med. 2017;27(1):27.
82. Qian Y, Wu Y, Rozman de Moraes A, Yi X, Geng Y, Dibaj S, Liu D, Naberhuis J, Bruera E. Fan therapy for the treatment of dyspnea in adults: a systematic review. J Pain Symptom Manage. 2019;58:481–6.
83. Simon ST, Weingartner V, Higginson IJ, Benalia H, Gysels M, Murtagh FE, Spicer J, Linde P, Voltz R, Bausewein C. "I can breathe again!" patients' self-management strategies for episodic breathlessness in advanced disease, derived from qualitative interviews. J Pain Symptom Manage. 2016;52(2):228–34.
84. Sharp JT, Drutz WS, Moisan T, Foster J, Machnach W. Postural relief of dyspnea in severe chronic obstructive pulmonary disease. Am Rev Respir Dis. 1980;122(2):201–11.
85. Wingårdh ASL, Göransson C, Larsson S, Slinde F, Vanfleteren L. Effectiveness of energy conservation techniques in patients with COPD. Respira Int Rev Thorac Dis. 2020;99(5):409–16.
86. Prieur G, Combret Y, Medrinal C, Arnol N, Bonnevie T, Gravier FE, Quieffin J, Lamia B, Reychler G, Borel JC. Energy conservation technique improves dyspnoea when patients with severe COPD climb stairs: a randomised crossover study. Thorax. 2020;75(6):510–2.
87. Wadell K, Webb KA, Preston ME, Amornputtisathaporn N, Samis L, Patelli J, Guenette JA, O'Donnell DE. Impact of pulmonary rehabilitation on the major dimensions of dyspnea in COPD. COPD. 2013;10(4):425–35.
88. Richardson CR, Franklin B, Moy ML, Jackson EA. Advances in rehabilitation for chronic diseases: improving health outcomes and function. BMJ. 2019;365:l2191.
89. Troosters T, Blondeel A, Janssens W, Demeyer H. The past, present and future of pulmonary rehabilitation. Respirology. 2019;24:830–7.
90. Jones S, Man WD, Gao W, Higginson IJ, Wilcock A, Maddocks M. Neuromuscular electrical stimulation for muscle weakness in adults with advanced disease. Cochrane Database Syst Rev. 2016;10:Cd009419.
91. Vanfleteren L, Gloeckl R. Add-on interventions during pulmonary rehabilitation; 2019.

92. Johnson M, Barbetta C, Currow D, Maddocks M, McDonald V, Mahadeva R, Mason M. Management of chronic breathlessness. In: Bausewein C, Currow D, Johnson M, editors. Palliative care in respiratory disease, vol. 73. Sheffield: ERS; 2016. p. 153–71.
93. Jennings AL, Davies AN, Higgins JP, Gibbs JS, Broadley KE. A systematic review of the use of opioids in the management of dyspnoea. Thorax. 2002;57(11):939–44.
94. Ben-Aharon I, Gafter-Gvili A, Leibovici L, Stemmer SM. Interventions for alleviating cancer-related dyspnea: a systematic review and meta-analysis. Acta Oncologica (Stockholm, Sweden). 2012;51(8):996–1008.
95. Simon ST, Higginson IJ, Booth S, Harding R, Bausewein C. Benzodiazepines for the relief of breathlessness in advanced malignant and non-malignant diseases in adults. Cochrane Database Syst Rev (Online). 2010;1:CD007354.
96. Simon ST, Koskeroglu P, Gaertner J, Voltz R. Fentanyl for the relief of refractory breathlessness: a systematic review. J Pain Symptom Manage. 2013;46(6):874–86.
97. Abernethy AP, McDonald CF, Frith PA, Clark K, Herndon JE 2nd, Marcello J, Young IH, Bull J, Wilcock A, Booth S, et al. Effect of palliative oxygen versus room air in relief of breathlessness in patients with refractory dyspnoea: a double-blind, randomised controlled trial. Lancet. 2010;376(9743):784–93.
98. Ekstrom M, Bajwah S, Bland JM, Currow DC, Hussain J, Johnson MJ. One evidence base; three stories: do opioids relieve chronic breathlessness? Thorax. 2018;73(1):88–90.
99. Vozoris NT, Wang X, Fischer HD, Bell CM, O'Donnell DE, Austin PC, Stephenson AL, Gill SS, Rochon PA. Incident opioid drug use and adverse respiratory outcomes among older adults with COPD. Eur Respir J. 2016;48(3):683–93.
100. Vozoris NT, O'Donnell DE, Bell C, Gill SS, Rochon PA. Incident opioid use is associated with risk of respiratory harm in non-palliative COPD. Eur Respir J. 2017;49(3):1602529.
101. Vozoris NT, Wang X, Austin PC, Lee DS, Stephenson AL, O'Donnell DE, Gill SS, Rochon PA. Adverse cardiac events associated with incident opioid drug use among older adults with COPD. Eur J Clin Pharmacol. 2017;73(10):1287–95.
102. Rocker G, Bourbeau J, Downar J. The new "opioid crisis": scientific bias, media attention, and potential harms for patients with refractory dyspnea. J Palliat Med. 2018;21(2):120–2.
103. Downar J, Colman R, Horton R, Hernandez P, Rocker G. Opioids in COPD: a cause of death or a marker of illness severity? Eur Respir J. 2016;48(5):1520–1.
104. Currow DC, McDonald C, Oaten S, Kenny B, Allcroft P, Frith P, Briffa M, Johnson MJ, Abernethy AP. Once-daily opioids for chronic dyspnea: a dose increment and pharmacovigilance study. J Pain Symptom Manage. 2011;42(3):388–99.
105. Jennings AL, Davies AN, Higgins JP, Broadley K. Opioids for the palliation of breathlessness in terminal illness. Cochrane Database Syst Rev. 2001;4:CD002066.
106. Rocker G. Harms of overoxygenation in patients with exacerbation of chronic obstructive pulmonary disease. CMAJ. 2017;189(22):E762–3.
107. Simon ST, Higginson IJ, Booth S, Harding R, Weingartner V, Bausewein C. Benzodiazepines for the relief of breathlessness in advanced malignant and non-malignant diseases in adults. Cochrane Database Syst Rev. 2016;10:CD007354.
108. Higginson IJ, Wilcock A, Johnson MJ, Bajwah S, Lovell N, Yi D, Hart SP, Crosby V, Poad H, Currow D, et al. Randomised, double-blind, multicentre, mixed-methods, dose-escalation feasibility trial of mirtazapine for better treatment of severe breathlessness in advanced lung disease (BETTER-B feasibility). Thorax. 2020;75(2):176–9.
109. Lovell N, Wilcock A, Bajwah S, Etkind SN, Jolley CJ, Maddocks M, Higginson IJ. Mirtazapine for chronic breathlessness? A review of mechanistic insights and therapeutic potential. Expert Rev Respir Med. 2019;13(2):173–80.
110. Lovell N, Bajwah S, Maddocks M, Wilcock A, Higginson IJ. Use of mirtazapine in patients with chronic breathlessness: a case series. Palliat Med. 2018;32(9):1518–21.

111. Farquhar MC, Prevost AT, McCrone P, Brafman-Price B, Bentley A, Higginson IJ, Todd CJ, Booth S. The clinical and cost effectiveness of a Breathlessness Intervention Service for patients with advanced non-malignant disease and their informal carers: mixed findings of a mixed method randomised controlled trial. Trials. 2016;17(1):185.
112. Rocker GM, Verma JY. 'INSPIRED' COPD Outreach Program: doing the right things right. Clin Invest Med. 2014;37(5):E311–9.
113. Farquhar MC, Prevost AT, McCrone P, Brafman-Price B, Bentley A, Higginson IJ, Todd C, Booth S. Is a specialist breathlessness service more effective and cost-effective for patients with advanced cancer and their carers than standard care? Findings of a mixed-method randomised controlled trial. BMC Med. 2014;12:194.
114. Costantini M, Romoli V, Leo SD, Beccaro M, Bono L, Pilastri P, Miccinesi G, Valenti D, Peruselli C, Bulli F, et al. Liverpool Care Pathway for patients with cancer in hospital: a cluster randomised trial. Lancet. 2014;383(9913):226–37.
115. Brighton LJ, Gao W, Farquhar M. Predicting outcomes following holistic breathlessness services: a pooled analysis of individual patient data. Palliat Med. 2019;33(4):462–6.
116. Booth S, Bausewein C, Higginson I, Moosavi SH. Pharmacological treatment of refractory breathlessness. Expert Rev Respir Med. 2009;3(1):21–36.
117. Horton R, Rocker G. Contemporary issues in refractory dyspnoea in advanced chronic obstructive pulmonary disease. Curr Opin Support Palliat Care. 2010;4(2):56–62.
118. Weingartner V, Scheve C, Gerdes V, Schwarz-Eywill M, Prenzel R, Otremba B, Muhlenbrock J, Bausewein C, Higginson IJ, Voltz R, et al. Characteristics of episodic breathlessness as reported by patients with advanced chronic obstructive pulmonary disease and lung cancer: results of a descriptive cohort study. Palliat Med. 2015;29(5):420–8.
119. Bowden JA, To TH, Abernethy AP, Currow DC. Predictors of chronic breathlessness: a large population study. BMC Public Health. 2011;11:33.
120. Currow D, Johnson M, White P, Abernethy A. Evidence-based intervention for chronic refractory breathlessness: practical therapies that make a difference. Br J Gen Pract. 2013;63(616):609–10.
121. Currow DC, Quinn S, Greene A, Bull J, Johnson MJ, Abernethy AP. The longitudinal pattern of response when morphine is used to treat chronic refractory dyspnea. J Palliat Med. 2013;16(8):881–6.
122. Johnson MJ, Currow DC. Chronic refractory breathlessness is a distinct clinical syndrome. Curr Opin Support Palliat Care. 2015;9(3):203–5.
123. Johnson MJ, Yorke J, Hansen-Flaschen J, Lansing R, Ekstrom M, Similowski T, Currow DC. Towards an expert consensus to delineate a clinical syndrome of chronic breathlessness. Eur Respir J. 2017;49(5):1602277.

# Chapter 7
# Preparatory and Anticipatory Grief, Anxiety and Depression in Life-Limiting Lung Disease

**Debra G. Sandford**

## Introduction

In the past decade or so, more attention is being given to the psychological impact of disease on the patient and their close family. Emotional distress is an almost universal experience for people given a diagnosis of a life-limiting lung disease. For some people, this distress is immediate and for others it may be a delayed response. An emotional distress response is not just limited to the person with the disease though, for their spouse or partner and other close family members (caregivers), they too can feel distress about these life-changing implications.

Within the academic literature that examines the patient and/or caregiver experience, the two most commonly referred to psychological conditions are anxiety and depression. The majority of people diagnosed with life-limiting lung disease do not meet criteria for a formal diagnosis of anxiety and/or depression, though they suffer from, at times, strong emotional distress.

Emotional distress is a normal, natural and to be expected reaction to 'bad news'. Being given a diagnosis of a terminal lung disease certainly meets criteria for 'bad news'. Indeed, one emotional response that is given much less attention within the literature about the psychological impact of life-limiting lung disease is grief, in particular anticipatory and/or preparatory grief.

Clinical practitioners should be mindful not to pathologise a normal, natural emotional reaction. Instead, the clinician should strive to better understand and develop skills to assist patients and their families to manage yet another aspect of living with and eventually dying from lung disease. This chapter is designed to

D. G. Sandford (✉)
The University of Adelaide, Adelaide Medical School, Adelaide, SA, Australia

The Royal Adelaide Hospital, Department of Thoracic Medicine, Adelaide, SA, Australia
e-mail: debra.sandford@adelaide.edu.au



K. O. Lindell, S. K. Danoff (eds.), *Palliative Care in Lung Disease*, Respiratory Medicine, https://doi.org/10.1007/978-3-030-81788-6_7

provide an overview of anticipatory and preparatory grief, anxiety and depression, as well as discuss some practical strategies that clinicians can utilise. Within this chapter, the term caregiver will be used to describe whomever the patient designates as the main support person, whether they be married, partnered or friend and family/families. Equally, the term clinician will be used to describe the medical, nursing, psychological and allied health practitioners who provide the professional care for the patient and caregivers/families.

| Glossary of Key Terms |
|---|
| *Anticipatory Grief* – the reaction of caregivers and family members who will lose someone they care about to a 'forewarned death'.<br>Also referred to in literature as *predeath grief, anticipatory mourning and pre-loss grief.* |
| *Preparatory Grief* – the reaction of the person diagnosed with a terminal disease. |
| *Physical Loss* – tangible loss, something lost or left behind and not recovered. |
| *Symbolic Loss* – psychosocial in nature, not tangible, can be associated with the physical loss but not always.<br>Also referred to in literature as *psychosocial loss.* |
| *Secondary Loss* – can be physical and/or symbolic in nature and develops as a consequence of the primary loss. |
| *Prolonged Grief Disorder (PGD) also known as Complicated Grief* – persistent and pervasive grief response characterised by persistent longing or yearning and/or preoccupation with the deceased accompanied by at least three of eight additional symptoms that include disbelief, intense emotional pain, feeling of identity confusion, avoidance of reminders of the loss, feelings of numbness, intense loneliness, meaninglessness or difficulty engaging in ongoing life [1]. |

## Loss and its Relationship to Grief and Lung Disease

### *Loss*

Loss has two categories: *physical* loss and *symbolic* loss (or psychosocial). Obviously, a physical loss is tangible (e.g. an amputated limb, items stolen, something lost or left behind and not recovered, miscarriage or stillbirth, the loss of income from losing a job), whereas a symbolic loss is psychosocial in nature and not tangible (e.g. a divorce or relationship breakdown, chronic or terminal illness, the shattered hopes and dreams associated with the physical loss).

Loss can leave people sad, bereft and grieving. Physical loss, because of its tangibility, is easier to recognise as needing to be mourned. The bereft person is 'given permission' by society and themselves to mourn. Conversely, with symbolic loss, often the person and those around them may not realise that a loss has occurred or downplay the impact of the loss and 'put on a brave face', which can result in the person amplifying the grief experience [2].

When a person is diagnosed with a life-limiting lung disease, they and their families will experience a symbolic loss as the implications of the diagnosis become understood and real. Many will experience a grief reaction at this point. However, what is little recognised and rarely written about are the secondary losses.

Secondary losses can be physical and symbolic in nature and develop as a consequence of the initial loss, in this case the diagnosis of the lung disease. Physical secondary losses might include some of the following: the patient needing supported living or hospice care, the need to 'downsize' or alter their residence to accommodate for their deteriorating health and the need to retire from work early and the subsequent loss of income, and the capacity to be as physically actove as they once were. Symbolic secondary losses are much more extensive and are especially so, the closer the patient is to their caregiver. In general, the patient and caregiver play numerous roles for each other: they may be each other's lover, best friend, travelling companion, cook, gardener, handyperson, business associate and the list goes on. These roles will all change as the lung disease progresses towards its inevitable end. We will discuss the implications of the secondary losses in more detail later in this chapter under 'Disease Progression and Role Changes'.

## Anticipatory and Preparatory Grief

Grief is the physical, cognitive, emotional, behavioural and social reaction(s) to loss.

Within academic literature terms used to describe predeath grief are differentiated into two categories. *Anticipatory grief* is predominantly used when describing the reaction of caregivers and family members who will lose someone they care about to a 'forewarned death', whereas *preparatory grief* is mainly used to describe the reaction of the person diagnosed with a terminal disease. These terms and others are used interchangeably within the literature. While these two reactions may 'look' similar to a clinician, the processes are quite different.

### *Anticipatory Grief*

Towards the end of World War II, the German-American psychiatrist Erich Lindemann wrote about his observations that wives were rejecting their soldier husband returning from the war. Lindemann based his theory on Freud's psychoanalytical theory of 'grief work', where the bereaved have to work through the emotional pain of loss in order to eventually relinquish the attachment bonds with the deceased to avoid an adverse bereavement outcome. Lindemann hypothesised that the wives had rejected their husbands because they had begun their *grief work* before the actual loss, he called this *anticipatory grief* [3].

Kubler-Ross' [4] early work which focused on anticipatory grief, and along with other grief theorists, Bowlby [5] and Parkes and Weiss [6], proposed that grief followed predictable stages or phases. In a later publication, Kubler-Ross [7] famously described five distinct but interconnected phases for post-death grief, where the grieving person eventually acquires 'final detachment' from the deceased person or 'acceptance' that a loss has occurred. One of the main tenets of these models was that in order to reach the final phase of acceptance or detachment, the grieving person had to 'complete' each stage. Failure to complete a stage could result in a variety of complications. For decades Kubler-Ross' model of grief was the most recognised model by lay and professional people alike and has become deeply entrenched within cultural beliefs. More recent however, academic theorists have empirically rejected the notion that individuals must progress through these stages.

More recently, anticipatory grief has been operationalised for research purposes with a focus on the thoughts, feelings and reactions that relate to the anticipated loss of a loved one [8, 9]. Another complication for researchers and those wishing to read widely on this subject is the manner in which the grief experienced by caregivers is referred to; terms that are also utilised within the literature are *predeath grief*, *anticipatory mourning* and *pre-loss grief* amongst others [10] which are often argued to be more appropriate and accurate terms in which to describe this emotional response.

Other authors [8, 11, 12] have suggested that the emotional response by caregivers towards the impending death of a loved one should not be called anticipatory grief at all, as it leads the reader to assume that anticipatory grief is the same as a post-death grief. Therese Rando [13] went as far as to call the term anticipatory grief a 'misnomer'. She argued that this term focuses too heavily on the anticipated death aspect without giving due consideration for all of the other past and current 'losses' the person has experienced.

Anticipatory grief differs from post-death grief in the following ways:

- Anticipatory grief is felt by both the caregiver(s) and patient (preparatory grief).
- It has a definite end point (the death of the patient).
- For some, the grief becomes more acute as the impending death becomes closer rather than eases over time as for post-death grief.

Additionally, anticipatory grief often includes hopefulness; and finally, the caregivers and patient are not able to fully take on the 'role' of a bereaved person [8, 11, 12, 14], thereby clearly establishing the processes that people go through predeath and post-death to be different.

The majority of anticipatory grief research has been conducted in hospice/palliative care units or similar, primarily utilising caregivers of dementia or cancer patients [15]. Johansson et al. [16] highlight that differences in disease trajectories will impact on anticipatory grief experienced by a caregiver. For example, grieving for someone with dementia will be different to that of someone with cancer, especially because the dementia patient and caregiver may have a different degree of emotional closeness. Further, these two distinct populations of caregivers and patients may not necessarily represent the emotional responses experienced by patients with lung diseases. Within the various lung disease populations, the emotional experiences can be widely different. For example, the emotional distress of lung cancer patients will be different from idiopathic pulmonary fibrosis (IPF) patients, who will be different again from chronic obstructive pulmonary disease (COPD) patients.

Within a palliative environment, Egerod et al. [17] conducted qualitative interviews in regard to grief (predeath and post-death) with 20 spouses of patients with fibrotic interstitial lung disease (f-ILD) prior to the patient's death and again after death, with a 6 to 12 months' period. They found that caregiver grief began around the time the patient was diagnosed and continued throughout the disease progression until death. At the time of the post-death interviews, only 1 spouse met criteria for prolonged grief disorder (PGD) as measured by the Prolonged Grief Disorder Questionnaire (PG-13), whereas the other 19 were assessed as having 'normal grief', with 5 of those showing elevated levels close to PGD [18].

Outside of the palliative environment, in a recent pilot study of idiopathic pulmonary fibrosis (IPF) patients and their caregivers, Sandford et al. [19] found, through a semi-structured clinical interview, that at the time of diagnosis, 72% of IPF patients and 77% of caregivers reported an emotional reaction that was consistent with grief. In the same study, at the time of interview, 58% of patients and 82% of caregivers reported a grief response, which was independent of lung function or disease progression. A possible extrapolation of this finding might indicate that as patients 'come to terms' with their disease, their grief response moderates, whereas as caregivers watch their loved ones deteriorate, their grief response actually increases.

## *Preparatory Grief*

Literature using the term 'preparatory grief' is far sparser than the literature using 'anticipatory grief', and while they share many features, they are different, mainly because the person diagnosed with the lung disease must go through a process where they prepare themselves for death [20]. Kubler-Ross further states that preparatory grief is the normal grief reaction to perceived losses experienced by persons who are dying.

Reflecting now, upon the loss perspective discussed above, the person diagnosed with lung disease will need to mourn the losses that are an unavoidable consequence of disease progression [21]. This will of course include the thoughts and sadness around leaving (through dying) their caregiver and other family members and missing out on things like grandchildren being born and growing up, weddings, graduations and other celebrations, as well as the simple pleasures that bring them joy, such as a cup of morning coffee, beautiful sunsets, fishing and catching up with friends.

Additionally, the person with lung disease will often undergo a transformation in self-image and self-confidence as they surrender the things that they could do before their lung disease took over their life [22]. Preparatory grief like other any grief will wax and wane, come in waves and tend to be more acute when there is a reason to remind the person that they have a terminal illness, such as an exacerbation in their disease process [23] (Fig. 7.1).

As the person's health deteriorates, they will become more dependent on others for a variety of needs; this will lead to not only a potential exacerbation in the grief response but also a further assault to their sense of self as their incapacity forces more role changes. For many patients who are prescribed oxygen therapy, the day that they are advised this is necessary is a day that for many is a 'watershed' moment. The inevitability of the terminality of their disease becomes unavoidable to ignore. Qualitative studies and interviews with patients about using oxygen therapy highlight that patients have mixed emotions in regard to using oxygen. Some feel embarrassed or self-conscious; others are afraid of becoming reliant. These negative connotations towards a helpful therapy only serve to increase a patient's sense of grief [24, 25].

Grief is not all sadness. Periyakoil [23] postulates that preparatory grief should be viewed through the dual-process model, which was outlined by Stroebe and Schut [26], where the patient experiences grief that can be broadly classified into loss-oriented or restoration-oriented grief. In this respect we again refer to our discussion of loss earlier in this chapter, where the loss-oriented grief refers to the persons experience of loss [lung disease] per se, whereas restoration-oriented grief is focused on the secondary losses that the person experiences. Further, and helpfully to clinicians, this model identifies grief as a dynamic process with the grieving person alternating between the loss-orientation and restoration-orientation, which fits nicely with a simpler explanation that patients might find easier to accept that grief comes in waves and isn't always focused on sadness.

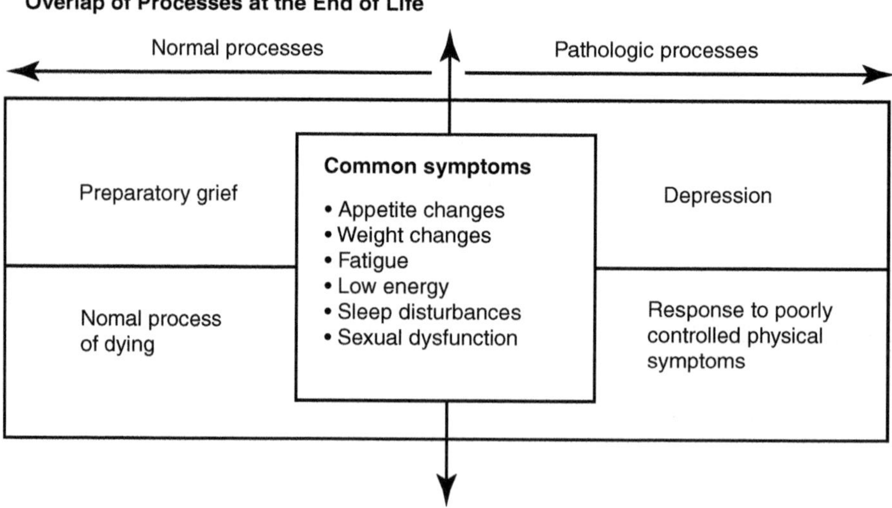


**Fig. 7.1** Commonly shared symptoms between depression and preparatory grief

## Relevance of Anticipatory and Preparatory Grief in Clinical Settings

Grief, whether it be preparatory, anticipatory or post-death, is an 'adjusting emotion'. Grief is an essential component of a person adjusting to their 'new normal', and with lung disease patients, this 'new normal' will continue to evolve as their disease progresses.

Patients and caregivers may not experience grief at the same time. This will depend on many things, disease progress, socio-economic circumstances, family dynamics, available support as well as all the normal variables that impact a person's psychological state. The fact that the patient and caregiver may be in a discordant state of emotional processing and adjusting is something that an astute clinician needs to be aware of, as this will certainly impact on the patients' sense of wellbeing and possibly their physical health and compliance to treatment. For clinicians, the impact of this emotional response and how best to support it should be of primary concern.

**Practical Clinical Advice**

The distress caused by watching someone you care about deteriorate is painful, regardless of what you call it. In my clinical practice, after giving them, the patient and caregivers, an explanation of anticipatory grief, thereafter, I call it simply 'grief'. Not one person, to date, has denied that what they feel is, just that, grief. How people experience 'grief' is subjective and is their experience alone. My belief is, in a clinical setting over a research setting, it is less important to give grief more defined names.

Most people after being assisted to name this emotion feel more empowered to work with the roller-coaster of emotions that will come and go throughout the period of illness. Once we have named these emotions and normalised this reaction for them, they often remark that they 'no longer feel like they are going crazy' or that they are 'reacting all wrong'.

Normalising grief reactions for patients and caregivers is of paramount importance. As is the explanation that these emotions come in waves, often in quiet moments or when they are doing familiar tasks. During these times when we 'let our minds wander', it is normal and natural for our minds to go down some dark paths, and that is when the grief wave will come crashing over them. Explaining this to caregivers and patients will empower them to recognise it when it comes and hopefully not be thrown off balance as much by the emotions when they hit.

Referring back to our earlier discussion on restoration-orientation grief, it is normal for patients and caregivers to seemingly ignore the evidence of the terminality of their disease and hope and pray for a cure. The capacity to not accept or believe that their diagnosis is one of a life-limiting lung disease will often occur when the person's symptoms are not impacting on their daily activities very much. As their disease progresses, and they experience an exacerbation, it is these times when restoration-oriented grief plays its role; as an example, this helps the patient and caregiver shift from hoping for a cure to hoping for effective symptom management [23]. It should be noted that patients, caregivers and families won't spend their entire time between diagnosis and death in a grief state. Grief will wax and wane and they may, depending upon their disease and its progression, spend periods of time in relative normality.

## Symptoms of Grief

Another important aspect for clinicians is being able to identify a 'grief' reaction by recognising the symptoms. These symptoms can be physical, emotional, cognitive and even spiritual. The table below lists some of the more commonly reported symptoms.

| *Physical* | *Spiritual* |
|---|---|
| Sleep changes – difficulty falling or staying asleep, or the opposite where extra sleep is needed<br>Headaches or muscle tension, especially in neck, shoulders and scalp<br>Nausea<br>Fatigue<br>Appetite changes – including poor appetite or 'comfort eating'<br>Decreased need or desire for sex | Spiritual beliefs might change<br>Angry with 'God' (whoever the person perceives God to be)<br>Renewing faith<br>Developing a faith<br>Seeking comfort from a faith<br>Seeking meaning through faith |
| *Emotional* | *Cognitive* |
| Denial<br>Disbelief<br>Worry<br>Anxiousness<br>Fear<br>Sadness<br>Anger<br>Helplessness<br>Guilt<br>Overwhelmed<br>Impatient<br>Distancing or isolating self from others who would normally support | Fogginess<br>Disorganised<br>Forgetful<br>Lack of patience<br>Difficulty recalling things<br>Difficulty keeping thoughts straight<br>Short-term memory difficulties<br>Difficulties making decisions<br>Difficulty concentrating |

Grief can also cause relationships to change within families as well as within social and work relationships. Grief can also magnify issues that already exist within relationships. Sadly, not every family has healthy, supportive and nurturing dynamics, and it is within the families that are already struggling that grief tends to exacerbate the negative aspects. Importantly, recognising that relationships have or are changing for your patient and their caregivers gives clinicians an opportunity to incorporate an appropriate mental health expert into the multidisciplinary team.

## Diagnosing a Grief Reaction

Diagnosing a grief reaction is not only important to do, but often empowering for the patient and/or caregivers, as it helps them feel more in charge of their emotional response(s). Grief can look a lot like anxiety and depression, and in fact feeling anxious and sad or depressed is a symptom of grief [22, 23, 27]. However, feeling anxious or depressed does not mean that we can be diagnosed with anxiety or depression. Feeling anxious and depressed is normal; we all feel anxious or depressed at times, when we experience things that cause a distressing emotional response. People who are clinically anxious and/or depressed feel these emotions in a pervasive way.

To diagnose clinical depression or anxiety, a person should feel depressed and/or anxious for most of the day nearly every day for at least 2 weeks or longer [1]. Grief, on the other hand, comes in waves. People suffering from a grief reaction can still feel pleasure at the things that usually bring them a sense of pleasure. Additionally, self-esteem is usually intact and not impacted by a grief response. A quick and easy question to ask your patient and/or their caregiver is 'does this feeling come in waves or is it there more pervasively?' If your patient answers pervasively, then it is more likely depression or anxiety and should be further investigated by clinical interview. If they answer, 'in waves', then it is more likely a grief reaction and should be treated with appropriate counselling.

## The Need to Find Meaning

Viktor Frankl wrote in *Man's Search for Meaning* [28], originally published in German in 1946 and since then translated into English and many other languages and reprinted many times, that 'man is not destroyed by suffering, he is destroyed by suffering without meaning'. As a person grieves, part of the process is to find meaning, which often leads to the person asking questions like 'why me?', 'what did I do to deserve this?', 'what am I going to tell the kids?', 'why now?' and a host of other meaning making questions. These questions when viewed in the light of a grief framework are meaning making questions which also assist the person to adjust to a 'new normal'. The need to make meaning out of our experiences is an almost universal human need [29]. Neimeyer and Sands [30] assert that the need to make meaning out of suffering is the critical and central issue in grief.

For some people, the quest to find meaning within their suffering will be a spiritual or religious undertaking [31].

Attempts to define spirituality have resulted in many concepts by academics; some believe that it is indefinable and purely subjective [32, 33]. Unruh et al. [34] found 92 definitions of spirituality in a comprehensive review. Walter [35] identified religious overtones to many definitions for spirituality associated with the founding figures and organisations in palliative care. Interestingly, a systematic review in 2007 found that only one fifth of the studies that they included differentiated between religious and spiritual beliefs and addressed the issue of definition [36]. This same review noted that most studies reported positive effects of religious or spiritual beliefs on bereavement, but those same studies had methodological flaws or were of weak design and were conducted primarily on white ethnical background females, of US origin with Protestant religious affiliation.

A study conducted in a palliative care centre in London found strong but not statistically significant positive influence on post-death grief. The same study found that people with low religiosity or spiritual beliefs had slower resolution with post-death grief at 9 months but had caught up on participants with stronger beliefs by 14 months [37].

Regardless of the attempts to develop theoretical models of spirituality and separate it from religion, for our patients and their caregivers, it is important that we are able to consider their needs, specifically using our knowledge and understanding if possible, to assist them with the quest to find meaning. From a clinical perspective, spiritual and/or religious beliefs will often provide an existential context to assist with predeath and post-death grief. Regardless of the religion, most religions and spiritual belief systems provide principals or doctrine about life and death, which our patients and caregivers might be able to draw strength from. Equally, those patients and caregivers who have low or no beliefs in religion or spirituality might not necessarily do worse than those patients with strong beliefs. It is up to the multidisciplinary care team to find ways of working with each and every patient and their families to offer the best possible support, using whatever coping and resiliency skills we can harness.

## Personality, Personal Differences, Culture, Age and Gender as a Factor

It should come as no surprise that the personality, personal differences, culture, age and gender are other factors to be mindful of when considering how caregivers and patients react. Given the sheer diversity of cultures, religions, personal backgrounds and experiences, personality traits, ages, genders, sexual orientations, customs and cultural rules to mention just a few, it is not surprising that researchers have had a difficult time conceptualising anticipatory and preparatory grief and of even less wonder that researchers have found such mixed results.

Research into the phenomenon that has been labelled anticipatory or preparatory grief has demonstrated that in some ways patients, caregivers and family members will react similarly despite individual differences. These 'commonalities' help clinicians and service providers plan for the services and treatments that may be needed. The challenge lays in appropriately offering the correct support or service at the time the individual needs it and/or modifying treatments or services as required.

Finally, despite all the research, reviews and experience gathered along the way, ultimately, each person, whether they be patient or caregiver, will react in their own way. This reaction will be based on factors such as their age, gender, support, previous loss experience, resiliency, their relationship with the person with the disease and the meaning they have been able to attach or make of the circumstances.

## Disease Progression and Role Changes

As lung disease progresses and the patient's health and quality of life deteriorate, the patient and their caregivers face the prospect of also undergoing many role changes. For some patients and caregivers, these role changes can be emotionally distressing and challenging. Not surprisingly, role changes may bring about a bout of anticipatory or preparatory grief, as the implications of disease trajectory become real [38]. Patients and their caregivers may be particularly vulnerable to emotional distress around the time a patient experiences an exacerbation or significant decline in lung function.

Many patients and their caregivers will be older and have developed set chores, jobs and images of self that result in greater difficulty adjusting to their 'new normal'. For example, a patient who has had a career or job where they feel respected and in charge and work long hours may find it difficult to retire from the work force early or reduce their hours. A patient who has kept house, cooked, cleaned and been the nurturing heart and soul of their family may find it difficult to relinquish these tasks to others as they become more debilitated by their disease. Both of these examples are of people who get a large sense of themselves through their 'careers'. Clinicians should be mindful of the possibility that with disease progression many of their patients and those who care for them will experience a renewed grief reaction or possibly exhibit depressive symptoms. At these times, referring patients and their caregiver to a psychologist may be helpful.

## Anticipatory Grief and Post-death Grief

The hypothesis that people who experience anticipatory grief will have better post-death grief adjustments is one that has received research attention for decades with mixed results [39]. Early studies [40–43] reported that anticipatory grief had a positive effect on post-death grief, whereas Levi [44] found that anticipatory grief correlated significantly with measures of depression and stress and suggested that anticipatory grief may be a risk factor for poor early post-death grief adjustment. In contrast, not having an opportunity for anticipatory grief was found to increase post-death grief of spouses [45]. Moon [38] cited three studies that found unresolved or unprocessed anticipatory grief can lead to distressful and extended post-death grief. Both Fan [39] and Moon [38] assert that anticipatory grief can have a potentially adaptive role to play in post-death grief.

## Grief and Its Relationship to Vicarious Trauma in Medical Staff

It is undisputed that providing hospice and palliative care is both a challenging and rewarding career. It provides the clinician with the opportunity to make meaningful differences to not only patients' lives but also to those of their families. However, these challenges and the frequent exposure to death and dying also provide a fertile environment for clinician burnout or vicarious trauma to manifest. Clinician burnout symptoms have been reported to impact up to 60% of primary care physicians [46, 47] and, in a recent study of palliative care clinicians, up around the 38% mark [48]. Clinicians suffering from vicarious trauma or burnout are more likely to express less empathy; make more medical errors; have higher dysfunction in their personal lives; experience feelings of depersonalisation, exhaustion and hopelessness; and feel unaccomplished in their workplace and also personally [46–49].

Grief of course has a role to play in the development of vicarious trauma and may even be bidirectional, meaning that the more a clinician exhibits symptoms of burnout, the more vulnerable they will be to experience a strong grief reaction when they lose a patient(s). Therefore, it is imperative that clinicians develop strategies around self-care that will assist them to decrease their likelihood of developing vicarious trauma or burnout and be better able to recognise their early warning signs and symptoms for when their 'emotional distress bucket is full'. Naturally, some signs and symptoms will be familiar to all of us, but we all will have our own level of how much we can cope with. Developing the capacity to reflect and be honest with ourselves about how we are feeling and coping is an invaluable tool that we all should aim to attain.

Swetz et al. [50] conducted a survey of 30 'seasoned' hospice and palliative medicine (HPM) physicians requesting they provide tried and tested methods for avoiding burnout. Sixty percent of respondents recommended promoting physical wellbeing, which included suggestions to exercise, eat well and healthily and get enough rest. Developing supportive, nurturing professional relationships was suggested by 57% of respondents. Other strategies that approximately 40% of respondents reported as being useful included taking a 'transcendental perspective' or in other words embracing our humanness, talking and debriefing to trusted others, participating in psychotherapy and making time for hobbies or non-medical activities outside of the work environment. Using humour, maintaining realistic expectations of outcomes and other aspects of the work environment, having breaks or time away from work and having a genuine passion for what you do were all suggested as useful.

Clinicians who work with patients and their families who have life-limiting disease will find themselves grieving. This is unavoidable and a natural and normal emotional response to forming a relationship with another person, even a professional one. Grief cannot be avoided, nor should we try to avoid it. Instead, one of the healthiest ways to process grief and the emotions it entails is to do the counter-intuitive and embrace those feelings that leave us feeling vulnerable – acknowledging we feel how we feel and letting those emotions sit with us for a while and then, when we are ready, letting them move off, knowing that they can come back, like waves crashing on the beach. Each time you sense grief, try to embrace it and let it sit. A psychologist can teach you mindfulness strategies to assist with this process. Letting ourselves feel grief, and acknowledging that, at times, we may feel overwhelmed, vulnerable and exhausted, is the first step in helping to safeguard ourselves from burnout or vicarious trauma.

## Anxiety and Feeling Anxious

It is easy to understand why people feel anxious when they can't breathe very well. It has been established beyond doubt that as dyspnoea increases, most patients will find themselves feeling increasingly anxious. Furthermore, as lung disease progresses, and the patient becomes more debilitated, anxiety has been reported to have a direct correlation with exercise tolerance and quality of life [51–53].

The *Diagnostic and Statistical Manual of Mental Disorders Fifth Edition* [1] lists six types of anxiety disorders ranging from generalised anxiety disorder, which is probably the most frequently diagnosed, to specific phobias. One that does not get a lot of mention in research papers and probably should is *anxiety disorder due to another medical condition 293.84 (ICD-10-CM multiple codes)*. In general, anxiety disorders manifest when a normal reaction to distress or stress becomes excessive. The state of fear or dread impacts a person's capacity to function in daily life in one or more domains most days, for most of the day for a period of time exceeding 2 weeks. With the diagnosis of *anxiety disorder due to another medical condition*, there must be evidence that the anxiety a person feels is due to the direct physiological effects of another medical condition [1]. Medical conditions such as COPD, ILDs and other lung diseases that cause dyspnoea and other distressing symptoms adequately meet this criterion.

In addition, the symptom overlap between lung disease symptoms and an anxiety or panic attack cannot be overlooked. Considering the pathophysiology of these symptoms is essential. Anxiogenic impact of hyperventilation, neurobiological sensitivity to Co2, lactate and other neurologic signals of suffocation along with misinterpreting respiratory symptoms such as dyspnoea have all been given as reasons why patients with lung disease may have a panic attack [54]. Chronic feelings of anxiety can result in the limbic system becoming hypersensitive. Both cortical structures (the hippocampus, the orbital frontal cortex, the insular cortex and other regions) and subcortical structures, such as the hypothalamus, the amygdala and other nuclei are all involved in these responses. An explanation for how this manifests came from Ziemann et al. [55] where they found in animal model that dyspnoea activates the right insular cortex and the amygdala. The amygdala elicits a fear response when it senses carbon dioxide and acidosis through its chemosensor. It is likely that anxiety and lung disease exacerbation and progression have a bidirectional relationship, at least for some lung diseases, such as chronic obstructive pulmonary disease (COPD) [54, 56].

Clinically, this is important to note as models such as the one mentioned above help the treating clinical team to be more understanding of why some of our patients actively avoid activity. Once this relationship between breathlessness and an anxiety or panic response becomes chronic, a phenomenon called kindling can mean that for some patients even a slight 'trigger' can lead to their brain anticipating the worst. Showing patients that they can exercise and move around safely, with or without oxygen therapy and other mobility aids, will help them accommodate to increasing breathlessness and hopefully reduce the limbic system activating as frequently [56]. The benefits of pulmonary rehabilitation programmes are well established and should be a source of regular referral for patients with chronic and life-limiting lung disease.

Another benefit to helping patients stay or become more active is that exercise, socialising and feeling connected with people and community are all fabulous ways of maintaining or increasing their quality of life. Exercise and staying active also helps to reduce depressive symptoms [51, 57].

## Depression and Feeling Depressed

Depression is characterised by low mood for most of the day, nearly every day for at least a 2-week period along with diminished interest and inability to find pleasure in things that the person used to find pleasure in, as well as possible weight loss or gain, a slowing down of thought and physical movement that is observable to others, fatigue or loss of energy, feelings of worthlessness or guilt, diminished ability to think and/or concentrate and possible suicidal ideation or plans [1]. To be diagnosed with major depressive disorder (MDD) or clinical depression a person must experience 5 or more of those symptoms. Depression is one of the most common mental health mood disorders with an estimated 322 million people globally suffering from the disorder. For people with lung disease, a world-wide prevelance of 4.4% has been widely reported [For example: 57, 59]. Further, in patient populations, depression has been acknowledged as causing significant distress, reduces treatment adherence, is aligned with longer inpatient stays and is correlated to higher morbidity and mortality [60–64].

In a comprehensive meta-analysis of 94 interview-based studies of cancer patients in oncological, haematological and palliative care settings, the authors found that in the first 5 years after diagnosis, approximately a sixth of patients met criteria for depression, with approximately a quarter having any type of depressed mood [64]. A recent study by Fernandez et al. [65] analysed results from 149 patients with interstitial lung disease (ILD) from Mexico and Argentina; they found that 18% (n = 27) of participants scored above 8 points (8–10 points, borderline abnormal; 0–7 points, normal) on the Hospital Anxiety and Depression Scale (HADS) for depressive symptoms, with 7% (n = 11) scoring between 11 and 21 points (11–21, abnormal), thus requiring further consideration for a depressive illness. They further identified that participants who were female and had a more recent diagnosis were more likely to score higher on the HADS.

It is difficult to tell if depression in patient populations is underestimated/underdiagnosed or overestimated/over-diagnosed [64]. This uncertainty around the diagnosis and estimation is due to several reasons. Firstly, in a clinical setting, many of the diagnoses are made by clinicians who are not specifically trained in mental health. Secondly, diagnosing depression takes time; the gold standard is using a clinical interview [66]. Even administering screening questionnaires to decide who may need a clinical interview can be burdensome, when added to an already busy clinical load. Thirdly, the criteria (listed above) for a diagnosis of depression as listed in the DSM-5 [1] or the International Classification of Diseases 10 (ICD-10) [67] are generic, especially the ICD-10, which does not mention the potential impact of disease. At least within the DSM-5, criteria for a diagnosis of depression has a limiting factor in that after meeting five or more of the common symptoms, one of the additional criteria states 'Episode not attributable to physiological effects of a substance or *another medical condition*'. Obviously, for clinicians working with patients who have a life-limiting lung disease, this criterion blurs the simplicity of a diagnosis.

Another complicating factor for clinicians is that our patients don't always use accurate language to describe what they are feeling. If a patient tells the clinician they feel depressed, it may mean they have depression, or it may mean that they are just feeling sad, overwhelmed and upset. Many people do not possess a wide emotional vocabulary, which means they might sometimes use 'umbrella' terms to describe how they feel. Most people, at some point in their lives, will feel depressed; it doesn't mean that they would meet criteria for a diagnosis of depression.

Lastly, and most importantly, much of the research into the prevalence of depression in people with chronic and life-limiting illness has been done using screening tools. It cannot be stated strongly enough that screening tools are not diagnostic tools. Researchers need to be very mindful of the potential to mislead and misrepresent the prevalence of depression within these patient populations. A good example of this is a 2005 study by Wagena et al. [63], where they rely on two self-report screening tools to assess the incidence of psychological distress and depression in patients with chronic obstructive pulmonary disease (COPD). Within the results and discussion sections, the authors refer to depressive symptoms as depression and refer to depressed COPD patients. Papers such as these get cited and referenced, and the potential myth of diagnosed depression that is found at higher than community levels within disease populations is perpetuated.

To add weight to the above criticism, Subica et al. [66] compared the Beck Depression Inventory II (BDI-II) as a diagnostic tool with a gold standard clinical interview with 1904 adult inpatients. They found that the BDI-II total score was a useful measure to screen patients for major depressive disorder (MDD) but not for presumptive diagnoses of clinical depression. Worryingly, they found that the

BDI-II was unsuccessful at distinguishing patients that had a clinical interview diagnosis of MDD from patients that had other mental disorders, where the BDI-II marginally exceeded chance performance.

Screening tools such as the BDI-II [68], the Hospital Anxiety and Depression Scale (HADS) [69] and other such screening tools can serve researchers and clinicians well, by alerting them to the psychological distress that their patients and participants might be experiencing [70], but relying on these tools to accurately diagnose mental health disorders is analogous to relying upon a chest x-ray to diagnose and specify the lung disease without the benefit of a bronchoscopy, high-resolution computed tomography (HRCT), pathology and other diagnostic procedures available to the clinician. Bunevicius and colleagues [70] conducted an interesting study assessing the diagnostic accuracy of two commonly utilised self-report scales (HADS and BDI-II) against the structured Mini International Neuropsychiatric Interview (MINI) with a group of patients with coronary artery disease. They found that the scales had low positive predictive value (PPV) in which some patients, who screened positive for depression using the scales, actually did not meet DSM criteria upon interview with the MINI. The researchers warn that relying solely on screening instruments can result in overburdening of available resources and patients possibly being poorly diagnosed and receiving anti-depressive treatment they do not need.

Despite the caveats noted above, there is evidence that depression and/or depressive symptoms are undertreated in palliative care settings. Care should be taken by all clinicians in palliative care, hospice, inpatient and outpatient settings to screen for low mood and be prepared to implement treatment or refer to appropriate clinicians to fully assess and incorporate psychological therapy into the multidisciplinary treatment plan.

## Distinguishing Between a Grief Reaction and Depression and/or Anxiety

At first glance, depression and/or anxiety and grief can present with similar and overlapping symptoms; indeed they can even coexist. Distinguishing between a grief reaction and depression and/or anxiety can be challenging for clinicians. The reason for this challenge is that many of the symptoms that have traditionally been used to diagnose depression or anxiety are also experienced by people who are grieving (predeath and post-death). However, we won't concentrate on post-death grief here; instead we will examine the similarities and differences in predeath grief, primarily looking at the patient reactions.

Distinguishing between these emotional reactions becomes even more challenging when overlaid with the physiological changes a patient can experience as their lung disease progresses. For example, weight loss (including anorexia), poor sleep, loss of appetite, fatigue and anhedonia are all symptoms of depression, anxiety and grief (*see box below*) [22]. These same symptoms can also be attributed to physiological deterioration associated with dying [27, 71]. Depressive symptoms in people nearing the end of their life can be associated with poorly controlled symptoms and should not be seen as part of the normal dying process, whereas preparatory grief will be experienced by most patients with a life-limiting lung disease and is a normal, natural and to be expected part of the dying process [22]. Depression and anxiety may respond well to pharmacotherapy; however for people who are experiencing preparatory grief, it is unlikely to be beneficial. Supportive strategies such as psychological therapy and other psychosocial supports are more likely to be effective [23].

*Symptoms that can be commonly shared by people suffering depression (pathalogical process) and also by people who expereince preparatory grief (normal process):*

Appetite changes
Weight changes
Fatigue
Low energy
Sleep disturbances
Sexual dysfunction

## Conclusion

It is important to distinguish between grief, anxiety and depression in terms of what treatment to pursue. More importantly, regardless of the mental health diagnosis, all of these patients and their caregivers will need support to manage the lung disease, their emotional response to the disease and the inevitable life changes and eventual death they will face. Support groups, such as the one trialled and refined by Lindell and her group [72], tackled difficult and emotionally challenging subjects like end-of-life decisions and increasing knowledge of disease. Numerous studies have shown that many patients if left to their own devices will not raise the subject of end-of-life planning and advance care directives, as they either assume that their physician understands their needs, they don't want to discuss a morbid subject or they don't want to face the inevitability of death, amongst other reasons [24, 72–74]. Physicians have also been shown to avoid some of these difficult and emotionally challenging conversations for reasons including not wanting to upset their patients and caregivers, not knowing when the 'best time' to bring up these subject is and being too busy with other medical aspects of their care [74].

Utilising as many members of the clinic's multidisciplinary team is one of the most efficient and effective ways of supporting your patient, their caregivers and yourself as you undertake this challenging and rewarding career. If there isn't a multidisciplinary team at your workplace, creating a network of private clinicians or organisations who will work together as a multidisciplinary team will work just as effectively.

Continuing to learn and develop skills that increase emotional intelligence will assist every clinician to have difficult and challenging conversations with their patients, be more empathic, be better at treating the 'whole' patient and have better outcomes. The additional benefit of increasing these skills is that you will develop greater resiliency and be less susceptible to burnout or vicarious trauma as these same skills help with recognising your own inner emotional state.

## References


1. American Psychiatric Association. Diagnostic and statistical manual of mental disorders: DSM-5. 5th ed. Washington: American Psychiatric Publishing Inc; 2013.
2. Rando, T.A., Grief and mourning: accommodating to loss. Dying: Facing the facts, 1995: p. 211–241.
3. Lindemann E. Symptomatology and management of acute grief. 1944. Am J Psychiatry. 1944/1994;151:155–60.
4. Kubler-Ross E. On death and dying. New York: Macmillan; 1969.
5. Bowlby J. Attachment and loss: Vol. 3. Loss: sadness and depression. New York, Basic Books; 1980.
6. Parkes CM, Weiss RS. Recovery from bereavement. New York: Basic Books; 1983.
7. Kubler-Ross E, Kessler D. On grief and grieving: finding the meaning of grief through the five stages of loss. New York: Scribner; 2005.
8. Sweeting HN, Gilhooly LM. Anticipatory grief: a review. Soc Sci Med. 1990;30(10):1073–80.
9. Nielsen MK, et al. Do we need to change our understanding of anticipatory grief in caregivers? A systematic review of caregiver studies during end-of-life caregiving and bereavement. Clin Psychol Rev. 2016;44:75–93.
10. Lindauer A, Harvath TA. Pre-death grief in the context of dementia caregiving: a concept analysis. J Adv Nurs. 2014;70(10):2196–207.
11. Aldrich CK. Some dynamics of anticipatory grief. In: Schonberg B, et al., editors. Anticipatory grief. New York: Columbia University Press; 1974.
12. Fulton R. Anticipatory mourning: a critique of the concept. Mortality. 2003;8(4):342–51.
13. Rando TA. Anticipatory grief: the term is a misnomer but the phenomenon exists. J Palliat Care. 1988;4(1–2):70–3.
14. Fulton R, Gottesman DJ. Anticipatory grief: a psychosocial concept reconsidered. Br J Psychiatry. 1980;137:45–54.
15. Coelho A, Barbosa A. Family anticipatory grief: an integrative literature review. Am J Hosp Palliat Med. 2017;34(8):774–85.
16. Johansson AK, et al. Anticipatory grief among close relatives of persons with dementia in comparison with close relatives of patients with cancer. Am J Hosp Palliat Med. 2012;30(1):29–34.
17. Egerod I, et al. Spousal bereavement after fibrotic interstitial lung disease: a qualitative study. Respir Med. 2019;146:129–36.
18. Prigerson HG, et al. Inventory of complicated grief: a scale to measure maladaptive symptoms of loss. Psychiatry Res. 1995;59(1–2):65–79.
19. Reynolds-Sandford D, et al. Differentiating between depression, anxiety and a grief reaction in idiopathic pulmonary fibrosis (IPF) patients and their caregivers. Is it time to rethink how and what we measure? Eur Respir J. 2019;54(suppl 63):PA1309.
20. Kubler-Ross E. On death and dying: what the dying have to teach doctors, nurses, clergy and their families. 1st ed. New York: Simon and Schuster; 1997.
21. Rando T. Clinical dimensions of anticipatory mourning: theory and practice in working with the dying, their loved ones and caregivers. Champaign, Illinois: Research Press; 2000.

22. Periyakoil VS, Hallenbeck J. Identifying and managing preparatory grief and depression at the end of life. Am Fam Physician. 2002;65(5):883–90.
23. Periyakoil VS, Kraemer HC, Noda A. Measuring grief and depression in seriously ill outpatients using the palliative grief depression scale. J Palliat Med. 2012;15(12):1350–5.
24. Sandford, D.G., et al., Lessons learnt from idiopathic pulmonary patients. University of Adelaide. 2020.
25. Kor YH, et al. Oxygen therapy for interstitial lung disease. A mismatch between patient expectations and experiences. Ann Am Thorac Soc. 2017;14(6):888–95.
26. Stroebe MS, Schut H. Models of coping and bereavement: a review. In: Stroebe MS, et al., editors. Handbook of bereavement research. Washington, DC: American Psychological Association; 2001.
27. Periyakoil VS. Differentiating grief from depression in patients who are seriously ill. Am Fam Physician. 2012;86(3):232–4.
28. Frankl VE. Man's search for meaning. Boston: Beacon Press; 1959.
29. Grey A. The spiritual component of palliative care. Palliat Med. 1994;8(3):215–21.
30. Neimeyer RA, Sands DC. Meaning reconstruction in bereavement: from principles to practice. In: Neimeyer RA, et al., editors. Grief and bereavement in contemporary society: bridging research and practice. New York: Routledge; 2011. p. 9–22.
31. Kellehear A. Spirituality and palliative care: a model of needs. Palliat Med. 2000;14(2):149–55.
32. Martsolf DS, Mickley JR. The concept of spirituality in nursing theories: differing world views and extent of focus. J Adv Nurs. 1998;27(2):294–303.
33. McSherry W, Draper P. The debates emerging from the literature surrounding the concept of spirituality as applied to nursing. J Adv Nurs. 1998;27(2):683–91.
34. Unruh AM, Versnel J, Kerr N. Spirituality unplugged: a review of the commonalities and contentions, and a resolution. Can J Occup Ther. 2002;69(1):5–19.
35. Walter T. The ideology and organization of spiritual care: three approaches. Palliat Med. 1997;11(1):21–30.
36. Becker G, et al. Do religious or spiritual beliefs influence bereavement? A systematic review. Palliat Med. 2007;21:2017–217.
37. Walsh K, et al. Spiritual beliefs may affect outcome of bereavement: a prospective study. Br Med J. 2002;324(7353):1551–5.
38. Moon PJ. Anticipatory grief: a mere concept? Am J Hosp Palliat Med. 2016;33(5):417–20.
39. Fan G. Anticipatory grief. In: Gu D, Dupre ME, editors. Encyclopedia of gerontology and population aging. Cham: Springer International Publishing; 2020. p. 1–4.
40. Rando T. In: Rando T, editor. *Loss and anticipatory grief.* Lexington: Lexington Books; 1986.
41. Fulton R, Fulton J. A psychosocial aspect of terminal care: anticipatory grief. Omega. 1971;2:91–9.
42. Natterson JM, Knudson AG. Observations concerning fear of death in fatally ill children and their mothers. Psychosom Med. 1960;22:456–65.
43. Friedman SB. Care of the family of the child with cancer. Pediatrics. 1967;40(3):498–504.
44. Levi L. Anticipatory grief: its measurement and proposed reconceptualization. Hosp J. 1991;7(4):1–28.
45. Stroebe W, Stroebe MS. Determinants of adjustment to bereavement in younger widows and widowers. In: Stroebe MS, Stroebe W, Hanson RO, editors. Handbook of bereavement: theory, research and intervention. Cambridge: Cambridge University Press; 1993. p. 208–26.
46. Shanafelt TD, et al. Burnout and self-reported patient care in an internal medicine program. Ann Intern Med. 2002;136(5):358–67.
47. Shanafelt TD, Sloan JA, Habermann TM. The well-being of physicians. Am J Med. 2003;114(6):513–9.
48. Kamal AH, et al. Prevalence and predictors of burnout among hospice and palliative care clinicians in the U.S. J Pain Symptom Manag. 2020;59(5):e6–e13.
49. Dyrbye LN, et al. A survey of U.S. physicians and their partners regarding the impact of work-home conflict. J Gen Intern Med. 2014;29:155–61.

50. Swetz KM, et al. Strategies for avoiding burnout in hospice and palliative medicine: peer advice for physicians on achieving longevity and fulfillment. J Palliat Med. 2009;12(9):773–7.
51. Holland AE, et al. Dyspnoea and comorbidity contribute to anxiety and depression in interstitial lung disease. Respirology. 2014;19(8):1215–21.
52. Kunik ME, et al. Surprisingly high prevalence of anxiety and depression in chronic breathing disorders. Chest. 2005;127(4):1205–11.
53. Nakazawa A, Cox NS, Holland AE. Current best practice in rehabilitation in interstitial lung disease. Ther Adv Respir Dis. 2017;11(2):115–28.
54. Smoller JW, et al. Panic anxiety, dyspnea, and respiratory disease. Theoretical and clinical considerations. Am J Respir Crit Care Med. 1996;154(1):6–17.
55. Ziemann E, et al. The amygdala is a chemosensor that detects carbon dioxide and acidosis to elicit fear behaviour. Cell. 2009;139:1012–21.
56. Amiri HM, Monzer K, Nugent K. The impact of anxiety on chronic obstructive pulmonary disease. Psychology. 2012;3(10):878–82.
57. Glaspole IN, et al. Health-related quality of life in idiopathic pulmonary fibrosis: data from the Australian IPF registry. Respirology. 2017;22(5):950–6.
58. Depression and other common mental health disorders: Global health estimates. 2017. Available from: https://apps.who.int/iris/bitstream/handle/10665/254610/WHO-MSD-MER-2017.2-eng.pdf.
59. Ryerson CJ, et al. Depression is a common and chronic comorbidity in patients with interstitial lung disease. Respirology. 2012;17(3):525–32.
60. Ruo B, et al. Depressive symptoms and health-related quality of life. The heart and soul study. JAMA. 2003;290(2):215–21.
61. Kalluri M, Luppi F, Ferrara G. What patients with idiopathic pulmonary fibrosis and caregivers want: filling the gaps with patient reported outcomes and experience measures. Am J Med. 2020;133(3):281–9.
62. Thrall G, et al. Depression, anxiety, and quality of life in patients with atrial fibrillation. Chest. 2007;132(4):1259–64.
63. Wagena EJ, et al. Are patients with COPD psychologically distressed? Eur Respir J. 2005;26:242–8.
64. Mitchell AJ, et al. Prevalence of depression, anxiety, and adjustment disorder in oncological, haematological, and palliative-care settings: a meta-analysis of 94 interview-based studies. Lancet Oncol. 2011;12(2):160–74.
65. Fernandez M, et al. Prevalence of anxiety and depression and their relationship with clinical characteristics in patients with interstitial lung disease. J Gerontol Geriatr Res. 2019;8(505):2.
66. Subica AM, et al. Factor structure and diagnostic validity of the Beck depression inventory-II with adult clinical inpatients: comparison to a gold-standard diagnostic interview. Psychol Assess. 2014;26(4):1106–15.
67. International classification of diseases and related health problems (ICD 10). 2019; 10th. Available from: https://icd.who.int/browse10/2019/en#/F30-F39.
68. Beck, A.T., R.A. Steer, and G. Brown, Beck depression inventory-II. 1996, San Antonio APA PsychTests.
69. Zigmond AS, Snaith RP. The hospital anxiety and depression scale. Acta Psychiatr Scand. 1983;67(6):361–70.
70. Bunevicius A, et al. Diagnostic accuracy of self-rating scales for screening of depression in coronary artery disease patients. J Psychosom Res. 2012;72(1):22–5.
71. Widera EW, Block SD. Managing grief and depression at the end of life. Am Fam Physician. 2012;86(3):259–64.
72. Lindell KO, et al. Impact of a disease-management program on symptom burden and health-related quality of life in patients with idiopathic pulmonary fibrosis and their care partners. Heart Lung. 2010;39(4):304–13.
73. Heffner JE, et al. Attitudes regarding advanced care directives among patients in pulmonary rehabilitation. Am J Crit Care Med. 1996;154(6):1735–40.
74. Jabbarian LJ, et al. Advance care planning for patients with chronic respiratory diseases: a systematic review of preferences and practices. Thorax. 2018;73:222–30.

# Chapter 8
# Symptom Management in Advanced Lung Disease

**Rebecca Anna Gersten and Sonye K. Danoff**

## Introduction

Patients with advanced lung disease often suffer from several poorly controlled symptoms. In fact, patients with chronic obstructive pulmonary disease (COPD) report a median of 11–14 uncontrolled symptoms at any given time [1]. Patients with interstitial lung disease (ILD) experience more breathlessness than do patients with lung cancer [2]. Depression is almost twice as likely to occur in patients with chronic illness than in the general population [3]. Patients with advanced lung disease have a higher symptom burden, worse quality of life, greater functional deterioration, and more social isolation when compared to those with cancer [4]. As symptom burden increases, patients with idiopathic pulmonary fibrosis (IPF) report worsening physical and emotional well-being [5]. At the end of life, patients with ILD are less likely to have medical record documentation of pain assessment [6] and are less likely to receive treatment for their symptoms [7] than patients with cancer.

Fortunately, a variety of pharmacologic and non-pharmacologic interventions are available for symptom management in patients with advanced lung disease. While opioids and benzodiazepines are the best-known pharmacologic agents, there is a rich supply of other medications to help with symptom control. Additionally, non-pharmacologic therapies are actually first-line treatment for many symptoms.

R. A. Gersten
Johns Hopkins University School of Medicine, Baltimore, MD, USA
e-mail: rgerste4@jhu.edu

S. K. Danoff (✉)
Division of Pulmonary & Critical Care Medicine, Johns Hopkins University School of Medicine, Baltimore, MD, USA
e-mail: sdanoff@jhmi.edu



K. O. Lindell, S. K. Danoff (eds.), *Palliative Care in Lung Disease*, Respiratory Medicine, https://doi.org/10.1007/978-3-030-81788-6_8

## Dyspnea

Dyspnea is a common and distressing symptom in patients with advanced lung disease of any cause and often results in disability and social isolation [8]. Refractory breathlessness is defined as breathlessness at rest or on minimal exertion that will persist chronically despite optimal treatment of the underlying cause(s) [9]. In patients with COPD, severity of breathlessness is a better indicator of prognosis than is lung function [10]. The IPF patient and caregiver journey is often dominated by uncontrolled dyspnea [11]. In one study, 88% of patients with IPF reported dyspnea [12].

Dyspnea may be assessed using any of the following tools: Saint George's Respiratory Questionnaire (SGRQ), Pulmonary Functional Status and Dyspnea Questionnaire, Medical Research Council (MRC) Dyspnea Scale, Chronic Respiratory Diseases Questionnaire, Dyspnoea-12 Score, Numerical Rating Scale (NRS), Visual Analogue Scale (VAS), Borg Dyspnea Scale, Transient Dyspnea Index (TDI)-Baseline Dyspnea Index (BDI), or UCSD Shortness of Breath (SOB) Questionnaire. The Respiratory Distress Observation Scale can be used for evaluating patients unable to self-report. In assessing dyspnea, it is important to screen for other underlying disorders that may not be optimally controlled and may contribute to this symptom. These may include pulmonary hypertension (PH), arrhythmia, pulmonary emboli, anemia, pleural effusions, or congestive heart failure [13]. Notably, 30–50% of patients with advanced IPF develop PH, and this often presents with worsening dyspnea [14]. Treatment should be targeted toward any detected contributing factor. Drainage of pleural effusion is recommended if present, and blood transfusion should be considered in the presence of severe anemia [13]. Oxygen needs, particularly with activity, should also be assessed and supplemented as appropriate.

There is a wide range of pharmacologic options for treatment of dyspnea. Patients should ideally have optimal management of their underlying pulmonary disease and may require additional "as needed" medications. For patients with underlying obstructive lung disease, beta-agonist bronchodilators may be helpful at relieving dyspnea. This population may also benefit from inhaled anticholinergic bronchodilators such as ipratropium.

Opioids remain the most effective pharmacologic treatment of dyspnea [15]. Opioids can be given orally in either an extended or immediate release formulation, rectally, transdermally, subcutaneously, or intravenously. Evidence is conflicting on the benefit of nebulized opioids, and systematic reviews have concluded that they are no more effective than placebo [13]. Epidural methadone in patients with severe COPD does show improvement in dyspnea [15]. While there is a theoretical concern for hypoventilation with the administration of opioids, this has not been demonstrated in clinical trials. Careful attention to prior exposure is important when selecting dosage, and the lowest effective dose should be used and titrated slowly to meet the individual patient's needs [1]. Concurrent use of a bowel regimen to prevent constipation is recommended. Patients may experience drowsiness, nausea, or vomiting as side effects.

Anxiolytics, such as benzodiazepines, may be helpful to reduce dyspnea and often have a synergistic effect with opioids. One study documented benefit for all ILD patients given opioids or benzodiazepines [16]. Benzodiazepines do reduce respiratory drive in a dose-dependent fashion, so these should be used judiciously. Additionally, they have a high potential for both physical and psychological dependency and can be difficult to withdraw from [1]. Buspirone is less sedative and also effective in treating breathlessness in patients with COPD [17].

Systemic glucocorticoids are often used in the treatment of both obstructive and restrictive lung disease. Dexamethasone is most frequently used in the palliative care setting given its reduced mineralocorticoid effects, increased potency, and higher solubility [15]. Tapering glucocorticoids is recommended as adrenal insufficiency may result following abrupt withdrawal. The role of nebulized furosemide remains controversial. There does appear to be a specific bronchodilator effect, but results have been inconsistent [15]. Promethazine has some evidence that it reduces dyspnea [17]. Selective serotonin reuptake inhibitors (SSRIs) may improve dyspnea irrespective of underlying anxiety [15]. Mirtazapine is an option to treat breathlessness with ongoing clinical trials evaluating its effectiveness [10]. In patients with excess secretions, mucolytics and occasional antibiotics may decrease dyspnea [13]. Theophylline may reduce dyspnea in patients with COPD. Sildenafil improves dyspnea in patients with IPF [18].

Non-pharmacologic interventions are very helpful in the treatment of dyspnea. One of the best-known interventions to improve dyspnea, exercise capacity, physical activity, and quality of life in all forms of advanced lung disease is pulmonary rehabilitation (PR) [13, 19]. PR optimally includes exercise training, psychosocial support, nutritional therapy, breathing strategies, inspiratory muscle training, and panic control [13]. It is recommended that all patients with advanced lung disease enroll in PR [19]. This may help avoid the vicious cycle of deconditioning leading to worsening dyspnea [10]. All patients with dyspnea should be assessed for use of walking aids as these can further increase level of physical activity [10]. Fans may have benefit in reducing dyspnea for patients with obstructive lung disease [20].

Hypoxia is thought to cause dyspnea in its own right, possibly by increasing work of breathing in its role as a respiratory stimulant [15]. Supplemental oxygen may, therefore, improve dyspnea but is only recommended in hypoxic patients [13]. Any benefit in symptomatology is usually seen in the first 72 hours of use [21]. In IPF patients with nocturnal hypoxia, supplemental oxygen actually improves daytime symptoms [14]. Supplemental oxygen is most commonly delivered via nasal cannula. Concentrators can deliver up to 10 L/min. It is recommended to add humidification as oxygen flow rate increases to avoid excessive drying of the airway mucosa. Some patients may require high-flow nasal cannula (HFNC), and HFNC may be particularly effective in ILD patients at the end of life [22]. Patients with severe dyspnea may experience relief with use of noninvasive positive pressure ventilation [13]. This can be especially beneficial in shortness of breath secondary to neuromuscular weakness. Heliox has also been shown to reduce dyspnea in patients with COPD [23].

Mental health is intimately tied to the sensation of dyspnea. It is quite important to treat psychosocial factors while treating dyspnea [13]. A written personal crisis plan outlining actions to help in the event of uncontrolled dyspnea is recommended [1]. Cognitive behavioral therapy, mindfulness-based stress reduction, relaxation, and acupuncture all provide dyspnea relief. Tai Chi and yoga may also be helpful [1]. Facial cooling by use of a fan or cold water spray may improve dyspnea [1, 13]. For some patients with severe emphysema, lung volume reduction may reduce dyspnea [23].

## Cough

Cough is a protective mechanism to clear the airway of foreign materials and secretions [23]. However, cough can be a very troubling symptom for many patients with advanced lung disease. A nonproductive cough can result from a hypersensitive reflex such that a trivial stimulation leads to an excessive response, while a productive cough can be caused by increased stimulation of physiologic cough reflex by endobronchial material [15]. Cough can disable patients socially and can sometimes result in complications such as rib fractures, pneumothorax, stress incontinence, and syncope [15]. In one study 85% of patients with IPF reported cough [12]. Chronic cough is particularly challenging in IPF and associated with poor sleep quality, limited exercise capacity, and decreased social interactions [19].

Symptom assessment can be performed using the Leicester Cough Questionnaire or Cough-Specific Quality of Life Questionnaire (CQLQ). The first step in symptom management is to evaluate for and treat any identified reversible causes of cough. It is important to evaluate for use of angiotensin-converting enzyme inhibitors. If gastroesophageal reflux disease (GERD) is suspected, consideration should be given to the prescription of a proton pump inhibitor or a histamine H2-receptor antagonist. Lifestyle modifications are recommended, including bed placement in reverse Trendelenburg position. Patients should be advised to avoid eating for 3 hours before bedtime. If upper airway cough (UAC) syndrome is suspected, a nasal corticosteroid or saline sinus rinse can be trialed. It is advisable to check for the presence of cerumen in the ear canal and to remove if present.

Once all reversible causes of cough are optimally treated, it is appropriate to trial other agents aimed to ameliorate cough. Opioids are centrally acting cough suppressants. Morphine and codeine are considered the most effective antitussives [15]. Dextromethorphan is a nonnarcotic synthetic morphine derivative with no sedative or analgesic qualities. Levodropropizine and moguisteine are peripheral cough suppressants. Benzonatate may be helpful. Nebulized lidocaine can relieve cough. Other options include baclofen, gabapentin, carbamazepine, or amitriptyline.

When cough is associated with mucus production, in conditions such as COPD or bronchiectasis, it may be helpful to introduce airway clearance. Nebulized acetylcysteine may help to break up secretions. Nebulized isotonic or hypertonic (3–7%) saline promotes expectoration, and pre-treatment with bronchodilators reduces risk of bronchoconstriction [23]. Short trials of antibiotics may be helpful as well. Anticholinergic medications, such as atropine and glycopyrrolate, may be helpful as treatment for cough in the setting of excessive secretions. There are some special considerations for patients with IPF. Nebulized sodium cromoglycate reduces cough [19]. Treatment with corticosteroids or thalidomide may also provide relief from cough [15].

New pharmacologic agents to reduce cough are currently under investigation. Gefapixant, a P2X3 receptor antagonist, has demonstrated efficacy in reducing objective cough frequency and improving patient-reported outcomes without any serious adverse events [24]. Aprepitant, a NK1 receptor antagonist, decreases awake cough frequency [25].

Non-pharmacologic interventions are particularly important in the setting of a productive cough. Chest physiotherapy can aid in expectoration of mucus. Cough assist devices can remove secretions in patients with an ineffective cough. Speech and language therapy evaluation and treatment may be helpful to reduce cough [10]. Additional non-pharmacologic interventions include hot tea and oral lozenges.

## Pain

Pain in patients with advanced lung disease is usually caused by infection or inflammation [23]. Dynamic hyperinflation in COPD or pneumothorax can also cause pain [23]. Treatment of pain is particularly important because thoracic pain may decrease respiration, contributing to dyspnea and anxiety.

Symptom assessment can be performed using the Numerical Rating Scale (NRS), Visual Analogue Scale (VAS), Faces Pain Scale, Categorical Likert Scale, Brief Pain Inventory (BPI), McGill Pain Questionnaire, or Memorial Pain Assessment Card. The Nonverbal Pain Scale (NVPS) can be used for patients who are unable to speak. The Behavioral Pain Scale (BPS) is traditionally used for intubated patients. Chest imaging may be necessary to evaluate for a treatable etiology for the patient's pain.

There are a variety of pharmacologic interventions to treat pain. The WHO "analgesic ladder" recommends trialing nonsteroidal anti-inflammatory drugs (NSAIDs) and acetaminophen prior to using opioids [13]. Caution should be used as NSAIDs may induce bronchospasm in susceptible patients [23]. Corticosteroids may provide pain relief by reduction of inflammation. Tricyclic antidepressants, anticonvulsants, neuroleptics, alpha2-adrenergic agonists such as clonidine, and baclofen may be helpful in the case of neuropathic pain [13]. Additionally, nerve blockades or intrathecal or epidural administration of neurolytic agents may be appropriate [23]. Consultation with a pain management or palliative care specialist may be necessary [13]. Non-pharmacologic interventions include acupuncture, physical therapy, cognitive behavioral therapy, and mindfulness-based stress reduction.

## Anxiety

Psychological distress is common in patients with advanced lung disease and is known to lower quality of life, decrease response to therapies during acute exacerbations, and increase frequency of hospitalizations [13]. Anxiety is inextricably linked to dyspnea and often associated with uncertainty regarding disease progression. Anxiety is present in 33–58% of patients with IPF[19] and increases as the pulmonary fibrosis progresses [26].

Symptom assessment can be performed using the Hospital Anxiety and Depression Scale (HADS), Patient Health Questionnaire (PHQ)-4, or Generalized Anxiety Disorder 7-item Scale (GAD-7). Careful assessment of medications is important as the use of steroids or methylphenidate may heighten anxiety.

Pharmacologic interventions include SSRI and buspirone. SSRIs are the drug of choice for patients with panic attacks [13]. Benzodiazepines can be helpful for breakthrough symptoms but have a high propensity for dependency.

Non-pharmacologic interventions are very important in the treatment of anxiety. Cognitive behavioral therapy should be an integral part of treatment. Relaxation techniques, panic control strategies, mindfulness training, distraction techniques, and breathing strategies may be helpful [13]. PR can alleviate anxiety even at the end of life [13]. Social work engagement may be particularly important in patients with social and financial stressors. Patients may benefit from support groups to feel more connected with those experiencing similar symptoms. Symptom management strategies and end-of-life preparedness may help reduce anxiety and depression in IPF patients [14].

## Depression

Depression is common in patients with advanced lung disease and associated with worse clinical outcomes [10]. Increased functional impairment over the course of an illness is associated with depression [13]. Depression is present in almost half of patients with IPF [3]. Depression is very common in patients with COPD and is often associated with self-blame for prior tobacco use [1].

Symptom assessment can be performed using the Wakefield Self-Assessment of Depression Inventory, Hospital Anxiety and Depression Scale (HADS), Patient Health Questionnaire (PHQ)-2, PHQ-9, Short Demoralization Scale (SDS), or Center for Epidemiologic Studies Depression Scale (CES-D). Pharmacologic interventions include SSRIs and tricyclic antidepressants. Methylphenidate can be used acutely if the patient does not suffer from concurrent anxiety [13]. Cognitive behavioral therapy in conjunction with pharmacologic therapy may be particularly helpful [13].

## Sleep Disturbances

There is an increased risk of sleep disturbances in patients with advanced lung disease [10]. Sleep disturbances are present in 47% of patients with IPF[14] and in 68% of patients with COPD [27]. In both populations, there is overlap between sleep disturbances and anxiety and depression [14, 27]. Insomnia, restless leg syndrome, and periodic limb movement in sleep are more common in patients with COPD than in the general population [27].

Symptom assessment can be performed using the Pittsburgh Sleep Quality Index, Epworth Sleepiness Scale, or Global Sleep Assessment Questionnaire (GSAQ). A detailed sleep history should be obtained. Timing and amount of caffeine consumption should be examined. Triggers for referral to a sleep specialist include severe daytime sleepiness, snoring or gasping during sleep, and morning headaches. The Berlin Questionnaire selectively screens for obstructive sleep apnea [27].

Pharmacologic interventions to treat sleep disturbances are generally not recommended in patients with advanced lung disease. Melatonin is a safe option, and ramelteon has been deemed safe for use in patients with mild to moderate COPD [28]. Tricyclic antidepressants can be effective in the treatment of insomnia [13]. Sedating antihistamines such as diphenhydramine can be used but are associated with some untoward anticholinergic side effects and should be used with caution in patients over age 65. Non-pharmacologic interventions are particularly important in the treatment of sleep disturbances. Good sleep hygiene should be encouraged, and cognitive behavioral therapy may be very effective.

## Fatigue

Fatigue is the most common symptom of every illness [10]. Greater than 90% of patients with IPF report fatigue [12]. Fatigue is common in patients with COPD and increases with disease severity (as measured by forced expiratory volume in one second [$FEV_1$]) [29]. Symptom assessment can be performed using the Brief Fatigue Inventory, Numerical Rating Scale (NRS), or Visual Analogue Scale (VAS). Although fatigue is characteristically not improved by sleep or rest, it is important to inquire about patients' sleep patterns and quality [10].

Pharmacologic interventions are usually not recommended. However, corticosteroids and methylphenidate are occasionally used in the acute period. Modafinil may be appropriate in certain patients. Non-pharmacologic interventions include exercise, nutrition, and cognitive behavioral therapy. PR is recommended [1].

## Anorexia

Anorexia often occurs later in the disease process. ILD patients on antifibrotic agents may experience anorexia as a side effect. It may be appropriate to discontinue these medications if significant weight loss ensues. It is important to continually assess dosage of other medications so as to not cause overdose, especially if there is rapid weight loss. Symptom assessment can be performed using the Functional Assessment of Anorexia/Cachexia Therapy (FAACT), Subjective Global Assessment of Nutrition instrument, or Visual Assessment Scale (VAS).

Pharmacologic interventions include mirtazapine and megestrol acetate. Non-pharmacologic interventions include PR, which can increase appetite by increasing level of physical activity. Consultation with a dietician may be very helpful. Nutritional supplements are recommended for interested patients with evidence of malnutrition [1]. Artificial nutrition or hydration should not be forced against patient will, and there is no evidence of suffering as a result of malnutrition or dehydration [13]. Wetting the patient's lips with the patient's beverage of choice may provide comfort, especially at the end of life.

## Delirium

Delirium may occur as a result of end-stage disease and may be hyper- or hypoactive. Symptom assessment can be performed using the Confusion Assessment Method (CAM), Memorial Delirium Assessment Scale (MDAS), or Mini-Mental Status Examination (MMSE). Pharmacologic interventions include the use of antipsychotic medications. However, non-pharmacologic interventions are recommended prior to initiation of medications. These include frequent reorientation, light during the day, presence of family or friends, minimization of environmental stimuli, and personal music choices through headphones [13].

## Spiritual Distress

Many patients with progressive, life-limiting illness experience spiritual distress. Questions often arise regarding existence, the meaning of life, regret, and destiny [15]. Resolution of spiritual questions may be especially important for patients closer to the end of life [13]. Symptom assessment can be performed using the Functional Assessment of Chronic Illness Therapy-Spiritual Well-Being (FACIT-Sp) or Spiritual Well-Being Scale.

Pharmacologic interventions are generally not recommended. In very rare and refractory cases, benzodiazepines or barbiturates can be used as palliative sedation. Non-pharmacologic interventions include active listening to patient fears and concerns and gentle reassurance. Involvement of family, pastoral care, and community and religious resources is particularly important. Watching loved ones suffer from spiritual distress may be extremely difficult, and it is particularly important to evaluate caregivers for burden and fatigue.

## Conclusions

Patients with advanced lung disease often suffer from a profound symptom burden that worsens physical and emotional well-being. Symptom management is key to improving patient quality of life. There are many validated tools to assess for the most common symptoms, including dyspnea, cough, pain, anxiety, depression, sleep disturbances, fatigue, anorexia, delirium, and spiritual distress. Fortunately, there is a large repertoire of pharmacologic and non-pharmacologic tools to help alleviate these symptoms. Initiation of therapy should be followed by constant reassessment of patient response. Adequate symptom control enables patients to live as long as possible with the best quality of life.

## References

1. Maddocks M, Lovell N, Booth S, Man WD-C, Higginson IJ. Palliative care and management of troublesome symptoms for people with chronic obstructive pulmonary disease. Lancet. 2017;390(10098):988–1002. https://doi.org/10.1016/S0140-6736(17)32127-X.
2. Ahmadi Z, Wysham NG, Lundström S, Janson C, Currow DC, Ekström M. End-of-life care in oxygen-dependent ILD compared with lung cancer: a national population-based study. Thorax. 2016;71(6):510–6. https://doi.org/10.1136/thoraxjnl-2015-207439.
3. Akhtar AA, Ali MA, Smith RP. Depression in patients with idiopathic pulmonary fibrosis. Chron Respir Dis. 2013;10(3):127–33. https://doi.org/10.1177/1479972313493098.
4. Barratt SL, Morales M, Spiers T, et al. Specialist palliative care, psychology, interstitial lung disease (ILD) multidisciplinary team meeting: a novel model to address palliative care needs. BMJ Open Resp Res. 2018;5(1):e000360. https://doi.org/10.1136/bmjresp-2018-000360.
5. Rajala K, Lehto JT, Sutinen E, Kautiainen H, Myllärniemi M, Saarto T. Marked deterioration in the quality of life of patients with idiopathic pulmonary fibrosis during the last two years of life. BMC Pulm Med. 2018;18(1):172. https://doi.org/10.1186/s12890-018-0738-x.
6. Brown CE, Engelberg RA, Nielsen EL, Curtis JR. Palliative care for patients dying in the intensive care unit with chronic lung disease compared with metastatic cancer. Annals ATS. 2016;13(5):684–9. https://doi.org/10.1513/AnnalsATS.201510-667OC.
7. Matsunuma R, Takato H, Takeda Y, et al. Patients with end-stage interstitial lung disease may have more problems with dyspnea than end-stage lung cancer patients. Indian J Palliat Care. 2016;22(3):282. https://doi.org/10.4103/0973-1075.185035.
8. Higginson IJ, Bausewein C, Reilly CC, et al. An integrated palliative and respiratory care service for patients with advanced disease and refractory breathlessness: a randomised controlled trial. Lancet Respir Med. 2014;2(12):979–87. https://doi.org/10.1016/S2213-2600(14)70226-7.
9. Reilly CC, Bausewein C, Garrod R, Jolley CJ, Moxham J, Higginson IJ. Breathlessness during daily activity: the psychometric properties of the London chest activity of daily living scale in

patients with advanced disease and refractory breathlessness. Palliat Med. 2017;31(9):868–75. https://doi.org/10.1177/0269216316680314.
10. Booth S, Johnson MJ. Improving the quality of life of people with advanced respiratory disease and severe breathlessness. Breathe. 2019;15(3):198–215. https://doi.org/10.1183/20734735.0200-2019.
11. Kalluri M, Claveria F, Ainsley E, Haggag M, Armijo-Olivo S, Richman-Eisenstat J. Beyond idiopathic pulmonary fibrosis diagnosis: multidisciplinary care with an early integrated palliative approach is associated with a decrease in acute care utilization and hospital deaths. J Pain Symptom Manag. 2018;55(2):420–6. https://doi.org/10.1016/j.jpainsymman.2017.10.016.
12. Rajala K, Lehto JT, Sutinen E, Kautiainen H, Myllärniemi M, Saarto T. mMRC dyspnoea scale indicates impaired quality of life and increased pain in patients with idiopathic pulmonary fibrosis. ERJ Open Res. 2017;3(4):00084–2017. https://doi.org/10.1183/23120541.00084-2017.
13. Lanken PN, Terry PB, DeLisser HM, et al. An official american thoracic society clinical policy statement: palliative care for patients with respiratory diseases and critical illnesses. Am J Respir Crit Care Med. 2008;177(8):912–27. https://doi.org/10.1164/rccm.200605-587ST.
14. Rozenberg D, Sitzer N, Porter S, et al. Idiopathic pulmonary fibrosis: a review of disease, pharmacological, and nonpharmacological strategies with a focus on symptoms, function, and health-related quality of life. J Pain Symptom Manag. 2020;59(6):1362–78. https://doi.org/10.1016/j.jpainsymman.2019.12.364.
15. Currow DC, Abernethy AP. Pharmacological management of dyspnoea. Curr Opin Support Palliat Care. 2007;1(2):96–101. https://doi.org/10.1097/SPC.0b013e3282ef5e03.
16. Bajwah S, Higginson IJ, Ross JR, et al. Specialist palliative care is more than drugs: a retrospective study of ILD patients. Lung. 2012;190(2):215–20. https://doi.org/10.1007/s00408-011-9355-7.
17. Awan S, Wilcock A. Nonopioid medication for the relief of refractory breathlessness. Curr Opin Support Palliat Care. 2015;9(3):227–31. https://doi.org/10.1097/SPC.0000000000000149.
18. Idiopathic Pulmonary Fibrosis Clinical Research Network, Zisman DA, Schwarz M, Anstrom KJ, Collard HR, Flaherty KR, Hunninghake GW. A controlled trial of sildenafil in advanced idiopathic pulmonary fibrosis. N Engl J Med. 2010;363(7):620–8. https://doi.org/10.1056/NEJMoa1002110.
19. Zou RH, Kass DJ, Gibson KF, Lindell KO. The role of palliative Care in Reducing Symptoms and Improving Quality of life for patients with idiopathic pulmonary fibrosis: a review. Pulm Ther. 2020;6(1):35–46. https://doi.org/10.1007/s41030-019-00108-2.
20. Morélot-Panzini C. Fooling the brain to alleviate dyspnoea. Eur Respir J. 2017;50(2):1701383. https://doi.org/10.1183/13993003.01383-2017.
21. Wiseman R, Rowett D, Allcroft P, Abernethy A, Currow D. Chronic refractory dyspnoea evidence based management. 4.
22. Koyauchi T, Hasegawa H, Kanata K, et al. Efficacy and tolerability of high-flow nasal cannula oxygen therapy for hypoxemic respiratory failure in patients with interstitial lung disease with do-not-intubate orders: a retrospective single-center study. Respiration. 2018;96(4):323–9. https://doi.org/10.1159/000489890.
23. Kreuter M, Herth FJF. Supportive and palliative Care of Advanced Nonmalignant Lung Disease. Respiration. 2011;82(4):307–16. https://doi.org/10.1159/000330730.
24. Muccino DR, Morice AH, Birring SS, et al. Design and rationale of two phase 3 randomised controlled trials (COUGH-1 and COUGH-2) of gefapixant, a P2X3 receptor antagonist, in refractory or unexplained chronic cough. ERJ Open Res. 2020;6(4):00284–2020. https://doi.org/10.1183/23120541.00284-2020.
25. Badri H, Smith JA. Emerging targets for cough therapies; NK1 receptor antagonists. Pulm Pharmacol Ther. 2019;59:101853. https://doi.org/10.1016/j.pupt.2019.101853.
26. Lindell KO, Liang Z, Hoffman LA, et al. Palliative care and location of death in decedents with idiopathic pulmonary fibrosis. Chest. 2015;147(2):423–9. https://doi.org/10.1378/chest.14-1127.

27. Vaidya S, Gothi D, Patro M. Prevalence of sleep disorders in chronic obstructive pulmonary disease and utility of global sleep assessment questionnaire: an observational case–control study. Ann Thorac Med. 2020;15(4):230. https://doi.org/10.4103/atm.ATM_85_20.
28. Kryger M, Roth T, Wang-Weigand S, Zhang J. The effects of ramelteon on respiration during sleep in subjects with moderate to severe chronic obstructive pulmonary disease. Sleep Breath. 2009;13(1):79–84. https://doi.org/10.1007/s11325-008-0196-4.
29. Baltzan MA, Scott AS, Wolkove N, et al. Fatigue in COPD: prevalence and effect on outcomes in pulmonary rehabilitation. Chron Respir Dis. 2011;8(2):119–28. https://doi.org/10.1177/1479972310396737.

# Chapter 9
# Communication in Palliative Care

**Taylor Lincoln and Jared Chiarchiaro**

## Introduction

Lung disease is a common cause of morbidity and mortality with care trajectories and symptom burden comparable to those associated with cancer [1, 2]. Despite these similarities, studies have shown that patients with lung disease, such as chronic obstructive pulmonary disease (COPD), lack an awareness of death and dying compared to those with cancer. Data indicates that frequency, timing, and quality of palliative care communication between clinicians and this patient population are poor. This is problematic because palliative care communication done well improves patients' symptoms and quality of life, leads to better concordance between patient goals and care delivered, and improves family psychosocial outcomes.

Communication surrounding palliative care rarely occurs in care of patients with advanced lung diseases [3]. As an example, a systemic review showed that most studies exploring palliative communication report rates of discussion regarding treatment preferences and end-of-life issues in less than 30% of patients with COPD [4]. Only a small proportion of patients with moderate to severe COPD have discussed treatment preferences and end-of-life care issues with their physicians, and the vast majority of these patients believe their physicians do not understand their preferences for end-of-life care [5]. When discussions do occur, the quality is often rated by patients as low [4] due to the absence of important elements such as prognosis,

T. Lincoln (✉)
Department of Internal Medicine, Division of Pulmonary, Critical Care, and Sleep Medicine, University of Pittsburgh School of Medicine, Pittsburgh, PA, USA
e-mail: lincolntb@upmc.edu

J. Chiarchiaro
Division of Pulmonary Allergy and Critical Care Medicine, Oregon Health & Science University, Portland, OR, USA
e-mail: chiarchi@ohsu.edu



K. O. Lindell, S. K. Danoff (eds.), *Palliative Care in Lung Disease*, Respiratory Medicine, https://doi.org/10.1007/978-3-030-81788-6_9

anticipatory guidance, and spirituality [6]. Patients with COPD are more likely than those with HIV/AIDS and cancer to express concern about the lack of education that they receive about their disease, treatment, prognosis, and advance care planning [7]. Clinicians acknowledge that discussion of goals of care and end-of-life preferences should occur early in the illness and when the patient is stable [8]. However, when discussions do occur, they often take place at advanced stages of the illness or hospitalization when patients may be unable to participate in decision-making, a situation that is burdensome to their surrogate decision-makers.

Herein we will review the existing literature on why effective palliative care communication is important for patients with advanced lung diseases, their families, and the healthcare system, discuss common barriers encountered by clinicians, and consider potential solutions to those barriers.

## Why communication is important for patients, their families, and the healthcare system:

Effective palliative care communication includes both a [1] discussion of the values and preferences that shape end-of-life care and [2] exploration of factors contributing to patient suffering and symptom management.

For patients with lung disease, discussions regarding end-of-life care frequently occur at advanced stages of illness when patients are often unable to participate in decision-making. In the absence of early goals of care discussions, patients are at risk to receive unwanted medical care resulting in prolongation of the dying process and undue burden on surrogate decision-makers. When patients are decisionally incapacitated, surrogate decision-makers are asked to collaborate with clinicians to assist in making emotionally and cognitively difficult decisions. This surrogate role has been associated with negative emotional outcomes, such as stress, guilt, or doubt, in at least one third of surrogate decision-makers [9]. Anxiety, depression, and post-traumatic stress disorder have all been described in surrogate decision-makers [10–13]. Families of patients who died in the ICU were found to have higher levels of both PTSD and depression when they experienced discordance between their preferred and actual decision-making roles [14]. Furthermore, a cross-sectional study of bereaved family members found that perceptions on quality of end-of-life care are associated with complicated grief [15] which is known to be associated with poor physical health due to diseases, such as cancer, heart disease, and hypertension, and poor psychosocial outcomes, including anxiety, depression, and suicide [16, 17].

These poor outcomes for surrogate decision-makers are largely due to the burden of making high stakes decisions without knowledge of patients' wishes. This burden may be alleviated by clarifying patients' preferences early in their disease course. One systematic review found that when surrogates knew which treatments were consistent with the patient's preferences, it reduced negative outcomes for surrogate decision-makers such as feelings of guilt and stress. In this study, surrogates who were confident in their loved one's treatment preferences felt as though they were simply reporting the patient's preferences as opposed to deciding on behalf of their loved one [9]. Other studies have demonstrated that end-of-life discussions were associated with better caregiver quality of life and bereavement adjustment at follow-up [18]. Additionally, terminally ill patient's prognostic awareness has been found to be associated with a higher quality of death reported by their caretakers who were also more physically and mentally healthy 6 months post-bereavement [19].

Physicians' ability to engage in goals of care discussions also contributes to outcomes for healthcare providers and the healthcare system. Caring for patients with advanced lung diseases who are seriously ill, suffer repeated exacerbations, and have limited treatment options makes clinicians vulnerable to moral distress and burnout. One study demonstrated that delivering bad news to patients can contribute to burnout among physicians who feel inadequately trained in communication skills [20]. Training interventions to improve end-of-life communication skills have shown significant improvements in confidence in communicating, attitudes toward psychosocial care, and sense of personal accomplishment [21]. Furthermore, the perception of providing harmful or futile care leads to moral distress and loss of empathy [22] which serves as a common cause of clinician burnout [23, 24]. Physician burnout has significant consequences on physician health with increased rates of depression [25], substance dependence [26], and suicidal ideation [27]. In addition to a moral and ethical cost, there is an economic cost to burnout. Cross-sectional studies have uncovered associations between physician burnout with decreased productivity, increased turnover, and increased medical errors resulting in poorer quality of care [28–30]. Each of these issues presents financial implications for healthcare organizations that subsequently incur significant losses [31, 32].

Early goals of care conversations have the potential to mitigate these patient, surrogate, and clinician outcomes. A substantial field of research has established that engaging patients in conversations about end-of-life care is associated with improvement in patient-centered outcomes. This is because a patient's values and preferences help to frame their medical decisions. When patients elect a surrogate decision-maker or complete an advanced directive, they are more likely to have their wishes known and followed [33]. One study found that end-of-life discussions were associated with less aggressive medical care near death and earlier referral to hospice, which in turn were associated with not only better patient but also caregiver quality of life and bereavement adjustment at follow-up [18]. As an example, in a multisite longitudinal study, patients with advanced cancer who reported awareness of their terminal prognosis had lower rates of psychological distress and higher rates of advance care planning [19]. Other studies show that patients with cancer are more likely to receive end-of-life care that is consistent with their preferences when they have had the opportunity to discuss their wishes with a physician. Patients aware of their terminal prognosis were more likely to desire symptom-focused care [34]. While most existing data focuses on patients with advanced cancer and COPD, patients with other advanced lung diseases and their families are likely to benefit as well.

Patients with advanced lung disease experience debilitating physical and emotional symptoms leading to loss of independence and the ability to fulfill social roles. Palliative medicine specialists approach symptoms as multifactorial, influenced not only by physical but also psychological, social, and spiritual suffering [35]. These symptoms are often best addressed by a multidisciplinary Palliative Medicine Team. However, nonspecialists with experience in the traditional biologic model for symptom assessment and treatment can begin the process of identifying symptoms and attempting treatment with both non-pharmacologic and pharmacologic therapies. When patients' symptoms are not assessed, distressing experiences such as breathlessness, fatigue, anorexia, pain, and mood disorders often go untreated with detrimental consequences on quality of life. A systematic review found that distressing symptoms present at end of life are equally prevalent for patients with end stage COPD as among advanced cancer patients. Specifically, among patients with COPD, 90–95% experience breathlessness, 68–80% fatigue, and 34–77% pain [36]. Early palliative care integration for seriously ill patients with lung cancer has been shown to be associated with improvements in both mood and quality of life [37]. In a meta-analysis, palliative care interventions delivered by a range of palliative care and non-palliative care specialists were found to be associated with improvements in symptom burden and quality of life [38].

The healthcare system also benefits from early, skillful palliative care communication. Clinicians who feel insufficiently trained in communication skills have been shown to have a higher prevalence of depersonalization and low personal accomplishment than those who perceived themselves to be sufficiently trained [39]. A qualitative study exploring oncology physicians' approach to end-of-life care found that those who viewed end-of-life communication and care as an important role reported increased job satisfaction and decreased burnout [40]. Communication skills training is associated with less burnout and work-related stress [20, 41]. Studies directly examining cost at end of life associated with early involvement of palliative care have shown mixed results. One study found that among patients with advanced cancer, those that reported discussing their end-of-life wishes with their physician had better quality of death and significantly lower healthcare costs in their final week of life [42]. A landmark study published in 2010 showed that among patients with metastatic non-small cell lung cancer, early palliative care referral led to less aggressive care at end of life and longer survival [37]. While the study did not measure costs, these findings suggest that timely introduction of palliative care has the potential to mitigate unnecessary societal costs [37].

In response to accumulating data, medical societies, such as the American Thoracic Society, recommend that clinicians who care for patients with chronic or advanced respiratory diseases should be trained in, and capable of, providing recommended basic competencies in palliative care which include communication in goals of care and symptom management [43].

## Barriers and Solutions

Palliative care communication including discussions about goals of care and symptom management has important consequences for patients, families, and healthcare providers. However, there are significant barriers to providing consistent, skillful communication in these areas. Herein we will present these barriers and discuss potential solutions.

### *Prognostication*

Clinicians view prognostication as one of the most difficult parts of their profession [44], and many are reluctant to provide patients and their families with prognostic information due to fear of erring or losing credibility [45]. Uncertainty regarding prognostication and, therefore, identification of which patients are most likely to benefit from end-of-life conversations are common challenges in patients with advanced lung diseases.

Many forms of advanced lung diseases follow the disease trajectory prior to death commonly seen in organ failure [46, 47]. Similarly to patients with heart failure, the course is one of overall functional declines punctuated by intermittent decompensation (Fig. 9.1). During each episode of decompensation, patients deteriorate significantly and either succumb to their disease or recover to a lower level of functioning. It is difficult to predict the outcome of each deterioration. Further complicating the clinical picture, chronic organ failure may represent a comorbidity

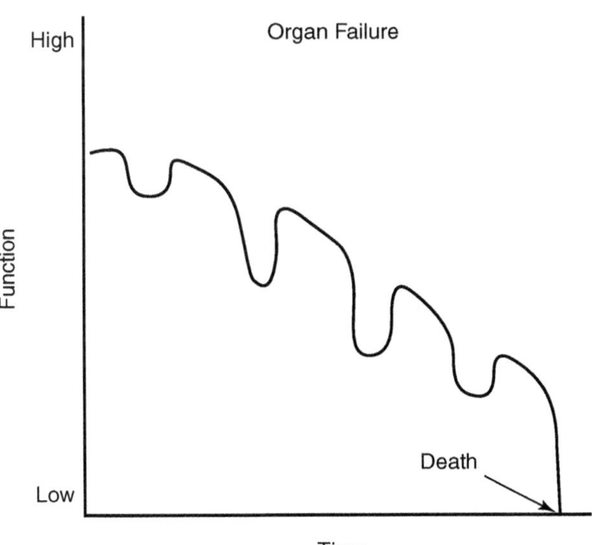


**Fig. 9.1** Functional decline prior to death due to organ failure. (Lunney et al. J Am Geriatr Soc) Acknowledgment wording: reproduced with permission of the © ERS 2020: Curtis [50]

that patients die with and not of. Physicians frequently cite difficulty in prognostication as a barrier to communication about palliative care and end of life in patients with organ failure [4, 48–51].

Findings from the SUPPORT study demonstrated the difficulty in prognostication of patients with chronic organ failure due to COPD compared to those with lung cancer. Using the Acute Physiology and Chronic Health Evaluation (APACHE) II model, they found that at 5 days prior to death, patients with lung cancer were predicted to have <10% chance of surviving 6 months and those with COPD were predicted to have >50% chance [52]. Despite the development of prognostic models specific to lung disease, prognostic accuracy remains challenging. One such prognostic model is the BODE (body mass index, airflow obstruction, dyspnea, exercise capacity) index. Of patients receiving the highest score on the BODE index, 62.3% were still alive at 3 years [53]. While this represents an improvement from broad prognostic models, such as APACHE II and FEV1 alone, it is still not predictive of 6-month prognosis.

One potential solution to the challenge of accurate prognostication is shifting focus away from survival estimates and toward identifying patients who are relatively well and may benefit from end-of-life conversations. Universal factors associated with ≥50% 6-month mortality in maximally treated disease include poor performance status, advanced age, malnutrition, comorbidities, organ dysfunction,

**Table 9.1** Characteristics that should prompt discussion of end-of-life preferences for patients with COPD

| |
|---|
| $FEV_1 < 30\%$ |
| Oxygen dependence |
| One or more hospital admission in the previous year for an acute exacerbation |
| Left heart failure or other comorbidities |
| Weight loss or cachexia |
| Decreased functional status |
| Increasing dependence on others |
| Age > 30 yrs |

*$FEV_1$* forced vital capacity at 1 second
Adapted from Curtis [50]

**Table 9.2** Disease-specific hospice eligibility criteria for patients with COPD (each criteria required)

| |
|---|
| 1. Severe chronic lung disease as documented by both A and B |
| A. Disabling dyspnea at rest, poorly responsive or unresponsive to bronchodilators, resulting in decreased functional capacity. $FEV_1$ after bronchodilators <30% predicted is objective evidence of disability dyspnea but it is not required |
| B. Progression evidenced by increasing visits to the hospital for pulmonary infections and/or respiratory infections or increasing physician home visits. Serial decrease of $FEV_1$ > 40 ml/yr is objective evidence of disease progression, but is not a requirement |
| 2. Hypoxemia at rest on room air, evidenced by $PO_2 \leq 55$ mmHg or oxygen saturation ≤ 88% on supplemental oxygen, or hypercapnea, evidenced by $PCO_2 \geq 50$ mmHg |
| 3. Right heart failure due to pulmonary disease |

and hospitalization for acute decompensation. Societies have proposed various options for identifying which patients are likely to benefit, all emphasizing the importance of early discussion. One such example was suggested by Curtis et al. to prompt discussion about end-of-life care for patients with COPD (Table 9.1) [50]. More broadly, clinicians can ask themselves "Would I be surprised if this patient died within the year?" An answer of "no" should prompt a discussion. This question has been shown to be moderately sensitive in predicting 1-year mortality, with a pooled sensitivity of 67% in meta-analysis [54]. Medicare eligibility for hospice is shown in Table 9.2. These criteria were found to have both poor sensitivity and specificity in identifying patients who would die within 6 months [55].

Each change in clinical status represents an opportunity to reassess the patient's quality of life, determine whether it remains acceptable, and consider with the patient what brings value to their life. In the absence of definitive prognostic information, which is nearly uniformly elusive in clinical medicine, it is important to acknowledge the uncertainty of each patient's future when communicating about end of life.

## *Perception or Fear of Harming the Patient or Provoking an Emotional Response*

Clinicians caring for patients with advanced illness report fear of harming the patient by sharing upsetting prognostic information or discussing end-of-life care. In one study, 23% of physicians caring for patients with COPD cited concerns that discussing end-of-life care will take away their patient's hope, and 21% felt the patient was not ready to talk about the care they would wish for if they got sicker [56]. Some patients do not wish to receive their physician's prognostic information or discuss advance care planning and end-of-life preferences. In some cultures, it is believed that communicating unfavorable prognoses to the patient becomes a self-fulfilling prophecy. However, existing data suggests that most patients wish to receive this information and expect their physician to initiate discussions [57]. Absence of communication about prognosis has been associated with prolongation of the dying process, undesired hospitalizations, and patient mistrust in the healthcare system [34]. Research has also demonstrated that clinicians' fear of removing patients' hope is largely unfounded. In fact, nondisclosure is associated with decreased quality of life and increased rate of depression in survivors [58]. Patients and families with overly optimistic prognostic estimates were more likely to die following receipt of aggressive medical interventions, such as intubation or cardiopulmonary resuscitation, with no difference in outcomes [59].

Prognostic information provides a framework for patients to make informed treatment decisions and consider important aspects of life care planning, such as legacy planning, addressing personal relationships, and saying goodbye. By

**Table 9.3** Discussing prognostic information

| *Recommendations* |
|---|
| Ask how much prognostic information the patient wants |
| For patients who want explicit information, ask what kind of information |
| Frame statistical information positively and negatively |
| Offer to describe survival range in addition to a specific period |
| Consider a separate conversation with a family member who wants more information, with the patient's permission |
| For patients who do not want explicit information, explore their perspective |

Adapted from Back [60]

balancing hope and reality, clinicians can potentially allow their patients to shift focus toward other, perhaps more attainable, goals while continuing to hold the hope for a better outcome. Clinicians can mitigate the potential for inflicting harm by eliciting patients' preferences for prognostic information. A proposed strategy is detailed in Table 9.3 [60].

Emotional distress associated with receipt of bad news can further be lessened by ensuring discussions take place in an appropriate setting, delivering the information tactfully, allowing the appropriate amount of time free of interruptions, and providing emotional support through verbal and nonverbal expressions of empathy. (See Section "Lack of Comfort with Palliative Care Topics")

## *Lack of Comfort with Palliative Care Topics*

Medical education has long been deficient in end-of-life care and improving physicians' competencies has increasingly become a topic of focus. In a national survey, both medical students and residents perceived preparation for providing care at end of life was worse than other common clinical tasks [61]. Additionally, a national survey of internists revealed that 56.8% reported inadequate training in prognostication [44]. Teaching of communication skills should include focused skills practice and be integrated with biomedical training. Most clinicians have not received the skills training required to provide high-quality palliative care communication or teach others how to do so.

### Symptom Management

Lung disease is a common cause of morbidity with similar symptom burden compared to cancer [1, 2]. However, patients with lung disease are less likely to have their symptoms elicited and, therefore, appropriately managed. Dyspnea is the most common symptom experienced by patients with advanced lung disease; however pain and mood disorders are also frequently encountered. The experience of dyspnea increases in frequency and severity as death approaches. The primary goal in managing dyspnea is optimizing treatment of the patient's underlying disease. For patients with refractory dyspnea, there are options for non-pharmacologic and pharmacologic therapies. When dyspnea is refractory to non-pharmacologic management, systemic low-dose opiates are the first-line medication, serving as a safe and effective pharmacologic treatment for refractory dyspnea.

Despite numerous studies documenting the safety of opiates for treatment of dyspnea in patients with advanced lung disease, there remains stigma associated with prescribing opiates, and patients suffer from poor control of their dyspnea [62–64]. Commonly cited source of discomfort in prescribing includes insufficient knowledge, lack of experience, and fear of adverse effects [62, 63]. In one of these studies, physicians with palliative care experience were more comfortable prescribing opiates [63]. Interestingly, a study from France showed that despite high rates of refractory breathlessness among COPD patients and reported comfort among the majority of clinicians in prescribing opiates, the rates of prescribing opiates within this population were low [64]. These findings may suggest assessment and treatment of dyspnea lies in a failure to assess breathlessness and provide treatment. Based on these findings, clinicians may benefit from a trigger during outpatient visits to assess common distressing symptoms in patients with advanced lung disease.

Empiric studies have demonstrated that short-term use of opiates reduces breathlessness in patients with a variety of conditions, including COPD and interstitial lung disease [65–67]. A randomized controlled trial showed that sustained-released morphine had a positive effect on disease-specific health status in patients with moderate to very severe breathlessness [68]. Importantly, opioids have not been shown to significantly reduce oxygen saturation, raise arterial carbon dioxide, or reduced respiratory rate; however patients retaining carbon dioxide were excluded in most of these studies [69]. In 2011, the American College of Chest Physicians released a consensus statement recommending the use of opiates for relief of dyspnea in patients with advanced cardiopulmonary disease in consideration of comorbidities and titrated to individual effect [70]. Knowledge about this literature may help clinicians feel more comfortable engaging their patients in conversations about symptom management. Additionally, providers may consider referral to specialty palliative care for patients with advanced lung disease with multiple comorbidities or a baseline elevation in carbon dioxide experiencing refractory dyspnea.

## Goals of Care Communication Skills

Specialized clinicians from a variety of fields that frequently care for patients with life-limiting illnesses report feeling inadequately trained to conduct end-of-life conversations [71–74]. Physicians specifically report difficulties with communicating prognoses, facilitating end-of-life decision-making, and managing the emotional responses these conversations naturally uncover [75, 76]. In response, national leaders and experts in communicating with seriously ill patients have developed multiple frameworks for approaching these core communication skills.

Each of these communication tasks is recommended to take place in a comfortable and private place. Every attempt should be made to minimize interruptions and allow an appropriate amount of time. Prior to engaging in the conversations, clinicians should ask whether the patient would like to have support persons present and assess preferences regarding receipt of prognostic information.

## Responding to Emotion

The experience of advanced illness and receipt of medical information challenging patient's hopes and expectations for the future evokes intense negative emotions. While clinicians may be unable to restore a patient's health, research demonstrates that providing support lessens the experience of emotional distress. Additionally, when patients are experiencing emotions, they are unable to process medical information effectively. Attending emotions will also bring them into the person's awareness and allow them to shift away from them toward a cognitive state capable of planning complex behaviors and decision-making. Lastly, studies demonstrate that patients have higher trust for the clinicians when they respond to emotion which leads to greater shared decision-making [77].

Clinicians can show emotional support by listening and expressing empathy both verbally and nonverbally. The acronym N-U-R-S-E [78] summarizes how to respond verbally to emotion (Table 9.4).

**Table 9.4** Verbal responses to emotion

| Recommendation | Example |
|---|---|
| N: *Name* the emotion | "This news is so shocking." |
| U: *Understand* the emotion | "I can't imagine what you are going through." |
| R: Respect (praise) the patient or surrogate | "I can see you have been here and advocated for your mother every step of the way." |
| S: *Support* the patient or surrogate | "You are not alone in this." |
| E: *Explore* the emotion | "Tell me more." |

**Table 9.5** Delivering serious news

| Recommendation | Example |
|---|---|
| *Ask*: Assess the patient's understanding of the situation | "What have you been told about your current medical condition?" "What is your sense of how things are going." |
| *Tell*: Provide medical information and frame how the information impacts outcomes meaningful to the patient | "We are worried she may not be able to return to living independently after this hospitalization." |
| *Ask*: Check understanding | "What questions do you have?" |

Table 9.6 Goals of care discussions

| Recommendation | Example |
|---|---|
| R: *Reframe* the situation, why the status quo is not working | "Things have changed over the past few months. Your lungs are getting sicker and I'm worried time is short." |
| E: Expect *emotion* and empathize | "This must be shocking news." |
| M: *Map* what is important | "Given this information, what worries you the most?" "What are you hoping for?" |
| A: *Align* with the patient and family values | "It sounds like you are hoping for more good time, interacting with family and being at home, and less time in the hospital." |
| P: *Plan* medical treatments that match patient values | "I recommend we continue treating your symptoms aggressively and work to keep you at home. When your body gets sicker, we will respect that and allow you to pass naturally." |

## Giving Serious News

Sharing serious news is difficult for clinicians who struggle with feelings of apprehension at the prospect of causing distress, fear of provoking an emotional response, and professional failure when unable to protect their patients from disease. Despite these difficulties, patients require an understanding of the medical situation to make value-based treatment decisions and plan for the future.

Evidence-based recommendations for giving serious news are organized into the Ask-Tell-Ask framework summarized in Table 9.5 [79]. The first "Ask" refers to eliciting the patient's understanding of the medical situation. This is followed by "Tell," consisting of labeling the news to give them a chance to emotionally prepare for the news. When the news or headline is then shared, clinicians should be concise, use simple language, and refer to outcomes that are meaningful to the patients. The last "Ask" is to check understanding or check in with the patient.

## Engaging in Decision-Making

VitalTalk designed REMAP as a road map for goals of care conversations to increase the quality and efficiency of conversations and make communication skills easier to learn [80]. The acronym serves a conversation guide toward reaching a patient-centered and shared decision. Table 9.6 details each step with accompanying example statements. The conversation begins with clinicians ensuring the patient or their surrogates are on the same page in terms of medical information. Sometimes, clinicians will have additional news to communicate (see sharing serious news above.) Throughout the conversation, clinicians will need to recognize and respond to emotion, particularly after communicating difficult news. If the patient or their surrogate is on the same page as clinicians and is prepared to talk further, the next step is to explore values and preferences in light of the medical situation. Throughout the conversation, it is also recommended to reflect what you are hearing to ensure you are aligned with the patient and family. Lastly, after gathering sufficient

**Table 9.7** Summary of barriers and potential solutions for clinicians when communicating about palliative care issues

| Barriers | Potential solutions |
|---|---|
| Difficulty with prognostication | Ensure early goals of care discussion by identifying patients at risk for death when patients are relatively well. When prognosis is uncertain, acknowledge uncertainty and focus on patient's values and goals<br>Consider using the following criteria to identify patients at risk for death and trigger conversations in the outpatient setting:<br>Universal factors associated with $\geq$50% 6-month mortality in maximally treated disease:<br>Poor performance status, advanced age, malnutrition, comorbidities, organ dysfunction, and hospitalization for acute decompensation<br>Characteristics recommended for patients with COPD:<br>$FEV_1 < 30\%$ predicted, oxygen dependence, one or more hospital admission in the previous year for an acute exacerbation of COPD, left heart failure or other comorbidities, weight loss or cachexia, decreased functional status, increasing dependence on others, age > 70 years (Curtis, Eur Resp J, 2008)<br>Surprise question: "Would I be surprised if this patient died within the year?" |
| Fear of destroying hope or provoking an emotional response | Existing data shows that most patients wish to receive prognostic information and expect their physician to initiate discussions [57]<br>Clinician's fear of removing hope is largely unfounded. Nondisclosure is associated with decreased quality of life and increased rate of depression in survivors [58]<br>Alleviate emotional distress associated with receipt of serious news by eliciting preferences for prognostic information and providing emotional support [60] |
| Lack of comfort with palliative care topics | *Symptom management:*<br>Include trigger for evaluation of distressing symptoms during outpatient visits for patients with advanced lung diseases<br>Knowledge of existing literature and experience with palliative care may mitigate clinicians' concerns regarding prescription of opiates for dyspnea<br>Physicians may consider referral to specialty palliative care providers for symptom management |
| | Frameworks exist to assist clinicians in navigating communication tasks (see Tables 9.3, 9.4, 9.5, 9.6, and 9.7) including:<br>Responding to emotion<br>Giving serious news<br>Goals of care discussions<br>Training programs emphasizing these frameworks allow clinicians to practice communication skills through interactive case-based sessions. These training programs have been shown to demonstrate improvement in clinician communication skills |
| Fragmented healthcare system | Collaborate with your patient's general and other subspecialty providers to decide who is primarily responsible for discussing end-of-life issues and symptom management<br>Designate a site within the electronic medical record where documentation regarding patients elected surrogate decision-maker, values, preferences, and goals of care conversations can be found and iteratively refined over the course of their illness. Healthcare systems should collaborate to make documentation readily accessible to providers from different systems |

information, VitalTalk recommends at least three mapping questions, you can offer a patient-centered recommendation based off the information provided.

## *Palliative Care Communication in a Fragmented Healthcare System*

Over the past decade, patient care has become increasingly complex. An individual's exposure to healthcare is likely to be spread across multiple providers, practice settings, and even healthcare systems. The resulting diffusion of responsibility and difficulty accessing prior medical documentation make iterative communication about goals of care and symptom management challenging and compound the barriers to communicating about palliative care (Table 9.7).

We know that patients often expect their providers to initiate discussions regarding prognosis and goals of care [51]. However, prior studies have demonstrated that a physician's decision to share prognosis is often based on whether the patient made a specific request [57]. A survey of general practitioners caring for patients with COPD in the United Kingdom found that 41% reported discussing prognosis often or always and 15% rarely or never and 30% left it for patients or their relatives to raise the subject [81]. There is also ambiguity among providers about who is responsible, specialists or general practitioners. A systematic review and narrative synthesis found that no single group of healthcare providers felt that their roles, relationships with patients, or work setting made them the most appropriate to have goals of care conversations with their patients with COPD [48]. Primary care physicians report uncertainty regarding their role in goals of care discussions when specialty providers are involved [51].

Further challenges arise with the documentation of goals of care conversations. A variety of clinicians may engage patients with advanced lung diseases in conversations about goals of care without communication or documentation to guide further discussions as the patient continues along the trajectory of their illness. Even if a clinician documents goals of care conversations, it may not be easily retrieved or accessible to providers from other healthcare systems. Among patients who had previously completed an advance directive, only 26% had it recognized during a hospitalization [82]. There is no standardization for the location of advance care planning or goals of care documentation [51]. A study exploring the location of advance care planning documentation within an electronic health record showed only 33.5% of patients with documentation had a scanned document and the remainder were within a progress note or problem list [83]. Lastly, the situation may be further complicated when visits with outpatient providers and hospital exposures occur across different healthcare systems with distinct EHR that do not communicate.

When multiple clinicians are caring for a patient, the oncologic literature recommends collaboration among providers to decide who will be primarily responsible for discussing prognosis and end-of-life care then ensuring the other providers are aware of the outcome of discussions [84]. Healthcare systems would benefit from a designated site within the EHR where an iterative account of the patient's wishes, values, and preferences in light of the current medical situation can be located. Ideally, this site would be readily accessible across healthcare systems.

## References


1. Gore JM, Brophy CJ, Greenstone MA. How well do we care for patients with end stage chronic obstructive pulmonary disease (COPD)? A comparison of palliative care and quality of life in COPD and lung cancer. Thorax. 2000;55(12):1000–6.
2. White P, White S, Edmonds P, et al. Palliative care or end-of-life care in advanced chronic obstructive pulmonary disease: a prospective community survey. Br J Gen Pract. 2011;61(587):e362–70.
3. Curtis JR, Engelberg RA, Wenrich MD, Au DH. Communication about palliative care for patients with chronic obstructive pulmonary disease. J Palliat Care. 2005;21(3):157–64.
4. Tavares N, Jarrett N, Hunt K, Wilkinson T. Palliative and end-of-life care conversations in COPD: a systematic literature review. ERJ Open Res. 2017;3(2):00068–2016.
5. Heffner JE, Fahy B, Hilling L, Barbieri C. Attitudes regarding advance directives among patients in pulmonary rehabilitation. Am J Respir Crit Care Med. 1996;154(6 Pt 1):1735–40.
6. Houben CH, Spruit MA, Schols JM, Wouters EF, Janssen DJ. Patient-clinician communication about end-of-life care in patients with advanced chronic organ failure during one year. J Pain Symptom Manag. 2015;49(6):1109–15.
7. Curtis JR, Wenrich MD, Carline JD, Shannon SE, Ambrozy DM, Ramsey PG. Patients' perspectives on physician skill in end-of-life care: differences between patients with COPD, cancer, and AIDS. Chest. 2002;122(1):356–62.
8. Quill TE. Perspectives on care at the close of life. Initiating end-of-life discussions with seriously ill patients: addressing the "elephant in the room". JAMA. 2000;284(19):2502–7.
9. Wendler D, Rid A. Systematic review: the effect on surrogates of making treatment decisions for others. Ann Intern Med. 2011;154(5):336–46.
10. A controlled trial to improve care for seriously ill hospitalized patients. The study to understand prognoses and preferences for outcomes and risks of treatments (SUPPORT). The SUPPORT Principal Investigators. JAMA 1995;274(20):1591–1598.
11. Cameron JI, Wittenberg E, Prosser LA. Caregivers and families of critically ill patients. N Engl J Med. 2016;375(10):1001.
12. Cameron JI, Chu LM, Matte A, et al. One-year outcomes in caregivers of critically ill patients. N Engl J Med. 2016;374(19):1831–41.
13. Kross EK, Engelberg RA, Gries CJ, Nielsen EL, Zatzick D, Curtis JR. ICU care associated with symptoms of depression and posttraumatic stress disorder among family members of patients who die in the ICU. Chest. 2011;139(4):795–801.
14. Gries CJ, Engelberg RA, Kross EK, et al. Predictors of symptoms of posttraumatic stress and depression in family members after patient death in the ICU. Chest. 2010;137(2):280–7.
15. Miyajima K, Fujisawa D, Yoshimura K, et al. Association between quality of end-of-life care and possible complicated grief among bereaved family members. J Palliat Med. 2014;17(9):1025–31.
16. Prigerson HG, Bierhals AJ, Kasl SV, et al. Traumatic grief as a risk factor for mental and physical morbidity. Am J Psychiatry. 1997;154(5):616–23.
17. Boelen PA, van den Bout J. Complicated grief and uncomplicated grief are distinguishable constructs. Psychiatry Res. 2008;157(1–3):311–4.
18. Wright AA, Zhang B, Ray A, et al. Associations between end-of-life discussions, patient mental health, medical care near death, and caregiver bereavement adjustment. JAMA. 2008;300(14):1665–73.

19. Ray A, Block SD, Friedlander RJ, Zhang B, Maciejewski PK, Prigerson HG. Peaceful awareness in patients with advanced cancer. J Palliat Med. 2006;9(6):1359–68.
20. Ramirez AJ, Graham J, Richards MA, et al. Burnout and psychiatric disorder among cancer clinicians. Br J Cancer. 1995;71(6):1263–9.
21. Clayton JM, Butow PN, Waters A, et al. Evaluation of a novel individualised communication-skills training intervention to improve doctors' confidence and skills in end-of-life communication. Palliat Med. 2013;27(3):236–43.
22. Dzeng E. Moral distress amongst physician trainees regarding futile treatments. J Gen Intern Med. 2016;31(8):830.
23. Rushton CH, Batcheller J, Schroeder K, Donohue P. Burnout and resilience among nurses practicing in high-intensity settings. Am J Crit Care. 2015;24(5):412–20.
24. Dzeng E, Curtis JR. Understanding ethical climate, moral distress, and burnout: a novel tool and a conceptual framework. BMJ Qual Saf. 2018;27(10):766–70.
25. Bianchi R, Schonfeld IS, Laurent E. Burnout-depression overlap: a review. Clin Psychol Rev. 2015;36:28–41.
26. Oreskovich MR, Kaups KL, Balch CM, et al. Prevalence of alcohol use disorders among American surgeons. Arch Surg. 2012;147(2):168–74.
27. Shanafelt TD, Balch CM, Dyrbye L, et al. Special report: suicidal ideation among American surgeons. Arch Surg. 2011;146(1):54–62.
28. Shanafelt T, Sloan J, Satele D, Balch C. Why do surgeons consider leaving practice? J Am Coll Surg. 2011;212(3):421–2.
29. Shanafelt TD, Balch CM, Bechamps G, et al. Burnout and medical errors among American surgeons. Ann Surg. 2010;251(6):995–1000.
30. West CP, Huschka MM, Novotny PJ, et al. Association of perceived medical errors with resident distress and empathy: a prospective longitudinal study. JAMA. 2006;296(9):1071–8.
31. Wright AA, Katz IT. Beyond burnout - redesigning care to restore meaning and sanity for physicians. N Engl J Med. 2018;378(4):309–11.
32. Dzau VJ, Kirch DG, Nasca TJ. To care is human – collectively confronting the clinician-burnout crisis. N Engl J Med. 2018;378(4):312–4.
33. Silveira MJ, Kim SY, Langa KM. Advance directives and outcomes of surrogate decision making before death. N Engl J Med. 2010;362(13):1211–8.
34. Mack JW, Weeks JC, Wright AA, Block SD, Prigerson HG. End-of-life discussions, goal attainment, and distress at the end of life: predictors and outcomes of receipt of care consistent with preferences. J Clin Oncol. 2010;28(7):1203–8.
35. Clark D. 'Total pain', disciplinary power and the body in the work of Cicely Saunders, 1958-1967. Soc Sci Med. 1999;49(6):727–36.
36. Solano JP, Gomes B, Higginson IJ. A comparison of symptom prevalence in far advanced cancer, AIDS, heart disease, chronic obstructive pulmonary disease and renal disease. J Pain Symptom Manag. 2006;31(1):58–69.
37. Temel JS, Greer JA, Muzikansky A, et al. Early palliative care for patients with metastatic non-small-cell lung cancer. N Engl J Med. 2010;363(8):733–42.
38. Kavalieratos D, Corbelli J, Zhang D, et al. Association between palliative care and patient and caregiver outcomes: a systematic review and meta-analysis. JAMA. 2016;316(20):2104–14.
39. Ramirez AJ, Graham J, Richards MA, Cull A, Gregory WM. Mental health of hospital consultants: the effects of stress and satisfaction at work. Lancet. 1996;347(9003):724–8.
40. Jackson VA, Mack J, Matsuyama R, et al. A qualitative study of oncologists' approaches to end-of-life care. J Palliat Med. 2008;11(6):893–906.
41. Graham J, Potts HW, Ramirez AJ. Stress and burnout in doctors. Lancet. 2002;360(9349):1975–6; author reply 1976
42. Zhang B, Wright AA, Huskamp HA, et al. Health care costs in the last week of life: associations with end-of-life conversations. Arch Intern Med. 2009;169(5):480–8.
43. Lanken PN, Terry PB, Delisser HM, et al. An official American Thoracic Society clinical policy statement: palliative care for patients with respiratory diseases and critical illnesses. Am J Respir Crit Care Med. 2008;177(8):912–27.

44. Christakis NA, Iwashyna TJ. Attitude and self-reported practice regarding prognostication in a national sample of internists. Arch Intern Med. 1998;158(21):2389–95.
45. Christakis NA. Death foretold : prophecy and prognosis in medical care. Chicago: University of Chicago; 1999.
46. Lunney JR, Lynn J, Hogan C. Profiles of older medicare decedents. J Am Geriatr Soc. 2002;50(6):1108–12.
47. Lunney JR, Lynn J, Foley DJ, Lipson S, Guralnik JM. Patterns of functional decline at the end of life. JAMA. 2003;289(18):2387–92.
48. Momen N, Hadfield P, Kuhn I, Smith E, Barclay S. Discussing an uncertain future: end-of-life care conversations in chronic obstructive pulmonary disease. A systematic literature review and narrative synthesis. Thorax. 2012;67(9):777–80.
49. Crawford A. Respiratory practitioners' experience of end-of-life discussions in COPD. Br J Nurs. 2010;19(18):1164–9.
50. Curtis JR. Palliative and end-of-life care for patients with severe COPD. Eur Respir J. 2008;32(3):796–803.
51. Bernacki RE, Block SD, American College of Physicians High Value Care Task F. Communication about serious illness care goals: a review and synthesis of best practices. JAMA Intern Med. 2014;174(12):1994–2003.
52. Claessens MT, Lynn J, Zhong Z, et al. Dying with lung cancer or chronic obstructive pulmonary disease: insights from SUPPORT. Study to understand prognoses and preferences for outcomes and risks of treatments. J Am Geriatr Soc. 2000;48(S1):S146–53.
53. Esteban C, Quintana JM, Moraza J, et al. BODE-index vs HADO-score in chronic obstructive pulmonary disease: which one to use in general practice? BMC Med. 2010;8:28.
54. Downar J, Goldman R, Pinto R, Englesakis M, Adhikari NK. The "surprise question" for predicting death in seriously ill patients: a systematic review and meta-analysis. CMAJ. 2017;189(13):E484–93.
55. Fox E, Landrum-McNiff K, Zhong Z, Dawson NV, Wu AW, Lynn J. Evaluation of prognostic criteria for determining hospice eligibility in patients with advanced lung, heart, or liver disease. SUPPORT investigators. Study to understand prognoses and preferences for outcomes and risks of treatments. JAMA. 1999;282(17):1638–45.
56. Knauft E, Nielsen EL, Engelberg RA, Patrick DL, Curtis JR. Barriers and facilitators to end-of-life care communication for patients with COPD. Chest. 2005;127(6):2188–96.
57. Hancock K, Clayton JM, Parker SM, et al. Truth-telling in discussing prognosis in advanced life-limiting illnesses: a systematic review. Palliat Med. 2007;21(6):507–17.
58. Hagerty RG, Butow PN, Ellis PM, et al. Communicating with realism and hope: incurable cancer patients' views on the disclosure of prognosis. J Clin Oncol. 2005;23(6):1278–88.
59. Weeks JC, Cook EF, O'Day SJ, et al. Relationship between cancer patients' predictions of prognosis and their treatment preferences. JAMA. 1998;279(21):1709–14.
60. Back AL, Anderson WG, Bunch L, et al. Communication about cancer near the end of life. Cancer. 2008;113(7 Suppl):1897–910.
61. Billings JA, Block S. Palliative care in undergraduate medical education. Status report and future directions. JAMA. 1997;278(9):733–8.
62. Janssen DJ, de Hosson SM, bij de Vaate E, Mooren KJ, Baas AA. Attitudes toward opioids for refractory dyspnea in COPD among Dutch chest physicians. Chron Respir Dis. 2015;12(2):85–92.
63. Young J, Donahue M, Farquhar M, Simpson C, Rocker G. Using opioids to treat dyspnea in advanced COPD: attitudes and experiences of family physicians and respiratory therapists. Can Fam Physician. 2012;58(7):e401–7.
64. Carette H, Zysman M, Morelot-Panzini C, et al. Prevalence and management of chronic breathlessness in COPD in a tertiary care center. BMC Pulm Med. 2019;19(1):95.
65. Ekstrom M, Nilsson F, Abernethy AA, Currow DC. Effects of opioids on breathlessness and exercise capacity in chronic obstructive pulmonary disease. A systematic review. Ann Am Thorac Soc. 2015;12(7):1079–92.

66. Allen S, Raut S, Woollard J, Vassallo M. Low dose diamorphine reduces breathlessness without causing a fall in oxygen saturation in elderly patients with end-stage idiopathic pulmonary fibrosis. Palliat Med. 2005;19(2):128–30.
67. Parshall MB, Schwartzstein RM, Adams L, et al. An official American Thoracic Society statement: update on the mechanisms, assessment, and management of dyspnea. Am J Respir Crit Care Med. 2012;185(4):435–52.
68. Verberkt CA, van den Beuken-van Everdingen MHJ, Schols J, Hameleers N, Wouters EFM, Janssen DJA. Effect of sustained-release morphine for refractory breathlessness in chronic obstructive pulmonary disease on health status: a randomized clinical trial. JAMA Intern Med. 2020;180(10):1306–14.
69. Barnes H, McDonald J, Smallwood N, Manser R. Opioids for the palliation of refractory breathlessness in adults with advanced disease and terminal illness. Cochrane Database Syst Rev. 2016;3:CD011008.
70. Mahler DA, Selecky PA, Harrod CG, et al. American College of Chest Physicians consensus statement on the management of dyspnea in patients with advanced lung or heart disease. Chest. 2010;137(3):674–91.
71. Buss MK, Lessen DS, Sullivan AM, Von Roenn J, Arnold RM, Block SD. Hematology/oncology fellows' training in palliative care: results of a national survey. Cancer. 2011;117(18):4304–11.
72. Kelley AS, Back AL, Arnold RM, et al. Geritalk: communication skills training for geriatric and palliative medicine fellows. J Am Geriatr Soc. 2012;60(2):332–7.
73. Arnold RM, Back AL, Barnato AE, et al. The critical care communication project: improving fellows' communication skills. J Crit Care. 2015;30(2):250–4.
74. Holley JL, Carmody SS, Moss AH, et al. The need for end-of-life care training in nephrology: national survey results of nephrology fellows. Am J Kidney Dis. 2003;42(4):813–20.
75. Jones L, Harrington J, Barlow CA, et al. Advance care planning in advanced cancer: can it be achieved? An exploratory randomized patient preference trial of a care planning discussion. Palliat Support Care. 2011;9(1):3–13.
76. Wenrich MD, Curtis JR, Ambrozy DA, Carline JD, Shannon SE, Ramsey PG. Dying patients' need for emotional support and personalized care from physicians: perspectives of patients with terminal illness, families, and health care providers. J Pain Symptom Manag. 2003;25(3):236–46.
77. Tulsky JA, Arnold RM, Alexander SC, et al. Enhancing communication between oncologists and patients with a computer-based training program: a randomized trial. Ann Intern Med. 2011;155(9):593–601.
78. Smith RC, Hoppe RB. The patient's story: integrating the patient- and physician-centered approaches to interviewing. Ann Intern Med. 1991;115(6):470–7.
79. Back AL, Arnold RM, Baile WF, Tulsky JA, Fryer-Edwards K. Approaching difficult communication tasks in oncology. CA Cancer J Clin. 2005;55(3):164–77.
80. Childers JW, Back AL, Tulsky JA, Arnold RM. REMAP: a framework for goals of care conversations. J Oncol Pract. 2017;13(10):e844–50.
81. Elkington H, White P, Higgs R, Pettinari CJ. GPs' views of discussions of prognosis in severe COPD. Fam Pract. 2001;18(4):440–4.
82. Pritchard RS, Fisher ES, Teno JM, et al. Influence of patient preferences and local health system characteristics on the place of death. SUPPORT investigators. Study to understand prognoses and preferences for risks and outcomes of treatment. J Am Geriatr Soc. 1998;46(10):1242–50.
83. Wilson CJ, Newman J, Tapper S, et al. Multiple locations of advance care planning documentation in an electronic health record: are they easy to find? J Palliat Med. 2013;16(9):1089–94.
84. Back AL, Young JP, McCown E, et al. Abandonment at the end of life from patient, caregiver, nurse, and physician perspectives: loss of continuity and lack of closure. Arch Intern Med. 2009;169(5):474–9.

# Chapter 10
# Palliative Care in COPD

**Anand S. Iyer and Dina Khateeb**

## Introduction

Chronic obstructive pulmonary disease (COPD) is a serious illness that affects an estimated 16 million Americans and is the fourth leading cause of death in the United States (US) [1, 2]. The broad array of COPD care needs in patients and their families is ideally suited for the comprehensive approach offered by palliative care. However, palliative care is rarely implemented for patients with COPD and is often only reserved for patients at the very end of life. This rare and late integration of palliative care misses a potential opportunity to help improve quality of life and deliver person-centered care for patients with COPD and their families earlier in the disease trajectory. This chapter builds the urgent case for palliative care in COPD. We describe barriers to its proactive integration into routine COPD practice and identify potential solutions through inter-professional care models and the fusion of palliative care into pulmonary medicine through a "palli-pulm" approach. In the end, we want to ensure that patients with COPD and their families receive proactive and comprehensive palliative care long before the end of life.

"The best time to plant a tree was 20 years ago. The next best time is now." – *Chinese Proverb*

A. S. Iyer (✉)
Division of Pulmonary, Allergy, and Critical Care Medicine, Birmingham, AL, USA

Department of Medicine, University of Alabama at Birmingham, Birmingham, AL, USA

Lung Health Center, Department of Medicine, University of Alabama at Birmingham, Birmingham, AL, USA

Center for Palliative and Supportive Care, Division of Gerontology, Geriatrics, and Palliative Care, University of Alabama at Birmingham, Birmingham, AL, USA
e-mail: aiyer@uabmc.edu

D. Khateeb
Berks Schuylkill Respiratory Specialists, Wyomissing, PA, USA



K. O. Lindell, S. K. Danoff (eds.), *Palliative Care in Lung Disease*, Respiratory Medicine, https://doi.org/10.1007/978-3-030-81788-6_10

# A Primer on COPD

## *COPD Diagnosis and Management*

COPD is predominately diagnosed in adults >40 years and is caused by years of cigarette smoking or other etiologies such as biomass exposure (e.g., wood-burning stoves) and alpha-1 antitrypsin deficiency, a rare genetic condition which leads to COPD in younger adults [3]. Though two primary clinical phenotypes of COPD, i.e., emphysema and chronic bronchitis, receive most of the focus in training, patients experience a spectrum of symptoms that impact quality of life and functional status and are rarely addressed at routine clinic visits.

COPD is diagnosed by a combination of exposure history, symptoms, and physical exam in addition to spirometry that demonstrates airflow limitation [forced expiratory volume/forced vital capacity ratio ($FEV_1/FVC$) <0.70] [4]. The Global Initiative for Chronic Obstructive Lung Disease (GOLD) defines COPD severity stages of worsening airflow obstruction using $FEV_1$ as mild, moderate, severe, and very severe (GOLD Stages I through IV, respectively) and also by letter grades to subclassify based on worsening symptom severity and exacerbation frequency (e.g., GOLD A through GOLD D in increasing severity) [4]. Patients may progress stepwise through each severity stage, remain within one stage for years, decline slowly, or progress rapidly [5]. The very severe stage is typically referred to as "end-stage COPD," when patients often require supplemental oxygen, experience frequent hospitalizations, and cope with severe limitations in functional status. However, COPD is heterogeneous and, it is not uncommon for a patient with very severe COPD to live for many years with limited to no symptoms or for someone with moderate COPD to be very symptomatic and frequently hospitalized. This heterogeneity makes planning for the future very difficult for clinicians.

COPD is typically managed by primary care physicians, as access to subspecialty pulmonologists varies substantially across the country, [6] especially in rural areas that have a higher prevalence of COPD and rising deaths due to COPD [7]. Beyond counseling on smoking cessation, primary therapies in COPD consist of bronchodilators delivered via inhalers or nebulizers and exertional or continuous supplemental oxygen [4]. As COPD becomes more severe and people experience more respiratory symptoms or increasingly frequent exacerbations, oral medications can be added that reduce symptoms and the risk for exacerbations. Patients can then be considered for advanced COPD therapies such as endobronchial valve placement, lung volume reduction surgery, and lung transplantation in select cases [8]. Finally, an essential component of comprehensive COPD care is cardiopulmonary rehabilitation, one of the most effective interventions that delivers sustained improvements in dyspnea and emotional symptoms and is associated with a reduction in 1-year mortality when initiated following hospitalization for an exacerbation [9, 10].

Compared to the relatively stable and then precipitous decline at the end of life for someone living with advanced cancer, the trajectory for someone living with

COPD is one of a long and slow decline punctuated by episodic exacerbations [11]. Exacerbations of COPD, or acute worsening of symptoms above baseline, require escalation of inhalers or antibiotics, oral steroids, emergency room visits, and hospitalizations where a patient could require noninvasive ventilation or invasive mechanical ventilation [12]. Hospitalizations due to severe exacerbations of COPD are sentinel events that occur every few years or multiple times yearly, i.e., frequent exacerbations, and are associated with reduced quality of life and an increased risk of mortality [13, 14]. An estimated one in five adults hospitalized for COPD dies in the year following a hospitalization for an exacerbation, and half die in 5 years [15].

## *Palliative Care Needs in COPD: The Broad Toll*

COPD has remained the third leading cause of global disability in those over 75 years during the past two decades [16]. In the next few decades, it is estimated that half of all adults who have COPD will be older than 75 years [17]. The last 2 years of life can be particularly complex in this population. In one cohort of older decedents with COPD in the last 2 years of life, nearly all had an emergency room visit, 80% were admitted to the hospital, 50% required an intensive care unit, 38% used a skilled nursing facility, and 12% used a long-term acute care facility [18]. In the past two decades, place of death for adults with COPD is also radically changing [19]. An increasing frequency of patients with COPD are dying at home, the preferred location of death for most as compared to the hospital. This signals a need to better prepare patients and their families for the end of life at home through earlier advance care planning.

COPD exerts a substantial toll on patients that extends far beyond the lungs (Fig. 10.1). Severe breathlessness is one of the most distressing symptoms experienced by patients with COPD and can be refractory to multiple medical therapies. The prevalence of breathlessness in people with COPD is higher than in those with advanced cancer and is frequently only partially relieved [20]. Breathlessness is a complex bidirectional process between pulmonary and neurological pathways [21]. Breathlessness in COPD can be defined objectively using a scale such as the modified Medical Research Council (mMRC) Dyspnea Scale (refer to Box 10.1) [22].

Anxiety and depression are also important comorbidities in COPD associated with poor outcomes, including exacerbations, readmissions, and mortality [23, 24]. As many as one-third of people living with COPD experience clinically elevated anxiety and depressive symptoms, which are prevalent across GOLD stages [25]. A high frequency of untreated anxiety and depressive symptoms exist in smokers with and without COPD – risk factors include African American race and male gender. Furthermore, anxiety symptoms, depressive symptoms, and psychiatric medication use increase in frequency by nearly two- to threefold across worsening GOLD letter grades (i.e., from A to D), suggesting greater symptom burden and exacerbation frequency influence emotional symptoms [25].

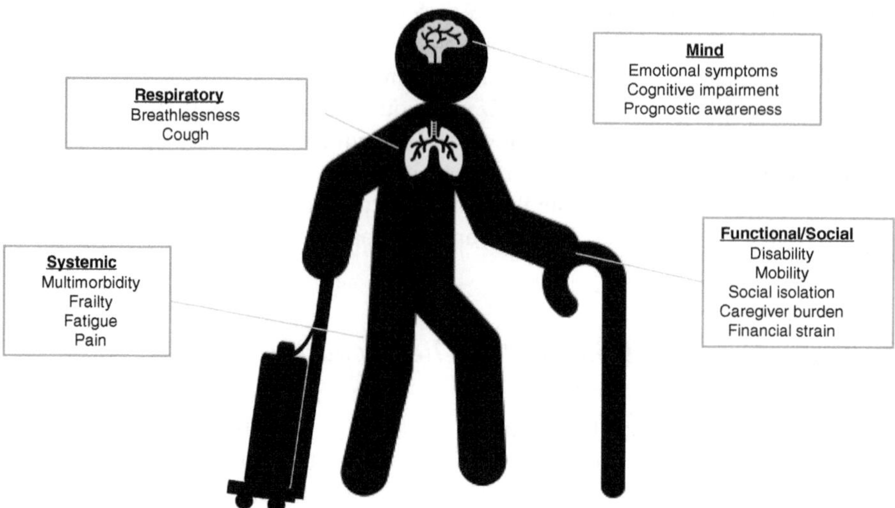


**Fig. 10.1** *The broad toll of COPD*. The impact of COPD extends far beyond the pulmonary system to include cognitive, systemic, functional, and social needs, especially evident in older adults with COPD

**Box 10.1 Measurement of Dyspnea – Modified Medical Research Council Dyspnea Scale**

- *Grade 0*: Breathless with strenuous exercise
- *Grade 1*: Breathless when hurrying on level ground or walking up a slight hill
- *Grade 2*: Walk slower than people of the same age because of breathlessness or stop for breath when walking at my own pace
- *Grade 3*: Stop for breath after walking about 100 yards or after a few minutes on level ground
- *Grade 4*: Too breathless to leave the house or breathless when dressing

Fatigue, sarcopenia, and frailty are also prevalent in COPD and difficult to manage. Fatigue, or the feeling of a lack of energy not relieved by rest, is prevalent in up to 71% of patients with COPD [26]. It has a significant impact on quality of life and activities of daily living and may be a strong predictor of hospitalization and length of hospital admission [27, 28]. The severity of fatigue has been associated with increased levels of other symptoms such as dyspnea, anxiety, and depression but is not correlated to severity of airflow limitation [29].

Sarcopenia includes low muscle strength, low muscle quantity or quality, and low physical performance [30] and is prevalent in 8–21% of patients with COPD. [31]

Sarcopenia is associated with reduced health status and quality of life in COPD [32]. While sarcopenia itself may exist independently, it often contributes to the disabling syndrome of frailty, defined as the presence of three or more of the following: unintentional weight loss, self-reported exhaustion, weak grip strength, slow walking speed, and low physical activity [33]. In older adults with COPD, the estimated prevalence of frailty is 10% and has been associated with increased rate of hospitalization, longer duration of hospitalization, and reduced quality of life [34, 35].

The physical and psychological symptoms of COPD can lead to restricted activities and reduced social interactions in as many as half of patients with COPD [36]. People living with COPD often report being restricted to their homes due to breathlessness and describe not being able to engage in activities that matter most to them [37]. This social isolation may trigger feelings of loneliness and has been associated with decreased exercise capacity, reduced health-related quality of life, and more emotional symptoms in COPD [38].

Beyond symptom burden, the trajectory of COPD is widely variable. This leads to significant prognostic uncertainty among clinicians who lack sufficient training to prognosticate in COPD, which is then further challenged when patients possess poor prognostic awareness about their illness [37, 39]. As COPD progresses, patients with COPD may become increasingly dependent on informal caregivers for activities of daily living, emotional support, and self-care needs. Involvement of informal caregivers in COPD care has been associated with improved patient adherence to therapies and may lead to reductions in professional home care costs [40]. However, data also illustrate that caregivers experience substantial emotional, physical, and financial burden [41]. Additionally, caregivers often experience similar levels of social isolation as their loved one [42]. The important relationships between a patient with COPD and his or her caregiver can become strained, and coping may become difficult [43].

## Palliative Care in COPD: Where Do Things Stand?

Palliative care is ideally suited to meet the many physical, emotional, spiritual, and prognostic awareness needs of people living with a COPD and their families. Palliative care can be delivered by board-certified specialists, i.e., *specialist palliative care*, or by clinicians who are not specialists in palliative care yet have received formal training in symptom management and values-based communication, i.e., *primary palliative care* [44]. Palliative care is appropriate at any point during the course of COPD and encompasses supportive care, hospice, end-of-life care, bereavement, and respite care [45]. Unlike hospice care, which is focused on the end of life, "early palliative care" is meant to be integrated into routine serious illness care long before the end of life – in cancer this is at the time of diagnosis [46]. People with COPD can and should receive proactive palliative care alongside disease-modifying therapies as appropriate. As COPD progresses and symptom burden changes or certain aspects become more severe, the intensity of palliative care can ebb and flow to align with care needs [47].

## *Specialist Palliative Care Success Stories in Cancer and Heart Failure*

The movement supporting early palliative care in serious illness grew out of the evidence demonstrating a benefit in patients with advanced cancer to improve quality of life, mood, and survival and to promote less aggressive care at the end of life [48–50]. In a nationwide cohort of veterans with advanced lung cancer, ambulatory palliative care reduced acute care utilization at the end of life [51]. Early palliative care also may improve survival in patients with advanced cancer [52]. Data further demonstrate a benefit for palliative care in non-cancer populations [53]. In one meta-analysis of palliative care in patients with advanced heart failure, home- and team-based palliative care was associated with improvements in patient-centered outcomes, documentation of preferences for the end of life, and reduced healthcare utilization [54]. Survival benefits have also been demonstrated in patients with heart failure receiving hospice care compared with those who do not [55].

## *Palliative Care Utilization in COPD*

Major national organizations such as the American Thoracic Society recognize the importance of palliative and end-of-life care in people living with COPD [56]. However, over a decade after this important statement, palliative care still remains exceedingly rare in COPD. In one study of hospitalized adults with COPD receiving supplemental oxygen, palliative care consultation occurred in only 2% of admissions [57]. Similarly, in one academic medical center, inpatient palliative care consultation remained low pre- and post-implementation of a comprehensive and multidisciplinary initiative focused on reducing hospital readmissions [58]. These results are troubling as patients with COPD frequently have more severe care needs than those with advanced cancer and yet receive palliative care much less frequently [59]. These data suggest that the inpatient setting may not be the ideal time to consult specialist palliative care. Regarding hospice, in one large analysis of older decedents with COPD, nearly half used hospice in the last 2 years of life [18]. Though this frequency of hospice use was higher than expected, its use varied substantially across the United States, with no geographic patterns. Notably, hospice use in this study was implemented for approximately 1 month, suggesting that older adults with COPD may not be engaging in critical advance care planning with their clinicians proactively in the ambulatory setting.

### *Barriers to Palliative Care in COPD*

Despite the many calls from international organizations, clinicians, patients, and their families, several barriers stand in the way of early integration of palliative care in COPD (refer to Box 10.2). Data from a cohort of patients with moderate to very severe COPD and their families support these national data and illustrate that few patients and their family members (approximately one-third) were aware of palliative care – most equated it with hospice and associated it as being end-of-life care [37, 60]. On the other hand, nearly all had knowledge of hospice care, drawn primarily from personal experiences with family members and loved ones. When presented with a standardized definition of early palliative care, patients with moderate to very severe COPD were eager to receive it before the end of life and certainly before end stage [37].

**Box 10.2 Barriers to Palliative Care in COPD: The 4 Ms**
- *M*isconceptions
- *M*isaligned goals
- *M*issed opportunities
- *M*echanisms for integration

The misconception of palliative care being only end-of-life care also extends to pulmonary clinicians, despite extensive experience with palliative care implementation in intensive care unit settings – in one descriptive study, pulmonologists frequently relegated palliative care to the end-of-life period only [61]. Pulmonary clinicians felt there could be misalignment between the specialties on the goals of care, and some feared the overuse of opioids and benzodiazepines in those with advanced COPD and chronic hypercapnia. Unclear referral criteria to specialist palliative care and practical implementation issues in busy clinical settings were also discussed as major barriers to palliative care implementation for people with COPD [61].

## Integrating Palliative Care in COPD

### *Who Should Receive Specialist Palliative Care in COPD?*

COPD is a chronic and progressively debilitating disease that can last for years, thus making it difficult for clinicians to draw the line on when to refer someone to specialist palliative care. Furthermore, patients often arrive and see specialist pulmonary clinics at various stages of severity, may be diagnosed late and already at end stages of the disease, or may have a highly variable and unpredictable illness trajectory that generates significant unknowns for pulmonary and primary care clinicians.

We propose that referral to specialist palliative care in COPD be based upon a combination of any or all of the following: [1] lung function; [2] needs; and/or [3] prognosis (Fig. 10.2). Think of each category as a dial that can be adjusted up or down as COPD progresses. At any point, one or all dials could pass a threshold for referral to specialist palliative care: more severe lung function, greater care needs, or worsening prognosis. In a lung-function-based model, all patients with a certain level of airflow limitation, e.g., moderate COPD or worse, could be considered as potential candidates for referral to specialist palliative care. The onus of exclusion then falls on the clinician to opt out of referral. Historically, palliative care has only been deemed appropriate in patients who have end-stage COPD, a point when it may be too late to improve quality of life. On the other hand, early palliative care needs exist in patients across COPD severity stages, extending into moderate COPD (GOLD Stage II), when patients and their families deem it was appropriate to refer [37]. Achieving consensus among pulmonologists and primary care clinicians on the appropriate threshold for referral using the lung-function-based model could be problematic. Another potential problem with this approach is that referral earlier in the disease trajectory for COPD may result in a large influx of patients to specialist palliative care clinics than can be handled by the current palliative care workforce. Furthermore, quality of life and lung function in COPD do not necessarily exist in a linear relationship, so patients may not understand their reason for referral if symptom burden is minimal despite having poor lung function [62].

An alternative approach to referral to specialist palliative care based on lung function is a needs-based model for referral. Priority specialist palliative care referral criteria in COPD include frequent hospitalizations, severe symptoms (e.g., respiratory or emotional), noninvasive ventilation, lack of social support, weight loss,

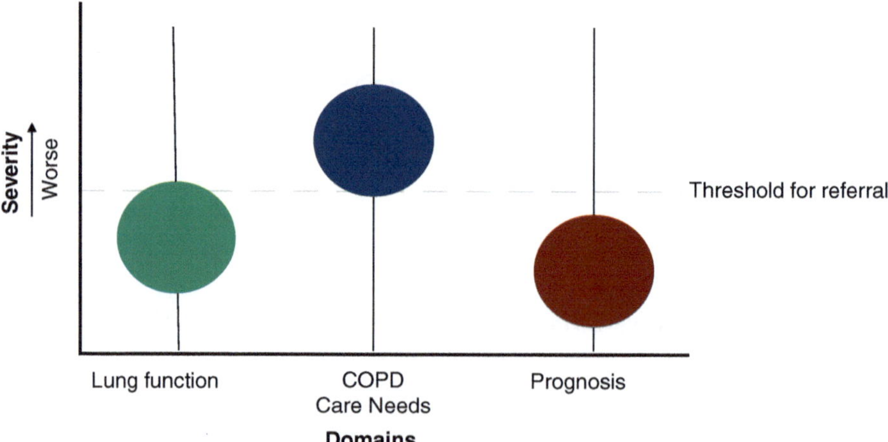


**Fig. 10.2** *Referring to specialist palliative care in COPD – adjusting the levers.* This figure illustrates three domains that could be considered for specialist palliative care referral in COPD. Each domain functions as a lever or dial that can be adjusted up or down as COPD progresses, eventually passing a threshold for referral. One or all of the levers can pass this hypothetical threshold

and others [61, 63] (Fig. 10.3). Many of these are typically used as criteria to refer a person with COPD to hospice [64, 65] (refer to Box 10.3). We believe that waiting to refer to specialist palliative care based upon criteria typically used for hospice referral would be too late and instead recommend that clinicians consider proactively referring their patients to specialist palliative care as patients approach these criteria.

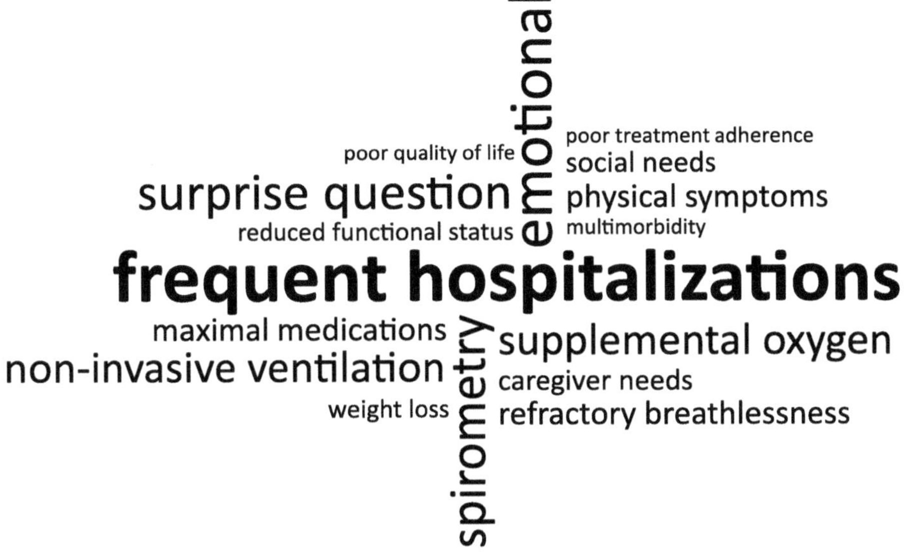


**Fig. 10.3** *Specialist palliative care referral criteria in COPD.* This word cloud displays criteria for potential referral to specialist palliative care in COPD

**Box 10.3. Potential Referral Criteria to Hospice in COPD**

- Cor pulmonale
- Very severe or end-stage COPD (GOLD Stage IV)
- Significant hypoxemia on supplemental oxygen
- Hypercapnia ($pCO_2 > 50$ mm Hg)
- Low albumin
- Dependence on oral steroids
- Disease progression
- Frequent exacerbations or care utilization (hospitalizations, emergency room visits, and outpatient visits)
- Weight loss in the preceding 6 months
- Inability to perform activities of daily living
- Breathlessness at rest or with minimal exertion
- Refractory breathlessness

Finally, a prognosis-based model could be implemented to increase referral of patients with COPD to specialist palliative care. Prognostic accuracy in COPD is made difficult by a variable disease trajectory and an inaccurate ability to predict when patients with COPD are nearing the end of their life [66]. The surprise question "Would I be surprised if this patient dies within 12 months?" is a simple tool that could be used to identify patients with COPD who might benefit from specialist palliative care but may oversimplify referral and exclude many patients with significant care needs [67]. COPD prognostic tools may better capture more patients who could benefit from palliative care. For example, the multidimensional BODE (*b*ody mass index, degree of airflow *o*bstruction, severity of *d*yspnea, and *e*xercise capacity) Index is a well-validated tool for the prediction of all-cause and respiratory-related mortality in COPD [68]. Another, the ProPal-COPD tool, predicts 1-year mortality and could be used to identify patients who may benefit from proactive palliative care by using the surprise question, mMRC Dyspnea Scale, clinical COPD questionnaire, airflow obstruction, body mass index, previous hospitalizations, and comorbidities [69]. In the end, we feel that an approach combining all three models may be the best way to ensure no gaps in referral to specialist palliative care exist.

## Successful Palliative Care Programs in COPD

Successful pragmatic models for integrating palliative care in the routine care of patients with COPD exist and share an inter-professional and team-based approach that harness healthcare professionals of varying disciplines and frequent assessments. A common thread appears to be a tailored approach to meet the individualized care needs of patients with COPD and their families. Additionally, many of the following programs reach out to patients in their homes.

### *INSPIRED COPD Outreach Program*

The INSPIRED (Implementing a Novel and Supportive Program of Individualized Care for Patients and Families Living With Respiratory Disease) COPD Outreach Program was implemented in 2010 by Rocker and colleagues in Nova Scotia to help meet the needs of patients with advanced COPD as they transition home following an emergency room visit or hospitalization [70]. This hospital-to-home-based program provides home visits by a certified respiratory educator focused on developing individualized action plans for the self-management of escalating symptoms, visits by a spiritual care practitioner to facilitate psychosocial support and advance care planning, and access to a daytime telephone support line. People who completed the full program and survived at least 6 months after enrollment had dramatic reductions in emergency room visits (by 60%), fewer hospital admissions, fewer days spent in the hospital, and significantly higher rates of home deaths compared to historical data outside of the program [71].

## *Nurse-Led Palliative Care*

Scheerens and colleagues have begun development and feasibility testing of an early integrated palliative home care intervention for adults with end-stage COPD in Belgium [72]. The intervention consists of regular visits performed by a palliative home care nurse trained in the care, symptom relief, and support of patients with end-stage COPD. Patients are provided informational leaflets with disease education and coping mechanisms to improve self-management. Additionally, palliative nurses use a written protocol to assess patient needs and symptoms to develop individualized action plans with involvement of other healthcare professionals as deemed necessary. Results of a Phase II pilot randomized controlled trial demonstrated feasibility and acceptability of this model among patients and healthcare professionals. While effectiveness analysis did not demonstrate an overall intervention effect, the intervention group demonstrated a trend toward higher perceived quality of care [73].

## *Breathlessness Services*

The breathlessness service of Higginson and colleagues in the United Kingdom is an innovative and well-tested program to bring palliative care to adults across various serious illnesses [74]. The service involves the use of a multidisciplinary team consisting of clinicians from palliative medicine, respiratory medicine, physiotherapy, and occupational therapy. After being evaluated by a pulmonary and palliative care clinician in the clinic, patients are given breathlessness "packs" that offer information and guidance on the management of dyspnea crisis along with tools to aid in self-management. Following the outpatient visit, physiotherapists visit patients' homes to evaluate for functional aids, provide training on pacing and exercises, and reinforce self-management. A month after the initial outpatient visit, patients return to the clinic with the palliative care clinician to develop action plans. In a randomized controlled trial of a breathlessness support service versus usual care for adults with refractory breathlessness and advanced disease, many of whom had COPD, patients enrolled in the breathlessness service had improved mastery of breathlessness and survival compared to controls [75].

## *Integrated Palliative Care Specialists in Pulmonary Clinic*

Recognizing the many unmet needs of patients with advanced lung disease, Smallwood and colleagues developed an integrated respiratory and palliative care service in Australia [76]. The Advanced Lung Disease Service offered visits in a clinic with pulmonary, palliative care, and psychology clinicians, nurse home visits, and telephone support. A majority of the enrolled patients had advanced COPD with severe breathlessness and were offered non-pharmacologic management and morphine if needed. The cohort study demonstrated a significant reduction in the mean number of emergency department visits for respiratory symptoms a year after enrolling in the program. Additionally, nearly 85%

of the patients had advance care planning or completed documents. Of the patients who died during the study, only about a quarter died in the hospital [76].

A similar multidisciplinary clinic that integrates pulmonary and palliative care clinicians was implemented in Wolverhampton, England, with the primary objectives of improving patient disease comprehension, clinician comprehension of prognosis, identification of opportunities for palliative care, management of symptoms, and support of patients and their caregivers [77]. Patients reported significant improvements in mobility and anxiety. Additionally, when compared to national reports, patients enrolled in the clinic were more likely to die at home.

## COPD Self-Management: The "Living Well with COPD" Program

To foster better partnerships between patients with COPD and their healthcare professionals, the McGill University Health Centre in Canada developed the "Living Well with COPD" program. While the self-management program did not include distinct palliative care clinician involvement, it did focus on many of the pillars of palliative care including optimizing quality of life, symptom management, and support for patients and caregivers. A multicenter, randomized clinical trial demonstrated that patients enrolled in the program had significantly improved quality of life and reduction in hospital admissions, emergency room visits, and unscheduled physician visits [78].

## Pulmonary Rehabilitation and Palliative Care in COPD

Pulmonary rehabilitation is often overlooked and underutilized as a potential venue for the delivery of palliative care in patients with COPD. Participants frequently complete a wide variety of guideline-directed symptom and functional assessments before and after completion of programs and are closely monitored multiple times weekly by healthcare professionals, thus situating pulmonary rehabilitation in the optimal position to introduce aspects of palliative care such as symptom monitoring and advance care planning [79].

## Palliative Care and Interventional Pulmonary

There may be some symptoms that patients with COPD encounter which do not respond to pharmacologic or non-pharmacologic management and require an interventional procedure with a palliative intent. An example includes endobronchial valves which can be inserted bronchoscopically into the airways of a select cohort of patients with COPD who have evidence of significant hyperinflation. The process is often referred to as bronchoscopic lung volume reduction as opposed to a surgical approach. In one analysis, endobronchial valves had multiple positive impacts on quality of life in COPD, including reduced breathlessness and improved functional status [80].

## A "Pallipulm" Approach to COPD Care

> "The greatest mistake in the treatment of diseases is that there are physicians for the body and physicians for the soul, although the two cannot be separated." – *Plato*

The domains of palliative care and pulmonary medicine may feel like opposing ends of the spectrum for a patient with COPD, which may generate a tension that hinders collaboration (Fig. 10.4). On the other hand, a "pallipulm" approach bridges the two fields and meets the significant and worsening gap in specialist palliative care clinician access [81]. We propose three steps to integrating pallipulm for COPD through the *3 A's approach* (refer to Box 10.4).

### *Step 1: Assess – Comprehensive COPD Care Needs Assessment*

First, a pallipulm program for COPD is personalized and tailored to the needs of the patient and their family. Elements of a pallipulm assessment for COPD are included in Box 10.5 and could be administered prior to a clinic visit in the waiting room. Focusing just on respiratory issues misses the breadth of problems and unmet needs that we have previously discussed and which also impact COPD outcomes (e.g., emotional symptoms, frailty, refractory breathlessness, caregiver burden, etc.). Rapid screens followed by a comprehensive palliative care assessment for those who screen positive are practical and can seamlessly integrate into busy clinic settings. The Support Needs Approach for Patients (SNAP) tool of Gardener and colleagues is undergoing validation and is an excellent pallipulm tool for

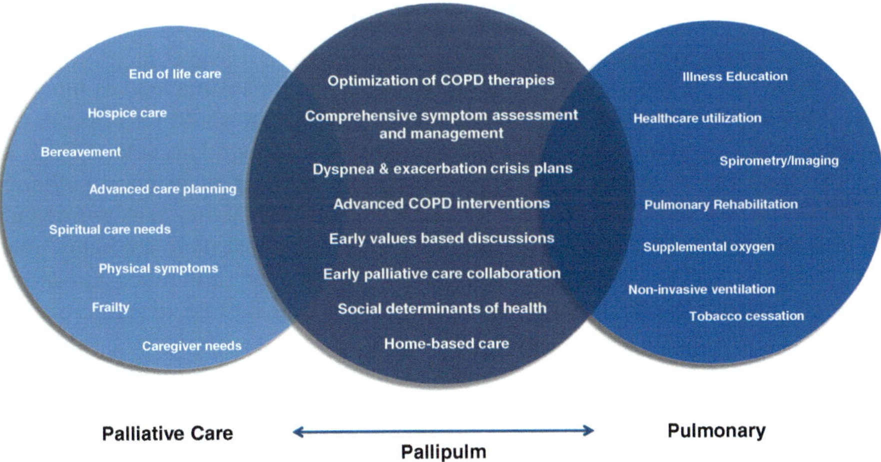


**Fig. 10.4** *Bridging the gap between palliative care and pulmonary medicine for COPD through pallipulm.* A pallipulm approach to COPD care bridges the gap between palliative care and pulmonary medicine to improve care for patients with COPD and to facilitate proactive referral to specialist palliative care when appropriate

**Box 10.4. Steps to Building a Pallipulm Program for COPD: The 3 A's**
- *Step 1.* Assess (rapid screening tools and comprehensive assessments)
- *Step 2.* Act (treat vs refer)
- *Step 3.* Adapt (reassess, adapt, and evolve)

comprehensive needs assessment and identification of unmet needs in patients with COPD [82].

**Box 10.5. Elements of a Standardized Pallipulm Assessment for COPD**
- Evaluate patient and family understanding of COPD, treatment plans, and prognosis
- Review and document all COPD interventions (pharmacologic and non-pharmacologic)
- Evaluate medical and psychological comorbidities
- Assess comprehensive symptom burden, including physical, emotional, and cognitive symptoms
- Review social determinants of health and support systems
- Identify surrogate decision-maker and key members of the decision-making team
- Review prior advance care plans
- Identify patient and family values about the end of life
- Discover caregiver bereavement concerns and needs

## *Step 2: Act – Pallipulm Management Tips for COPD*

Once unmet needs have been identified, pallipulm clinicians manage as much on their own and have a clear sense of when dials pass the threshold for referral, and a collaborative approach with specialist palliative care may be necessary. Such an approach clearly demands more opportunities for training in primary palliative care; fortunately, multiple programs offering this type of training exist nationwide [83, 84]. Central to the pallipulm tenet is the knowledge that there are many treatable traits in COPD, even in patients with end-stage disease, and much can still be done to improve a patient's quality of life and mood despite disease severity. Optimizing as many of these as possible and ensuring that each intervention aligns with the values and wishes of the patient and her family form the pallipulm focus [8].

The pallipulm clinician carefully navigates the many complex physical and emotional symptoms of COPD. This begins with a comprehensive and stepwise approach to manage refractory breathlessness [85] by optimizing disease-directed regimens followed by evidence-based non-pharmacologic therapies such as breathing training, walking aids, neuroelectrical muscle stimulation, and chest wall vibration based on availability [86]. Other interventions could include the development of an individual dyspnea crisis action plan [87] or the delivery of airflow in the form of a fan or medical airflow via cannula which have demonstrated significant relief of breathlessness for some patients [88]. If breathlessness remains a distressing symptom after optimization of disease-directed therapies and non-pharmacologic interventions, pharmacologic therapies should be considered. The mainstay pharmacologic treatment for refractory breathlessness is low-dose oral or parenteral opioids [89]. Despite fears of adverse respiratory effects, a recent meta-analysis has demonstrated no evidence of significant adverse effects when opiates are titrated and used appropriately [90]. A recent randomized controlled trial found that sustained-release morphine in COPD was safe and did not appear to worsen hypercapnia [91]. Current guidelines support the use of opioids in the treatment of refractory breathlessness in advanced COPD and provide guidance on initiating doses and maintenance regimens [56]. Other pharmacologic therapies have limited data; there is insufficient evidence to support the use of nebulized furosemide or opioids in the management of dyspnea. Additionally, the use of benzodiazepines alone for the management of dyspnea is not recommended and can have adverse effects when used in combination with opioids [92].

As with the management of dyspnea, reversible causes of cough should be explored and treated in addition to optimizing disease-directed therapies. One non-pharmacologic strategy that has demonstrated some positive results in managing refractory chronic cough is speech and language therapy [93]. When combined with pregabalin, speech therapy has been shown to reduce symptoms and improve quality of life for patients with chronic cough [94]. A trial of gabapentin may be considered if there are no contraindications and may help to reduce the impact of refractory cough on quality of life [95].

Depression and anxiety are prevalent in COPD and independently associated with poor outcomes yet rarely assessed or managed. The challenge with these symptoms is the limited training that specialist pulmonary clinicians receive in managing depressive and anxiety symptoms. Additionally, many pulmonary clinicians may not have the requisite time in pulmonary practices to schedule close follow-up to reassess symptoms and side effects as well as adjust doses of antidepressants or anxiolytics. Thus, a pallipulm approach to anxiety and depressive symptom management centers on increased awareness of these important comorbidities, assessment using validated screening tools, and close collaboration with palliative care and primary care. There have been several mechanisms proposed to screen for depression or anxiety in COPD [96]. Regarding treatment, insufficient evidence exists to support any one antidepressant for the treatment of COPD-related depression, and no guidelines have been published of which we are aware [97]. Cognitive behavioral therapy may be effective in treating depression in COPD but requires further study [98]. The strongest evidence for the treatment of COPD-related anxiety and depression is for pulmonary rehabilitation which has been shown to significantly improve emotional symptoms [99].

Finally, a pallipulm clinician is ideally suited to begin proactive advance care planning in COPD [100]. She/he begins by having proactive open and honest conversations centered on patient values. These discussions identify surrogate decision-makers, describe what may happen during an acute exacerbation including detailed discussions on invasive mechanical ventilation and noninvasive ventilation, and ensure that values and wishes are documented for the end of life that includes wishes for place of death. Finally, a pallipulm clinician works hand in hand with a patient suffering with COPD to identify ways to improve self-care and educate about COPD and on how to live and age well despite functional limitations. Some considerations include discussions on adapting to changes and progressive dyspnea or fatigue, self-management plans for exacerbations, coping with functional decline, goal setting, and ways to reduce burden on care partners [101].

### *Step 3: Adapt*

Once an initial assessment has been made that identifies unmet COPD care needs and interventions have been implemented, a pallipulm approach includes routine check-ins to measure responses to interventions and to adapt the approach to the ever-changing trajectory of COPD. This may include reassessment of pulmonary and extrapulmonary symptoms, interdisciplinary team discussions with specialist palliative care clinicians for complex cases, and adapting to the changing care needs of patients and their families. Given the unpredictable trajectory of COPD, especially following exacerbations, the pallipulm clinician evolves the approach after patients experience these sentinel events and stands ready to address high symptom burden and caregiver needs that may or may not return to baseline. This may trigger changes in the prognosis and should prompt values-based discussion surrounding end-of-life care.

## Conclusion

Palliative care is just the right thing to do for patients with COPD and their families. Not only does palliative care improve outcomes, its integration has been associated with cost savings, mostly realized through the reduction in acute care utilization near the end of life [102]. The British Thoracic Society proposed a pyramid of value that illustrated the estimated impact on cost per quality-adjusted life years across five categories of routine COPD interventions from most to least cost-effective: flu vaccine, smoking cessation, pulmonary rehabilitation, inhalers, and telehealth [103] (Fig. 10.5). Palliative care deserves a place in this pyramid of value for COPD. We hope that this chapter has inspired further research in the field and has compelled the reader to reserve a place for palliative care on the table when thinking about interventions for patients with COPD.

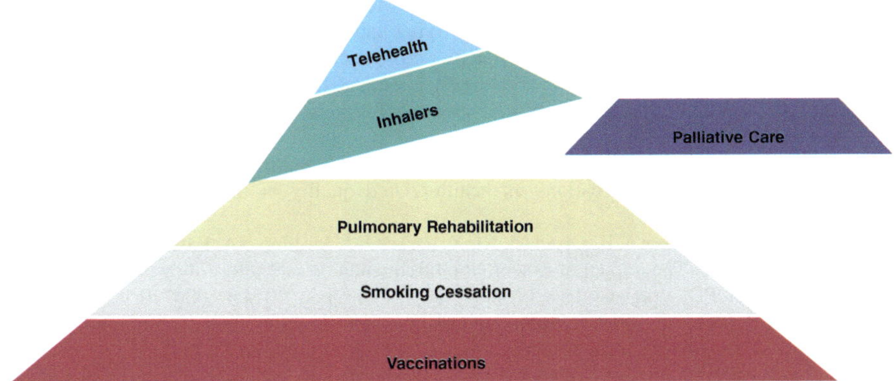


**Fig. 10.5** *A place for palliative care in the COPD pyramid of value.* This figure compares the relative cost-effectiveness of five interventions in COPD, with those at the bottom considered highly cost-effective compared to those at the top. Palliative care deserves a place in this pyramid

# References

1. Biener AI, Decker SL, Rohde F. Prevalence and treatment of chronic obstructive pulmonary disease (COPD) in the United States. JAMA. 2019;322:602.
2. Han MK, Martinez CH, Au DH, Bourbeau J, Boyd CM, Branson R, Criner GJ, Kalhan R, Kallstrom TJ, King A, Krishnan JA, Lareau SC, Lee TA, Lindell K, Mannino DM, Martinez FJ, Meldrum C, Press VG, Thomashow B, Tycon L, Sullivan JL, Walsh J, Wilson KC, Wright J, Yawn B, Zueger PM, Bhatt SP, Dransfield MT. Meeting the challenge of COPD care delivery in the USA: a multiprovider perspective. Lancet Respir Med. 2016;4:473–526.
3. Barnes PJ, Burney PG, Silverman EK, Celli BR, Vestbo J, Wedzicha JA, Wouters EF. Chronic obstructive pulmonary disease. Nat Rev Dis Primers. 2015;1:15076.
4. Singh D, Agusti A, Anzueto A, Barnes PJ, Bourbeau J, Celli BR, Criner GJ, Frith P, Halpin DMG, Han M, Lopez Varela MV, Martinez F, Montes de Oca M, Papi A, Pavord ID, Roche N, Sin DD, Stockley R, Vestbo J, Wedzicha JA, Vogelmeier C. Global strategy for the diagnosis, management, and prevention of chronic obstructive lung disease: the GOLD science committee report 2019. Eur Respir J. 2019;53:1900164.
5. Young KA, Strand M, Ragland MF, Kinney GL, Austin EE, Regan EA, Lowe KE, Make BJ, Silverman EK, Crapo JD, Hokanson JE, Investigators CO. Pulmonary subtypes exhibit differential global initiative for chronic obstructive lung disease spirometry stage progression: The COPDGene(R) Study. Chronic Obstr Pulm Dis. 2019;6:414–29.
6. Croft JB, Lu H, Zhang X, Holt JB. Geographic accessibility of pulmonologists for adults with COPD: United States, 2013. Chest. 2016;150:544–53.
7. Iyer AS, Cross SH, Dransfield MT, Warraich HJ. Urban-rural disparities in deaths from chronic lower respiratory disease in the United States. Am J Respir Crit Care Med. 2020.
8. van Dijk M, Gan CT, Koster TD, Wijkstra PJ, Slebos DJ, Kerstjens HAM, van der Vaart H, Duiverman ML. Treatment of severe stable COPD: the multidimensional approach of treatable traits. ERJ Open Res. 2020;6:00322.
9. Yohannes AM, Dryden S, Casaburi R, Hanania NA. Long-term benefits of pulmonary rehabilitation in COPD patients: a 2-year follow-up study. Chest. 2020.
10. Lindenauer PK, Stefan MS, Pekow PS, Mazor KM, Priya A, Spitzer KA, Lagu TC, Pack QR, Pinto-Plata VM, ZuWallack R. Association between initiation of pulmonary rehabilitation after hospitalization for COPD and 1-year survival among Medicare beneficiaries. JAMA. 2020;323:1813–23.

11. Amblas-Novellas J, Murray SA, Espaulella J, Martori JC, Oller R, Martinez-Munoz M, Molist N, Blay C, Gomez-Batiste X. Identifying patients with advanced chronic conditions for a progressive palliative care approach: a cross-sectional study of prognostic indicators related to end-of-life trajectories. BMJ Open. 2016;6:e012340.
12. Burge S, Wedzicha JA. COPD exacerbations: definitions and classifications. Eur Respir J Suppl. 2003;41:46s–53s.
13. Xu W, Collet JP, Shapiro S, Lin Y, Yang T, Wang C, Bourbeau J. Negative impacts of unreported COPD exacerbations on health-related quality of life at 1 year. Eur Respir J. 2010;35:1022–30.
14. Schmidt SA, Johansen MB, Olsen M, Xu X, Parker JM, Molfino NA, Lash TL, Sorensen HT, Christiansen CF. The impact of exacerbation frequency on mortality following acute exacerbations of COPD: a registry-based cohort study. BMJ Open. 2014;4:e006720.
15. McGhan R, Radcliff T, Fish R, Sutherland ER, Welsh C, Make B. Predictors of rehospitalization and death after a severe exacerbation of COPD. Chest. 2007;132:1748–55.
16. Global Burden of Disease Collaborators. Global burden of 369 diseases and injuries in 204 countries and territories, 1990-2019: a systematic analysis for the Global Burden of Disease Study 2019. Lancet. 2020;396:1204–22.
17. Khakban A, Sin DD, FitzGerald JM, McManus BM, Ng R, Hollander Z, Sadatsafavi M. The projected epidemic of chronic obstructive pulmonary disease hospitalizations over the next 15 years. A population-based perspective. Am J Respir Crit Care Med. 2017;195:287–91.
18. Iyer AS, Goodrich CA, Dransfield MT, Alam SS, Brown CJ, Landefeld CS, Bakitas MA, Brown JR. End-of-life spending and healthcare utilization among older adults with chronic obstructive pulmonary disease. Am J Med. 2020;133:817–824 e811.
19. Cross SH, Ely EW, Kavalieratos D, Tulsky JA, Warraich HJ. Place of death for individuals with chronic lung disease: trends and associated factors from 2003 to 2017 in the United States. Chest. 2020;158:670–80.
20. Ahmadi Z, Lundstrom S, Janson C, Strang P, Emtner M, Currow DC, Ekstrom M. End-of-life care in oxygen-dependent COPD and cancer: a national population-based study. Eur Respir J. 2015;46:1190–3.
21. Jolley CJ, Luo YM, Steier J, Rafferty GF, Polkey MI, Moxham J. Neural respiratory drive and breathlessness in COPD. Eur Respir J. 2015;45:355–64.
22. Munari AB, Gulart AA, Dos Santos K, Venancio RS, Karloh M, Mayer AF. Modified Medical Research Council dyspnea scale in GOLD classification better reflects physical activities of daily living. Respir Care. 2018;63:77–85.
23. Vikjord SAA, Brumpton BM, Mai XM, Vanfleteren L, Langhammer A. The association of anxiety and depression with mortality in a COPD cohort. The HUNT study, Norway. Respir Med. 2020;171:106089.
24. Xu W, Collet JP, Shapiro S, Lin Y, Yang T, Platt RW, Wang C, Bourbeau J. Independent effect of depression and anxiety on chronic obstructive pulmonary disease exacerbations and hospitalizations. Am J Respir Crit Care Med. 2008;178:913–20.
25. Iyer AS, Holm KE, Bhatt SP, Kim V, Kinney GL, Wamboldt FS, Jacobs MR, Regan EA, Armstrong HF, Lowe KE, Martinez CH, Dransfield MT, Foreman MG, Shinozaki G, Hanania NA, Wise RA, Make BJ, Hoth KF, Investigators CO. Symptoms of anxiety and depression and use of anxiolytic-hypnotics and antidepressants in current and former smokers with and without COPD - a cross sectional analysis of the COPDGene cohort. J Psychosom Res. 2019;118:18–26.
26. Blinderman CD, Homel P, Billings JA, Tennstedt S, Portenoy RK. Symptom distress and quality of life in patients with advanced chronic obstructive pulmonary disease. J Pain Symptom Manag. 2009;38:115–23.
27. Kouijzer M, Brusse-Keizer M, Bode C. COPD-related fatigue: impact on daily life and treatment opportunities from the patient's perspective. Respir Med. 2018;141:47–51.
28. Paddison JS, Effing TW, Quinn S, Frith PA. Fatigue in COPD: association with functional status and hospitalisations. Eur Respir J. 2013;41:565–70.

29. Kapella MC, Larson JL, Patel MK, Covey MK, Berry JK. Subjective fatigue, influencing variables, and consequences in chronic obstructive pulmonary disease. Nurs Res. 2006;55:10–7.
30. Cruz-Jentoft AJ, Bahat G, Bauer J, Boirie Y, Bruyere O, Cederholm T, Cooper C, Landi F, Rolland Y, Sayer AA, Schneider SM, Sieber CC, Topinkova E, Vandewoude M, Visser M, Zamboni M. Writing Group for the European Working Group on Sarcopenia in Older P, the Extended Group for E. Sarcopenia: revised European consensus on definition and diagnosis. Age Ageing. 2019;48:16–31.
31. Benz E, Trajanoska K, Lahousse L, Schoufour JD, Terzikhan N, De Roos E, de Jonge GB, Williams R, Franco OH, Brusselle G, Rivadeneira F. Sarcopenia in COPD: a systematic review and meta-analysis. Eur Respir Rev. 2019;28
32. Sepulveda-Loyola W, Osadnik C, Phu S, Morita AA, Duque G, Probst VS. Diagnosis, prevalence, and clinical impact of sarcopenia in COPD: a systematic review and meta-analysis. J Cachexia Sarcopenia Muscle. 2020;11:1164–76.
33. Fried LP, Tangen CM, Walston J, Newman AB, Hirsch C, Gottdiener J, Seeman T, Tracy R, Kop WJ, Burke G, McBurnie MA. Cardiovascular health study collaborative research G. frailty in older adults: evidence for a phenotype. J Gerontol Series A Biol Sci Med Sci. 2001;56:M146–56.
34. Lahousse L, Ziere G, Verlinden VJ, Zillikens MC, Uitterlinden AG, Rivadeneira F, Tiemeier H, Joos GF, Hofman A, Ikram MA, Franco OH, Brusselle GG, Stricker BH. Risk of frailty in elderly with COPD: a population-based study. J Gerontol A Biol Sci Med Sci. 2016;71:689–95.
35. Kennedy CC, Novotny PJ, LeBrasseur NK, Wise RA, Sciurba FC, Benzo RP. Frailty and clinical outcomes in chronic obstructive pulmonary disease. Ann Am Thorac Soc. 2019;16:217–24.
36. Iyer AS, Wells JM, Bhatt SP, Kirkpatrick DP, Sawyer P, Brown CJ, Allman RM, Bakitas MA, Dransfield MT. Life-space mobility and clinical outcomes in COPD. Int J Chron Obstruct Pulmon Dis. 2018;13:2731–8.
37. Iyer AS, Dionne-Odom JN, Ford SM, Crump Tims SL, Sockwell ED, Ivankova NV, Brown CJ, Tucker RO, Dransfield MT, Bakitas MA. A formative evaluation of patient and family caregiver perspectives on early palliative care in COPD across disease severity. Ann Am Thor Soc. 2019.
38. Reijnders T, Schuler M, Jelusic D, Troosters T, Janssens W, Schultz K, von Leupoldt A. The impact of loneliness on outcomes of pulmonary rehabilitation in patients with COPD. COPD. 2018;15:446–53.
39. Christakis NA, Iwashyna TJ. Attitude and self-reported practice regarding prognostication in a national sample of internists. Arch Intern Med. 1998;158:2389–95.
40. Trivedi RB, Bryson CL, Udris E, Au DH. The influence of informal caregivers on adherence in COPD patients. Ann Behav Med. 2012;44:66–72.
41. Figueiredo D, Gabriel R, Jacome C, Cruz J, Marques A. Caring for relatives with chronic obstructive pulmonary disease: how does the disease severity impact on family carers? Aging Ment Health. 2014;18:385–93.
42. Strang S, Osmanovic M, Hallberg C, Strang P. Family Caregivers' heavy and overloaded burden in advanced chronic obstructive pulmonary disease. J Palliat Med. 2018;21:1768–72.
43. Gabriel R, Figueiredo D, Jacome C, Cruz J, Marques A. Day-to-day living with severe chronic obstructive pulmonary disease: towards a family-based approach to the illness impacts. Psychol Health. 2014;29:967–83.
44. Spiker M, Paulsen K, Mehta AK. Primary palliative care education in U.S. residencies and fellowships: a systematic review of program leadership perspectives. J Palliat Med. 2020;23:1392–9.
45. Munday D, Boyd K, Jeba J, Kimani K, Moine S, Grant L, Murray S. Defining primary palliative care for universal health coverage. Lancet. 2019;394:621–2.
46. Bakitas MA, Tosteson TD, Li Z, Lyons KD, Hull JG, Li Z, Dionne-Odom JN, Frost J, Dragnev KH, Hegel MT, Azuero A, Ahles TA. Early versus delayed initiation of concurrent

palliative oncology care: patient outcomes in the ENABLE III randomized controlled trial. J Clin Oncol. 2015;33:1438–45.
47. Lloyd A, Kendall M, Starr JM, Murray SA. Physical, social, psychological and existential trajectories of loss and adaptation towards the end of life for older people living with frailty: a serial interview study. BMC Geriatr. 2016;16:176.
48. Temel JS, Greer JA, Muzikansky A, Gallagher ER, Admane S, Jackson VA, Dahlin CM, Blinderman CD, Jacobsen J, Pirl WF, Billings JA, Lynch TJ. Early palliative care for patients with metastatic non-small-cell lung cancer. N Engl J Med. 2010;363:733–42.
49. Bakitas M, Lyons KD, Hegel MT, Balan S, Barnett KN, Brokaw FC, Byock IR, Hull JG, Li Z, McKinstry E, Seville JL, Ahles TA. The project ENABLE II randomized controlled trial to improve palliative care for rural patients with advanced cancer: baseline findings, methodological challenges, and solutions. Palliat Support Care. 2009;7:75–86.
50. Bakitas M, Lyons KD, Hegel MT, Balan S, Brokaw FC, Seville J, Hull JG, Li Z, Tosteson TD, Byock IR, Ahles TA. Effects of a palliative care intervention on clinical outcomes in patients with advanced cancer: the project ENABLE II randomized controlled trial. JAMA. 2009;302:741–9.
51. Vranas KC, Lapidus JA, Ganzini L, Slatore CG, Sullivan DR. Association of Palliative Care use and setting with health-care utilization and quality of care at the end of life among patients with advanced lung cancer. Chest. 2020;158:2667–74.
52. Sullivan DR, Chan B, Lapidus JA, Ganzini L, Hansen L, Carney PA, Fromme EK, Marino M, Golden SE, Vranas KC, Slatore CG. Association of early palliative care use with survival and place of death among patients with advanced lung cancer receiving care in the veterans health administration. JAMA Oncol. 2019;
53. Quinn KL, Shurrab M, Gitau K, Kavalieratos D, Isenberg SR, Stall NM, Stukel TA, Goldman R, Horn D, Cram P, Detsky AS, Bell CM. Association of receipt of palliative care interventions with health care use, quality of life, and symptom burden among adults with chronic noncancer illness: a systematic review and meta-analysis. JAMA. 2020;324:1439–50.
54. Diop MS, Rudolph JL, Zimmerman KM, Richter MA, Skarf LM. Palliative care interventions for patients with heart failure: a systematic review and meta-analysis. J Palliat Med. 2017;20:84–92.
55. Connor SR, Pyenson B, Fitch K, Spence C, Iwasaki K. Comparing hospice and nonhospice patient survival among patients who die within a three-year window. J Pain Symptom Manag. 2007;33:238–46.
56. Lanken PN, Terry PB, Delisser HM, Fahy BF, Hansen-Flaschen J, Heffner JE, Levy M, Mularski RA, Osborne ML, Prendergast TJ, Rocker G, Sibbald WJ, Wilfond B, Yankaskas JR, Force ATSE-o-LCT. An official American Thoracic Society clinical policy statement: palliative care for patients with respiratory diseases and critical illnesses. Am J Respir Crit Care Med. 2008;177:912–27.
57. Rush B, Hertz P, Bond A, McDermid RC, Celi LA. Use of palliative care in patients with end-Stage COPD and receiving home oxygen: national trends and barriers to care in the United States. Chest. 2017;151:41–6.
58. Bhatt SP, Wells JM, Iyer AS, Kirkpatrick DP, Parekh TM, Leach LT, Anderson EM, Sanders JG, Nichols JK, Blackburn CC, Dransfield MT. Results of a medicare bundled payments for care improvement initiative for chronic obstructive pulmonary disease readmissions. Ann Am Thorac Soc. 2017;14:643–8.
59. Moens K, Higginson IJ, Harding R, Euro I. Are there differences in the prevalence of palliative care-related problems in people living with advanced cancer and eight non-cancer conditions? A systematic review. J Pain Symptom Manag. 2014;48:660–77.
60. Lane T, Ramadurai D, Simonetti J. Public awareness and perceptions of palliative and comfort care. Am J Med. 2019;132:129–31.
61. Iyer AS, Dionne-Odom JN, Khateeb DM, O'Hare L, Tucker RO, Brown CJ, Dransfield MT, Bakitas MA. A qualitative study of pulmonary and palliative care clinician perspectives on early palliative care in chronic obstructive pulmonary disease. J Palliat Med. 2020;23:513–26.

62. Brien SB, Lewith GT, Thomas M. Patient coping strategies in COPD across disease severity and quality of life: a qualitative study. NPJ Prim Care Respir Med. 2016;26:16051.
63. Disler RT, Green A, Luckett T, Newton PJ, Inglis S, Currow DC, Davidson PM. Experience of advanced chronic obstructive pulmonary disease: metasynthesis of qualitative research. J Pain Symptom Manag. 2014;48:1182–99.
64. Fox E, Landrum-McNiff K, Zhong Z, Dawson NV, Wu AW, Lynn J. Evaluation of prognostic criteria for determining hospice eligibility in patients with advanced lung, heart, or liver disease. SUPPORT Investigators. Study to Understand Prognoses and Preferences for Outcomes and Risks of Treatments. JAMA. 1999;282:1638–45.
65. Healthcare V. Hospice eligibility: end-stage copd and other forms of lung disease. 2020 [cited 2020 December 1]. Available from: https://www.vitas.com/for-healthcare-professionals/hospice-and-palliative-care-eligibility-guidelines/hospice-eligibility-guidelines/copd-and-lung-disease.
66. Christakis NA, Lamont EB. Extent and determinants of error in doctors' prognoses in terminally ill patients: prospective cohort study. BMJ. 2000;320:469–72.
67. Noppe D, Veen HI, Mooren K. COPD patients in need of palliative care: identification after hospitalization through the surprise question. Chron Respir Dis. 2019;16:1479972318796219.
68. Celli BR, Cote CG, Marin JM, Casanova C, Montes de Oca M, Mendez RA, Pinto Plata V, Cabral HJ. The body-mass index, airflow obstruction, dyspnea, and exercise capacity index in chronic obstructive pulmonary disease. N Engl J Med. 2004;350:1005–12.
69. Duenk RG, Verhagen C, Bronkhorst EM, Djamin RS, Bosman GJ, Lammers E, Dekhuijzen P, Vissers K, Engels Y, Heijdra Y. Development of the ProPal-COPD tool to identify patients with COPD for proactive palliative care. Int J Chron Obstruct Pulmon Dis. 2017;12:2121–8.
70. Rocker GM, Verma JY. 'INSPIRED' COPD Outreach Program: doing the right things right. Clin Invest Med. 2014;37:E311–9.
71. Blackman R, Demmons J, Gillis D, Rocker G. Dying at home from COPD: feasible or fantasy. Chest. 2016;150:951A.
72. Scheerens C, Chambaere K, Pardon K, Derom E, Van Belle S, Joos G, Pype P, Deliens L. Development of a complex intervention for early integration of palliative home care into standard care for end-stage COPD patients: a phase 0-I study. PLoS One. 2018;13:e0203326.
73. Scheerens C, Pype P, Van Cauwenberg J, Vanbutsele G, Eecloo K, Derom E, Van Belle S, Joos G, Deliens L, Chambaere K. Early-integrated palliative home care and standard care for end-stage COPD (EPIC): a phase II pilot RCT testing feasibility, acceptability and effectiveness. J Pain Symptom Manag. 2019;
74. Reilly CC, Bausewein C, Pannell C, Moxham J, Jolley CJ, Higginson IJ. Patients' experiences of a new integrated breathlessness support service for patients with refractory breathlessness: results of a postal survey. Palliat Med. 2016;30:313–22.
75. Higginson IJ, Bausewein C, Reilly CC, Gao W, Gysels M, Dzingina M, McCrone P, Booth S, Jolley CJ, Moxham J. An integrated palliative and respiratory care service for patients with advanced disease and refractory breathlessness: a randomised controlled trial. Lancet Respir Med. 2014;2:979–87.
76. Smallwood N, Thompson M, Warrender-Sparkes M, Eastman P, Le B, Irving L, Philip J. Integrated respiratory and palliative care may improve outcomes in advanced lung disease. ERJ Open Res. 2018;4
77. Ward H. Improving access and coordination to palliative care for patients with end stage respiratory disease – The Royal Wolverhampton NHS Trust and Compton Care. 2020 [cited 2020 December 1]. Available from: https://www.england.nhs.uk/ourwork/clinical-policy/respiratory-disease/improving-access-and-coordination-to-palliative-care/.
78. Bourbeau J, Julien M, Maltais F, Rouleau M, Beaupre A, Begin R, Renzi P, Nault D, Borycki E, Schwartzman K, Singh R, Collet JP, Chronic Obstructive Pulmonary Disease axis of the Respiratory Network Fonds de la Recherche en Sante du Q. Reduction of hospital utilization in patients with chronic obstructive pulmonary disease: a disease-specific self-management intervention. Arch Intern Med. 2003;163:585–91.

79. Janssen DJ, McCormick JR. Palliative care and pulmonary rehabilitation. Clin Chest Med. 2014;35:411–21.
80. Dransfield MT, Garner JL, Bhatt SP, Slebos DJ, Klooster K, Sciurba FC, Shah PL, Marchetti NT, Sue RD, Wright S, Rivas-Perez H, Wiese TA, Wahidi MM, Goulart de Oliveira H, Armstrong B, Radhakrishnan S, Shargill NS, Criner GJ, Group LS. Effect of Zephyr endobronchial valves on dyspnea, activity levels, and quality of life at one year. Results from a randomized clinical trial. Ann Am Thorac Soc. 2020;17:829–38.
81. Kamal AH, Wolf SP, Troy J, Leff V, Dahlin C, Rotella JD, Handzo G, Rodgers PE, Myers ER. Policy changes key to promoting sustainability and growth of the specialty palliative care workforce. Health Aff. 2019;38:910–8.
82. Gardener AC, Ewing G, Mendonca S, Farquhar M. Support needs approach for patients (SNAP) tool: a validation study. BMJ Open. 2019;9:e032028.
83. Grudzen CR, Brody AA, Chung FR, Cuthel AM, Mann D, McQuilkin JA, Rubin AL, Swartz J, Tan A, Goldfeld KS, Investigators P-E. Primary palliative care for emergency medicine (PRIM-ER): Protocol for a pragmatic, cluster-randomised, stepped wedge design to test the effectiveness of primary palliative care education, training and technical support for emergency medicine. BMJ Open. 2019;9:e030099.
84. Pelayo-Alvarez M, Perez-Hoyos S, Agra-Varela Y. Clinical effectiveness of online training in palliative care of primary care physicians. J Palliat Med. 2013;16:1188–96.
85. Marciniuk DD, Goodridge D, Hernandez P, Rocker G, Balter M, Bailey P, Ford G, Bourbeau J, O'Donnell DE, Maltais F, Mularski RA, Cave AJ, Mayers I, Kennedy V, Oliver TK, Brown C, Canadian Thoracic Society CCDEWG. Managing dyspnea in patients with advanced chronic obstructive pulmonary disease: a Canadian Thoracic Society clinical practice guideline. Can Respir J. 2011;18:69–78.
86. Bausewein C, Booth S, Gysels M, Higginson I. Non-pharmacological interventions for breathlessness in advanced stages of malignant and non-malignant diseases. Cochrane Database Syst Rev. 2008. CD005623.
87. Mularski RA, Reinke LF, Carrieri-Kohlman V, Fischer MD, Campbell ML, Rocker G, Schneidman A, Jacobs SS, Arnold R, Benditt JO, Booth S, Byock I, Chan GK, Curtis JR, Donesky D, Hansen-Flaschen J, Heffner J, Klein R, Limberg TM, Manning HL, Morrison RS, Ries AL, Schmidt GA, Selecky PA, Truog RD, Wang AC, White DB, Crisis ATSAHCoPMoD. An official American Thoracic Society workshop report: assessment and palliative management of dyspnea crisis. Ann Am Thorac Soc. 2013;10:S98–106.
88. Swan F, Newey A, Bland M, Allgar V, Booth S, Bausewein C, Yorke J, Johnson M. Airflow relieves chronic breathlessness in people with advanced disease: an exploratory systematic review and meta-analyses. Palliat Med. 2019;33:618–33.
89. Barnes H, McDonald J, Smallwood N, Manser R. Opioids for the palliation of refractory breathlessness in adults with advanced disease and terminal illness. Cochrane Database Syst Rev. 2016;3:CD011008.
90. Verberkt CA, van den Beuken-van Everdingen MHJ, Schols J, Datla S, Dirksen CD, Johnson MJ, van Kuijk SMJ, Wouters EFM, Janssen DJA. Adverse respiratory effects of opioids for chronic breathlessness: to what extent can we learn lessons from chronic pain? Eur Respir J. 2018;52:1800882.
91. Verberkt CA, van den Beuken-van Everdingen MHJ, Schols J, Hameleers N, Wouters EFM, Janssen DJA. Effect of sustained-release morphine for refractory breathlessness in chronic obstructive pulmonary disease on health status: a randomized clinical trial. JAMA Intern Med. 2020;180:1306–14.
92. Ekstrom MP, Bornefalk-Hermansson A, Abernethy AP, Currow DC. Safety of benzodiazepines and opioids in very severe respiratory disease: national prospective study. BMJ. 2014;348:g445.
93. Chamberlain Mitchell SA, Garrod R, Clark L, Douiri A, Parker SM, Ellis J, Fowler SJ, Ludlow S, Hull JH, Chung KF, Lee KK, Bellas H, Pandyan A, Birring SS. Physiotherapy,

and speech and language therapy intervention for patients with refractory chronic cough: a multicentre randomised control trial. Thorax. 2017;72:129–36.
94. Vertigan AE, Kapela SL, Ryan NM, Birring SS, McElduff P, Gibson PG. Pregabalin and speech pathology combination therapy for refractory chronic cough: a randomized controlled trial. Chest. 2016;149:639–48.
95. Ryan NM, Birring SS, Gibson PG. Gabapentin for refractory chronic cough: a randomised, double-blind, placebo-controlled trial. Lancet. 2012;380:1583–9.
96. Maurer J, Rebbapragada V, Borson S, Goldstein R, Kunik ME, Yohannes AM, Hanania NA. Anxiety AWPo, depression in C. anxiety and depression in COPD: current understanding, unanswered questions, and research needs. Chest. 2008;134:43S–56S.
97. Pollok J, van Agteren JE, Carson-Chahhoud KV. Pharmacological interventions for the treatment of depression in chronic obstructive pulmonary disease. Cochrane Database Syst Rev. 2018;12:CD012346.
98. Pollok J, van Agteren JE, Esterman AJ, Carson-Chahhoud KV. Psychological therapies for the treatment of depression in chronic obstructive pulmonary disease. Cochrane Database Syst Rev. 2019;3:CD012347.
99. Gordon CS, Waller JW, Cook RM, Cavalera SL, Lim WT, Osadnik CR. Effect of pulmonary rehabilitation on symptoms of anxiety and depression in COPD: a systematic review and meta-analysis. Chest. 2019;156:80–91.
100. Meehan E, Sweeney C, Foley T, Lehane E, Burgess Kelleher A, Hally RM, Shanagher D, Korn B, Rabbitte M, Detering KM, Cornally N. Advance care planning in COPD: guidance development for healthcare professionals. BMJ Support Palliat Care. 2019.
101. Carpentieri JD, Elliott J, Brett CE, Deary IJ. Adapting to aging: older people talk about their use of selection, optimization, and compensation to maximize Well-being in the context of physical decline. J Gerontol B Psychol Sci Soc Sci. 2017;72:351–61.
102. Enguidanos SM, Cherin D, Brumley R. Home-based palliative care study: site of death, and costs of medical care for patients with congestive heart failure, chronic obstructive pulmonary disease, and cancer. J Soc Work End Life Palliat Care. 2005;1:37–56.
103. Tinelli M, Kanavos P, Efthymiadou O, Visintin E, Grimaccia F, Mossman J. Using IMPRESS to guide policy change in multiple sclerosis. Mult Scler. 2018;24:1251–5.

[illegible]

# Chapter 11
# Palliative Care in Interstitial Lung Disease

**Marlies S. Wijsenbeek and Catharina C. Moor**

Interstitial lung diseases (ILDs) are a large, heterogeneous group of more than 200 diseases, which diffusely affect the lungs. These diseases are characterized by interstitial inflammation, interstitial fibrosis, or a combination of both [1]. ILDs can broadly be classified in four groups. The first group encompasses ILDs with a known cause, such as underlying connective tissue disease or drug-induced ILD. The second and largest group is the idiopathic interstitial pneumonias (IIPs); the most common IIP is idiopathic pulmonary fibrosis (IPF). The third group consists of granulomatous disorders, of which sarcoidosis is the most prevalent entity. The last group comprises rare ILDs [2]. The disease courses of different ILDs vary considerably. Some ILDs may be reversible, some have the potential to stabilize, and others, particularly fibrotic ILDs, can be progressive and ultimately fatal [3]. IPF is by definition progressive and has the worst prognosis of all ILDs, with a median survival of 3–5 years after diagnosis if untreated [4]. Even though the individual diseases are rare, ILD is the 40th most common cause of death worldwide, and mortality is still rising [5, 6].

Most common symptoms of ILDs are cough, dyspnea, and fatigue [7]. Symptoms often deteriorate over time in patients with progressive disease [8]. Living with a chronic disease, with a high symptom burden and uncertain prospects, has a major impact on the daily lives of patients with ILD and their families [9]. Consequently, most ILD patients have an increasingly impaired (health-related) quality of life ((HR)QOL) [3, 10–12].

For IPF, two antifibrotic drugs (nintedanib and pirfenidone) are available [13, 14]. These drugs slow down disease progression and may prolong survival, but have

M. S. Wijsenbeek (✉) · C. C. Moor
Academic Centre of Excellence for Interstitial Lung Diseases and Sarcoidosis, Department of Respiratory Medicine, Erasmus MC, University Medical Centre Rotterdam, Rotterdam, Netherlands
e-mail: m.wijsenbeek-lourens@erasmusmc.nl; c.moor@erasmusmc.nl



K. O. Lindell, S. K. Danoff (eds.), *Palliative Care in Lung Disease*, Respiratory Medicine, https://doi.org/10.1007/978-3-030-81788-6_11

no convincing effect on health-related quality of life. For other fibrotic ILDs, immunosuppressive medication has been the mainstay of treatment until now, often based on limited evidence. Recently, the antifibrotic drug nintedanib was also approved for the treatment of progressive fibrotic ILDs other than IPF, based on the results of phase III clinical trials [15, 16]. Although this is a major step forward, current pharmacological treatments do not reverse or halt fibrosis. The only curative treatment option in progressive fibrotic ILDs is lung transplantation, which is only a possibility for a selected subgroup of patients [17]. Importantly, mortality on the waiting list for lung transplantation is also substantial and higher for ILDs than for other lung diseases [18].

Despite the often poor prognosis and high symptom burden, structured integration of palliative care into the care pathway in ILD is still in its infancy. This chapter provides an overview of the current knowledge on palliative care in ILD.

## Palliative Care in ILD

Similar to other chronic life-limiting conditions, the goal of palliative care in ILD is to reduce symptoms and improve the quality of life of patients and their families, using a multidisciplinary approach [19, 20]. Even though the importance of palliative care in ILD has been increasingly acknowledged in recent years, palliative care services are still underused in clinical practice [6]. Moreover, prospective studies on palliative care in ILD are limited. Consequently, evidence-based palliative care guidelines for ILD do not exist. The 2011 ATS/ERS/JRS/ALAT IPF treatment guideline states that palliative care should be considered in addition to disease-modifying therapies but provides no further details [21]. The UK guideline (NICE) on diagnosis and management of IPF recommends that best supportive care should be offered from the point of diagnosis [22]. Because of the absence of specific palliative care guidelines, an international expert working group recently developed a consensus statement about palliative care in ILD and proposed important topics for future research in this area [6].

## Barriers

Referral of ILD patients to palliative care services is generally low, ranging from 0% to 38% in the literature [23–28]. Different barriers for referral to specialist palliative care have been observed in ILD. Some barriers are ILD-related, and some are related to specific healthcare system, religious, or cultural differences [6, 25]. Other barriers to palliative care are more universal, such as the misconception that palliative care is the same as end-of-life care; confusion about the role of palliative care among the general public, patients, and healthcare providers; fear of talking about the future; and the wish to focus on more positive aspects [6, 23, 29–31]. An important and ILD-specific problem is the unpredictable nature and prognostic uncertainty of ILDs. Moreover, healthcare providers report organizational gaps, lack of time, and lack of specific training about palliative care [31, 32]. In a qualitative European study, patient representatives mentioned that access to palliative care was highly variable between and within countries [33]. Barriers for patients on the lung transplant waiting list are similar and mainly concern the poor understanding of the role of palliative care in this patient group [34].

## Timing and Initiation of Palliative Care

In patients with progressive fibrotic ILDs, palliative care should be discussed early in the disease course, preferably at the time of diagnosis [6, 33, 35, 36]. Studies in oncology show that early referral to palliative care improves quality of life for patients and caregivers and prolongs survival [37–39]. Until now, this has never been convincingly demonstrated in ILD. Although early palliative care is widely recommended, studies indicate that timing of palliative care referral is highly variable. Acute exacerbations occur in a subgroup of patients with different ILDs and are associated with high mortality. Many times, advance care planning and treatment limitations are not discussed with patients and families, leading to futile medical interventions and patients dying in places that they did not desire. A study in the United States found that only 3.8% of patients received palliative care before admission to the intensive care unit (ICU), while 77% of patients died in the ICU [27]. In another retrospective cohort, only 13.7% of 277 deceased IPF patients had received a palliative care referral [24]. Most patients (71%) were referred within 1 month prior to death [24]. In a European-wide survey, one-third of healthcare providers answered that they start palliative care at an early disease stage, if desired by patients [40]. In contrast, the vast majority of healthcare providers stated that palliative care is usually initiated late in the disease course. In a recent study among healthcare professionals, the most common indications for referral of patients to specialist palliative care were disease progression, high symptom burden, psychological support, hospitalizations, and end of life [41].

Importantly, palliative care can be initiated alongside pharmacological interventions and should not lead to discontinuation of disease-modifying treatment. Nevertheless, in many patients, there will be a transition from more disease-centered to symptom-centered care as the disease progresses [42]. The unpredictable nature and heterogeneous disease course of ILDs may hamper early palliative care interventions. A disease behavior-based algorithm can be used to assess in which patients palliative care is needed [6]. In patients with inevitably progressive fibrosis (e.g., IPF), there is an immediate need for palliative care. In other forms of pulmonary fibrosis, palliative care needs have to be structurally evaluated during follow-up visits to determine the right timing for palliative care referral [6, 35]. Various experts have argued that palliative care should be based on needs, rather than on diagnosis or prognosis [6, 43].

## Palliative Care Needs of Patients with ILD

During the last decade, many studies evaluated patient and caregiver needs [40]. Even though similar needs have emerged in several studies, care needs can obviously differ between patients. Moreover, care needs will likely change during the disease trajectory in individual patients [9]. Thorough assessment of patients' needs and goals of care throughout the disease course is thus essential to enhance personalized supportive care [42, 44]. The 2019 annual report of the British Thoracic Society ILD registry reported that palliative care needs were not routinely assessed in clinical practice. In 62% of patients, palliative care needs were evaluated at the first clinic visit. At follow-up visits, this dropped to 40% [45].

Overall, many patients expressed the wish for timely information about their disease, in general, and, more specifically, future perspectives and prognosis [9, 29, 33, 36, 40, 46–53]. However, some patients mentioned that they wish to be informed more gradually as the disease progresses [9, 49]. Consequently, providing accurate information and education is a complex task for healthcare providers and should be tailored to individual patients' needs and wishes [36]. Patients often experience an increasing symptom burden and deteriorating quality of life over time, especially in advanced disease stages [8, 11, 54]. Symptoms as cough, dyspnea, depression, and fatigue have a significant negative impact on quality of life [10, 11, 55, 56]. Consequently, (better) symptom relief is one of the major care needs reported by patients. Besides, partners of ILD patients also report a high symptom burden, social isolation, frustration, and emotional distress [9, 29, 53, 57, 58]. In one study, more than 50% of partners mentioned that they would appreciate the possibility for psychological support [53]. Thus, palliative care interventions should particularly focus on improving symptom burden and reducing psychological distress, for patients as well as their partners [6]. Other frequently reported (unmet) needs of ILD patients are emotional and practical support throughout the disease course, access to ILD specialists, and access to palliative and end-of-life care support [40].

Structured tools may help to identify palliative care needs and facilitate early palliative care interventions in clinical practice. Several questionnaires for palliative care needs assessment have been developed for patients with cancer, but most have not yet been validated in ILD [59–62]. The needs assessment tool:progressive disease-cancer (NAT:PD-C) has been adapted and validated for patients with ILD (NAT:PD-ILD) [62]. The NAT:PD-ILD is a communication and decision tool which comprises sections on patients well-being, caregivers' needs and well-being, and priority for referral to specialist palliative care [63]. This tool seems valid and reliable in ILD, but implementation studies are still ongoing [64]. In a single-center study, the introduction of a simple "supportive care decision aid tool" resulted in better identification of patients with palliative care needs and seemed to increase referral rates to specialist palliative care [65].

## Palliative Care Organization

Palliative care is an integral part of comprehensive care for patients with ILD throughout the disease course. The optimal composition of a multidisciplinary palliative care team for ILD patients has not been studied and depends on various factors, such as cultural aspects and local resources [6]. In some centers, palliative care is mostly provided by ILD specialists, and in other centers, palliative care specialists have a more prominent role [41]. To cover all aspects of supportive care, psychologists, physiotherapists, dieticians, and social workers may also be involved. Respondents of a recent survey suggested that dedicated ILD nurse specialists should follow palliative care training programs and function as the main contact for patients to optimize supportive care and ensure continuity of care [41]. Other studies also indicated that the involvement of ILD nurse specialists is much appreciated by patients and can improve quality of care [47, 53]. However, it should be noted that ILD nurse specialists are not available in all countries and mainly work in ILD specialist centers [41, 53].

## Supportive Measures

### *Supplemental Oxygen*

Oxygen therapy is an important component of supportive care for patients with ILD [66]. Current guidelines recommend long-term oxygen therapy (LTOT) for patients with severe resting hypoxemia, though based on limited evidence. These recommendations are mainly based on data from chronic obstructive pulmonary disease (COPD), due to the lack of ILD-specific studies [21]. However, it can be questioned if data from COPD can be extrapolated to patients with ILD, as patient populations are significantly different. For example, a retrospective study found that exertional hypoxemia was more frequent and severe in patients with fibrotic ILD compared to a matched cohort of COPD patients [67]. Moreover, survival after initiation of LTOT is significantly worse for patients with ILD compared to COPD [68].

The main goals of supplemental oxygen in ILD are to improve functional capacity and physical symptoms (e.g., dyspnea, fatigue, impaired exercise tolerance) and to prolong survival [66, 69]. The decision whether to start supplemental oxygen should always be made together with patients and caregivers, balancing the potential benefits and burden. Several qualitative studies revealed that patients may have mixed feelings regarding oxygen therapy. The initiation of oxygen is regarded as an important marking of disease deterioration for patients, where also disease becomes more visible for the outside world [46]. Besides this, practical limitations and acceptance issues may play a role [9, 46, 70]. On the other hand, patients mentioned that the use of supplemental oxygen improved physical symptoms and exercise tolerance and helped them to feel more in control [46, 70, 71].

One crossover randomized trial investigated the effect of ambulatory oxygen on quality of life in ILD patients with exertional hypoxemia. Ambulatory oxygen reduced dyspnea scores and improved health-related quality of life after 2 weeks [71]. In a recent Delphi study, the majority of ILD experts recommended ambulatory oxygen for patients with exertional hypoxemia and impaired exercise tolerance [66]. Resting hypoxemia can be defined as partial pressure of arterial oxygen (PaO2) of <55 mmHg, oxygen saturation measured by pulse oximetry <89%, or PaO2 of <60 mmHg in combination with cor pulmonale and/or polycythemia [66]. Further studies are needed to assess long-term effects of supplementary oxygen on symptoms and quality of life. A pilot study recently demonstrated that a triple-blinded randomized trial, using portable oxygen concentrators for a longer period of time, seems feasible in patients with fibrotic ILD [72]. A randomized trial (PFOX) is currently being conducted to evaluate whether ambulatory oxygen will increase physical activity, HRQOL, and symptoms in patients with pulmonary fibrosis after 6 months [73]. Whether nocturnal oxygen has beneficial effects on quality of life and survival remains to be elucidated [69]. Nevertheless, in the abovementioned Delphi study, there was consensus among ILD experts to recommend oxygen suppletion for patients with nocturnal hypoxemia, after exclusion of other potential causes [66].

## *Pulmonary Rehabilitation*

Pulmonary rehabilitation aims at reducing symptoms, improving physical activity, and optimizing quality of life in patients with chronic respiratory diseases [74]. Pulmonary rehabilitation is a comprehensive and multidisciplinary intervention. Besides exercise training, pulmonary rehabilitation often includes education, psychosocial support, and nutrition advices [21, 69, 74]. Current guidelines in IPF provide a weak recommendation for pulmonary rehabilitation in the majority of patients, based on low-quality evidence [21]. The 2013 ATS/ERS statement on pulmonary rehabilitation states that pulmonary rehabilitation can lead to meaningful improvement in quality of life for patients with ILD, but observed changes are usually smaller than seen in patients with COPD [74].

A 2014 Cochrane review found that pulmonary rehabilitation improved exercise capacity, symptoms, and quality of life in patients with ILD [75]. Effects were comparable in a subgroup of patients with IPF [75]. None of the included randomized controlled trials reported any adverse events, implying that pulmonary rehabilitation is a safe option for patients with ILD. These results have been confirmed by more recent randomized trials. A study in a range of ILDs (IPF, asbestosis, ILD associated with connective tissue disease) showed that health-related quality of life, dyspnea, and 6-minute walking distance improved after an 8-week supervised exercise program [76]. In patients with relatively mild disease, these effects sustained after 6 months. A randomized controlled trial in 54 patients with IPF demonstrated that a 3-week inpatient pulmonary rehabilitation program improved quality of life and 6-minute walking distance compared to usual care. After 3 months, quality of life and exercise capacity remained better in the intervention group [77]. Pulmonary rehabilitation seems to have more profound effects in early disease stages in patients with IPF [77, 78]. Referral to pulmonary rehabilitation should not be discouraged in advanced disease stages, but potential benefits and burden need to be discussed together with patients. Current pulmonary rehabilitation programs are mainly focused on COPD. Both patients and clinicians highlighted the need for ILD-specific pulmonary rehabilitation programs [50, 79], especially with regard to the educational content. The optimal content, duration, and long-term effects of pulmonary rehabilitation programs in ILD have not been extensively studied and need further research.

## *Symptom Relief (Table 11.1)*

### Dyspnea

Dyspnea is present in almost all patients with ILD [7]. Severe breathlessness is associated with a poor quality of life and prognosis [10, 56]. As discussed above, supplemental oxygen and pulmonary rehabilitation can both have beneficial effects on dyspnea in ILD [71, 75, 76]. Unfortunately, further treatment options are limited, and studies focusing on relief of dyspnea in patients with ILD are scarce.

Comorbidities such as obstructive sleep apnea, cardiac disease, pulmonary hypertension, infections, and anxiety may worsen dyspnea and should be optimally managed [6]. Antifibrotic drugs do not have significant beneficial effects on dyspnea in IPF [69]. Moreover, a combination of nintedanib and sildenafil did not improve dyspnea or quality-of-life scores in a randomized trial of IPF patients with advanced functional impairment (diffusion capacity of the lungs for carbon monoxide <35%) [80]. Widely used pharmacological treatment options for dyspnea are low-dose opioids and benzodiazepines. Patients and clinicians may be hesitant to use opioids because of fear of opioid dependency or respiratory drive depression [6]. A large longitudinal cohort study among 1600 patients with oxygen-dependent fibrotic ILDs showed an acceptable safety profile of opioids and low-dose benzodiazepines [81]. Both drugs were not associated with increased hospital admissions or mortality when used in low doses. The use of high-dose benzodiazepines (≥15 mg oral oxazepam equivalent) was associated with increased mortality, whereas the use of high-dose opioids (≥30 mg oral morphine equivalent) was not. This study supports the use of opioids and low-dose benzodiazepines to manage dyspnea in patients with advanced fibrotic ILD from a safety perspective, but does not draw any

**Table 11.1** Overview of potential management options for symptom relief in ILD

| | Pharmacological management | Non-pharmacological management |
|---|---|---|
| Dyspnea | Treat any reversible causes, e.g., infection or pulmonary hypertension | Cool air fan |
| | Low-dose opioids | Relaxation and breathing exercises |
| | Benzodiazepines if anxiety-related breathlessness is present | Pulmonary rehabilitation |
| | Supplemental oxygen | Positioning |
| | Bronchodilators if airflow limitation present | Reassurance |
| | | Cognitive behavioral therapy or psychotherapy |
| | | Energy conservation or pacing activities |
| | | Loose clothing |
| | | Mouth care |
| | | Breathlessness intervention service |
| Cough | Treat any reversible causes or comorbidities, e.g., infection, COPD, or angiotensin- converting enzyme inhibitors | Lifestyle advice – eat small meals and earlier in day |
| | Rhinitis therapy if indicated – oral antihistamine with or without decongestant | Speech therapy |
| | Anti-reflux therapy (high-dose proton pump inhibitor and H2 antagonists) | |
| | Prokinetic therapy, if esophageal dysfunction is suspected | |
| | Low-dose opioids, including codeine | |
| | Gabapentin | |
| | Low-dose prednisolone | |
| | Antifibrotic treatment | |
| | Simple linctus or codeine linctus | |
| Fatigue | Treat secondary underlying causes such as sleep apnea, anemia, venous thromboembolism, infection, dehydration, diabetes mellitus, or hypothyroidism | Pulmonary rehabilitation |
| | Supplemental oxygen | Cognitive behavioral or mindfulness-based therapy |
| Depression and anxiety | Antidepressants | Psychological counseling and cognitive behavioral therapy |
| | Anxiolytics | Pulmonary rehabilitation |
| | | Patient and partner support program |
| | | Multidisciplinary palliative care intervention |
| | | Guided self-help program |
| Weight loss | Low-dose prednisolone | Dietary evaluation including protein supplementation |
| | | Pulmonary rehabilitation |

**Table 11.1** (continued)

| | Pharmacological management | Non-pharmacological management |
|---|---|---|
| Pain | Paracetamol | Pulmonary rehabilitation |
| | Codeine | |
| | Low-dose opioids | |
| Miscellaneous | | Patient education |
| | | Patient support groups |
| | | Family reassurance |
| | | Assess patients' coping strategies, where necessary facilitate the development of new effective strategies to help patients regain a sense of control (e.g., staying active, taking a walk, engaging in social relationships) |
| | | Advise patients and families where to seek financial and practical support |
| | | Arrange support from appropriate spiritual advisers |
| | | Participation in research programs |
| | | Individualized case conference model of care |

Adapted with permission from Kreuter et al. [6]

conclusions regarding efficacy [81]. In a small retrospective study, all ILD patients who used opioids and benzodiazepines in a palliative setting experienced beneficial effects [28]. A recent single-center RCT analyzed the safety and efficacy of low-dose morphine on dyspnea and cough in 36 patients with pulmonary fibrosis. The first results of this study showed that 1 week of low-dose morphine improved cough scores and tended to improve 6-minute walking distance, but did not reduce dyspnea [82]. Larger trials evaluating the efficacy of benzodiazepines and morphine on symptom relief in ILD are needed. A recent feasibility study evaluated the safety of mirtazapine in patient with COPD or ILD and severe breathlessness. Outcomes of this study indicate that mirtazapine is safe and well-tolerated; a phase III efficacy study is currently ongoing [83]. A randomized study in 105 patients with dyspnea due to advanced disease (19 ILD patients) found that a breathlessness support service improved breathlessness mastery and survival after 6 months compared to usual care [84]. The multidisciplinary breathlessness support service integrated palliative care assessment and management, respiratory care, physiotherapy, and occupational therapy and included both hospital and home visits. Even though the number of ILD patients in this study was small, these data support early integration of respiratory and palliative care services in ILD; the impact on survival needs further study. Other recommended non-pharmacological treatment options for dyspnea are handheld air fans, relaxation therapy, and cognitive behavioral therapy [6].

## Cough

Chronic cough is one of the most debilitating symptoms in ILD patients, with a reported prevalence of up to 94% [7, 69, 85]. Cough has a major impact on quality of life of patients and their partners and may lead to social isolation and psychological distress. Until now, no effective therapies exist. Comorbidities such as gastroesophageal reflux, obstructive sleep apnea, rhinosinusitis, postnasal drip, and infections can induce or perpetuate cough. Moreover, medication use (i.e., angiotensin-converting enzyme inhibitors) is also a known cause of chronic cough. Thus, the first step in the evaluation and treatment of cough in ILD is to treat any reversible causes and/or comorbidities, if present [6, 86]. Nonetheless, treatment of comorbidities may not always lead to reduction of cough. Studies evaluating the effects of anti-acid therapy on gastroesophageal reflux-related cough showed conflicting results. An observational study in a small number of patients found that the use of a proton pump inhibitor decreased acid reflux. Surprisingly, no changes in objective and subjective cough measures were observed, which may be related to the paradoxical increase in non-acid reflux [87]. One randomized trial revealed that omeprazole reduced objective cough frequency, but did not improve cough-related quality of life. Besides, the incidence of lower respiratory tract infections seemed to increase in patients using omeprazole [88].

Cough in ILD is often refractory to conventional antitussive therapies, such as linctus or codeine tablets. Nevertheless, antitussives are frequently prescribed as they have beneficial effects in some patients [86]. Furthermore, low-dose prednisolone or neuromodulators such as gabapentin may be considered, although it is important to note that studies in ILD are lacking. A small single-center randomized trial conducted in 2012 found that thalidomide reduced cough and improved cough-related quality of life in IPF [89]. However, the use of thalidomide was associated with a high incidence of adverse events. Since then, no follow-up studies have been performed to validate these findings and evaluate the balance between effects and side effects; consequently, thalidomide should not be used as therapy for cough in IPF or other ILDs. An observational non-randomized trial in IPF indicated that pirfenidone may improve cough-related quality of life and decrease objective cough counts [90]. The effects of nintedanib on cough have never been prospectively studied. Inhaled sodium cromoglicate (PA101) has emerged as another promising pharmacological treatment option for chronic cough in IPF; a phase II trial showed that PA101 reduced cough frequency by 31% after 2 weeks and was well-tolerated by patients [91]. In patients with systemic sclerosis-associated ILD, long-term treatment with mycophenolate mofetil and cyclophosphamide seemed to reduce cough frequency, but had no effects on cough-related quality of life [92]. Speech and language therapy has shown to reduce cough frequency and improve cough-related quality of life in patients with chronic cough [93]. Although not specifically evaluated in patients with ILD, speech therapy could be considered in patients who do not respond to antitussive medication [86].

## Fatigue

Fatigue is one of the most frequent and burdensome symptoms in ILD, present in up to 95% of patients [94]. In most patients, the cause of fatigue is multifactorial; fatigue has both physical and mental components (perceived fatigability) [95]. Behavioral and social aspects, psychological distress, physical factors, comorbidities, and side effects of medication can all play a role [95–97]. Moreover, fatigue seems to be related to disease severity in some ILDs [98, 99]. Hence, evaluation and treatment of fatigue should target multiple domains. Common comorbidities associated with fatigue are obstructive sleep apnea, thyroid disorders, diabetes mellitus, and anemia [94]. Two studies in IPF patients with obstructive sleep apnea showed that treatment with continuous positive airway pressure (CPAP) significantly improved fatigue, quality of life, and activities of daily living [100, 101]. As discussed previously, pulmonary rehabilitation can also lead to a reduction in fatigue in patients with ILD [76, 102]. In patients with concurrent anxiety, stress, or depressive symptoms, referral to a psychologist can be considered. Cognitive behavioral or mindfulness-based therapies have also been proposed as treatment option for fatigue in ILD, but prospective studies are currently lacking [94, 103]. Furthermore, no pharmacological interventions exist for treatment of fatigue in ILD. Because of the high prevalence and negative impact of fatigue on daily lives of patients and their families, assessment and treatment of fatigue need to be integrated in palliative care programs.

## Depression, Anxiety, and General Well-being

Depression and anxiety may occur in up to 50% of patients with ILD [7, 69]. Both are significantly associated with other symptoms, especially dyspnea, cough and fatigue, comorbidities, and functional status [94, 104–107]. Dyspnea is related to anxiety in a bidirectional way; anxiety can cause increasing dyspnea, but dyspnea can also lead to more anxiety and depression [10, 69, 104, 106]. No specific interventions for anxiety and depression have been studied in ILD. Anxiolytics and antidepressants are rarely prescribed but could be a reasonable treatment option, preferably after an appropriate psychiatric evaluation [6].

Other proposed treatment options are psychological counseling and cognitive behavioral therapy [69]. A patient and partner empowerment program for IPF, consisting of three group sessions led by a psychologist, improved short-term health-related quality of life and tended to reduce anxiety and depressive symptoms compared to usual care in a single-center study [108]. A randomized feasibility trial in patients with advanced fibrotic ILD evaluated a case conference intervention (Hospital2Home) led by a palliative care nurse specialist [109]. The multidisciplinary Hospital2Home intervention included assessment of palliative care needs and concerns and discussion of end-of-life preferences. During a case conference at the patient's home, involved healthcare providers, patients, and caregivers agreed upon an individualized care plan. Subsequently, regular follow-up phone calls were conducted. This intervention significantly improved palliative care concerns, anxiety, depression, and quality of life after 4 weeks [109]. In contrast, a recent pilot study in 22 IPF patients found that referral to a palliative care clinic had no beneficial effects on quality of life, anxiety, and depression after 6 months and may even lead to worsening of symptoms [110]. However, as this was a pilot study in a small number of patients, no conclusions can be drawn regarding efficacy of the palliative care intervention. Moreover, the majority of patients only received one palliative care visit during the 6-month study period. Thus, it could be hypothesized that patients with IPF may benefit from a more longitudinal follow-up [110]. The authors further concluded that palliative care interventions are often heterogeneous and difficult to standardize. Relatively similar results were found in a 6-week disease management program for patients and caregivers, led by an ILD specialist nurse. Patients who participated in the program tended to have higher anxiety levels and lower health-related quality-of-life scores than patients who received standard care [111]. Nevertheless, patient satisfaction was high; patients felt less lonely, were able to put their disease better into perspective, and considered the sessions very beneficial. Besides, caregivers had decreased stress levels after 6 weeks. The main goal of this study was to obtain data to inform the design and sample size of a future trial; hence, this study was underpowered to reliably evaluate between-group differences [111]. A larger randomized controlled trial of a multidisciplinary palliative care intervention for patients with IPF and their caregivers (SUPPORT) is currently ongoing and will hopefully provide a more definite answer on the effects of early palliative care on quality of life, symptom burden, stress, advance care planning, and healthcare resource use [112].

## End-of-Life Care

Palliative care aims at optimizing quality of life as well as quality of dying. To facilitate a dignified death, timely advance care planning is essential. Advance care planning includes conversations about end-of-life issues, such as treatment limitations and preferred place of death. Patient preferences and wishes should be well-documented and regularly evaluated at outpatient clinic visits [35]. As mentioned previously, this process should be tailored to individual patients' needs, as some patients wish to receive more gradual information about end-of-life care during the disease course [9].

Several studies found that the majority of IPF patients worldwide currently die in the hospital, even though most patients prefer to die at home [24, 26, 113, 114]. The reported percentage of patients dying in the ICU varies from 7% to 33% [24, 113]. It is likely that cultural differences play a role in the location of death, as it seems that fewer patients in Europe die in the ICU and more patients die at home than in the United States [113]. One retrospective study in IPF showed that a multidisciplinary integrated palliative care approach, including early advance care planning discussions, was associated with fewer hospitalizations and emergency room visits in the last year of life [115]. Moreover, implementation of the program significantly increased the percentage of patients who died at home. In a UK ILD center, the implementation of a decision aid tool in daily practice significantly increased the documentation of end-of-life decisions (from 15.7% to 91.8%) [65]. Two studies indicated that end-of-life decisions are less frequently reported in ILD compared to cancer patients [20, 116]. Furthermore, ILD patients had a higher symptom burden at the end of life and were less likely to die in a palliative care setting [116]. A potential reason is that death is more likely to be unexpected in ILD patients, due to the heterogeneous and sometimes unpredictable disease course also including acute exacerbations [116]. This further emphasizes the importance of early advance care planning, especially in patients with progressive fibrotic ILD.

## Conclusion

Patients with progressive fibrotic ILD have a high and increasing symptom burden with dyspnea, cough, fatigue, and anxiety being the most important symptoms. Disease course is often unpredictable, and survival may be similar or worse to many oncological conditions. Nevertheless, there is a paucity of evidence to support specific palliative care interventions in ILD, though awareness and ILD-specific studies are increasing. Timely conversations and explanation about the role of palliative care measures, together with advance care planning, are key to improve quality of life and quality of dying for patients with ILD and their families.

## References

1. Wijsenbeek M, Cottin V. Spectrum of fibrotic lung diseases. N Engl J Med. 2020;383(10):958–68.
2. Travis WD, Costabel U, Hansell DM, King TE Jr, Lynch DA, Nicholson AG, et al. An official American Thoracic Society/European Respiratory Society statement: update of the international multidisciplinary classification of the idiopathic interstitial pneumonias. Am J Respir Crit Care Med. 2013;188(6):733–48.
3. Cottin V, Wollin L, Fischer A, Quaresma M, Stowasser S, Harari S. Fibrosing interstitial lung diseases: knowns and unknowns. Eur Respir Rev. 2019;28(151)
4. Lederer DJ, Martinez FJ. Idiopathic pulmonary fibrosis. N Engl J Med. 2018;378(19):1811–23.
5. Mortality GBD, Causes of Death C. Global, regional, and national life expectancy, all-cause mortality, and cause-specific mortality for 249 causes of death, 1980-2015: a systematic analysis for the Global Burden of Disease Study 2015. Lancet. 2016;388(10053):1459–544.
6. Kreuter M, Bendstrup E, Russell AM, Bajwah S, Lindell K, Adir Y, et al. Palliative care in interstitial lung disease: living well. Lancet Respir Med. 2017;5(12):968–80.
7. Carvajalino S, Reigada C, Johnson MJ, Dzingina M, Bajwah S. Symptom prevalence of patients with fibrotic interstitial lung disease: a systematic literature review. BMC Pulm Med. 2018;18(1):78.

8. Rajala K, Lehto JT, Sutinen E, Kautiainen H, Myllärniemi M, Saarto T. Marked deterioration in the quality of life of patients with idiopathic pulmonary fibrosis during the last two years of life. BMC Pulm Med. 2018;18(1):172.
9. Sampson C, Gill BH, Harrison NK, Nelson A, Byrne A. The care needs of patients with idiopathic pulmonary fibrosis and their carers (CaNoPy): results of a qualitative study. BMC Pulm Med. 2015;15:155.
10. Glaspole IN, Chapman SA, Cooper WA, Ellis SJ, Goh NS, Hopkins PM, et al. Health-related quality of life in idiopathic pulmonary fibrosis: data from the Australian IPF Registry. Respirology. 2017;22(5):950–6.
11. Kreuter M, Swigris J, Pittrow D, Geier S, Klotsche J, Prasse A, et al. Health related quality of life in patients with idiopathic pulmonary fibrosis in clinical practice: insights-IPF registry. Respir Res. 2017;18(1):139.
12. Natalini JG, Swigris JJ, Morisset J, Elicker BM, Jones KD, Fischer A, et al. Understanding the determinants of health-related quality of life in rheumatoid arthritis-associated interstitial lung disease. Respir Med. 2017;127:1–6.
13. King TE Jr, Bradford WZ, Castro-Bernardini S, Fagan EA, Glaspole I, Glassberg MK, et al. A phase 3 trial of pirfenidone in patients with idiopathic pulmonary fibrosis. N Engl J Med. 2014;370(22):2083–92.
14. Richeldi L, du Bois RM, Raghu G, Azuma A, Brown KK, Costabel U, et al. Efficacy and safety of nintedanib in idiopathic pulmonary fibrosis. N Engl J Med. 2014;370(22):2071–82.
15. Distler O, Highland KB, Gahlemann M, Azuma A, Fischer A, Mayes MD, et al. Nintedanib for systemic sclerosis-associated interstitial lung disease. N Engl J Med. 2019;
16. Flaherty KR, Wells AU, Cottin V, Devaraj A, Walsh SLF, Inoue Y, et al. Nintedanib in progressive fibrosing interstitial lung diseases. N Engl J Med. 2019;381(18):1718–27.
17. Brown AW, Kaya H, Nathan SD. Lung transplantation in IIP: a review. Respirology. 2016;21(7):1173–84.
18. Kourliouros A, Hogg R, Mehew J, Al-Aloul M, Carby M, Lordan JL, et al. Patient outcomes from time of listing for lung transplantation in the UK: are there disease-specific differences? Thorax. 2019;74(1):60–8.
19. World Health Organization. WHO Definition of Palliative Care: World Health Organizaiton; 2019. Available from: https://www.who.int/cancer/palliative/definition/en/.
20. Brown CE, Engelberg RA, Nielsen EL, Curtis JR. Palliative care for patients dying in the intensive care unit with chronic lung disease compared with metastatic cancer. Ann Am Thorac Soc. 2016;13(5):684–9.
21. Raghu G, Collard HR, Egan JJ, Martinez FJ, Behr J, Brown KK, et al. An official ATS/ERS/JRS/ALAT statement: idiopathic pulmonary fibrosis: evidence-based guidelines for diagnosis and management. Am J Respir Crit Care Med. 2011;183(6):788–824.
22. NICE Guidance. Idiopathic pulmonary fibrosis in adults: quality standard; 2015. Available from: https://www.nice.org.uk/guidance/qs79/chapter/Quality-statement-5-Palliative-care.
23. Kim JW, Atkins C, Wilson AM. Barriers to specialist palliative care in interstitial lung disease: a systematic review. BMJ Support Palliat Care. 2019;9(2):130–8.
24. Lindell KO, Liang Z, Hoffman LA, Rosenzweig MQ, Saul MI, Pilewski JM, et al. Palliative care and location of death in decedents with idiopathic pulmonary fibrosis. Chest. 2015;147(2):423–9.
25. Rush B, Berger L, Anthony CL. Access to palliative care for patients undergoing mechanical ventilation with idiopathic pulmonary fibrosis in the United States. Am J Hosp Palliat Care. 2018;35(3):492–6.
26. Rajala K, Lehto JT, Saarinen M, Sutinen E, Saarto T, Myllarniemi M. End-of-life care of patients with idiopathic pulmonary fibrosis. BMC Palliat Care. 2016;15(1):85.
27. Liang Z, Hoffman LA, Nouraie M, Kass DJ, Donahoe MP, Gibson KF, et al. Referral to palliative care infrequent in patients with idiopathic pulmonary fibrosis admitted to an intensive care unit. J Palliat Med. 2017;20(2):134–40.
28. Bajwah S, Higginson IJ, Ross JR, Wells AU, Birring SS, Patel A, et al. Specialist palliative care is more than drugs: a retrospective study of ILD patients. Lung. 2012;190(2):215–20.

29. Lindell KO, Kavalieratos D, Gibson KF, Tycon L, Rosenzweig M. The palliative care needs of patients with idiopathic pulmonary fibrosis: a qualitative study of patients and family caregivers. Heart Lung. 2017;46(1):24–9.
30. Mc Veigh C, Reid J, Larkin P, Porter S, Hudson P. The experience of palliative care service provision for people with non-malignant respiratory disease and their family carers: an all-Ireland qualitative study. J Adv Nurs. 2018;74(2):383–94.
31. Sørensen AR, Marsaa K, Prior TS, Bendstrup E. Attitude and barriers in palliative care and advance care planning in nonmalignant chronic lung disease: results from a Danish National Survey. J Palliat Care. 2020;825859720936012
32. Barril S, Alonso A, Rodríguez-Portal JA, Viladot M, Giner J, Aparicio F, et al. Palliative Care in Diffuse Interstitial Lund Disease: Results of a Spanish Survey Cuidados paliativos en la enfermedad pulmonar intersticial difusa: resultados de una encuesta de ámbito nacional. Arch Bronconeumol. 2018;54(3):123–7.
33. Bonella F, Wijsenbeek M, Molina-Molina M, Duck A, Mele R, Geissler K, et al. European IPF Patient Charter: unmet needs and a call to action for healthcare policymakers. Eur Respir J. 2016;47(2):597–606.
34. Colman R, Singer LG, Barua R, Downar J. Outcomes of lung transplant candidates referred for co-management by palliative care: a retrospective case series. Palliat Med. 2015;29(5):429–35.
35. Danoff SK, Schonhoft EH. Role of support measures and palliative care. Curr Opin Pulm Med. 2013;19(5):480–4.
36. Bajwah S, Koffman J, Higginson IJ, Ross JR, Wells AU, Birring SS, et al. 'I wish I knew more …' the end-of-life planning and information needs for end-stage fibrotic interstitial lung disease: views of patients, carers and health professionals. BMJ Support Palliat Care. 2013;3(1):84–90.
37. Temel JS, Greer JA, Muzikansky A, Gallagher ER, Admane S, Jackson VA, et al. Early palliative care for patients with metastatic non-small-cell lung cancer. N Engl J Med. 2010;363(8):733–42.
38. Bakitas MA, Tosteson TD, Li Z, Lyons KD, Hull JG, Li Z, et al. Early versus delayed initiation of concurrent palliative oncology care: patient outcomes in the ENABLE III randomized controlled trial. J Clin Oncol. 2015;33(13):1438–45.
39. Dionne-Odom JN, Azuero A, Lyons KD, Hull JG, Tosteson T, Li Z, et al. Benefits of early versus delayed palliative care to informal family caregivers of patients with advanced cancer: outcomes from the ENABLE III randomized controlled trial. J Clin Oncol. 2015;33(13):1446–52.
40. Moor CC, Wijsenbeek MS, Balestro E, Biondini D, Bondue B, Cottin V, et al. Gaps in care of patients living with pulmonary fibrosis: a joint patient and expert statement on the results of a Europe-wide survey. ERJ Open Res. 2019;5:4.
41. Kim JW, Olive S, Jones S, Thillai M, Russell AM, Johnson MJ, et al. Interstitial lung disease and specialist palliative care access: a healthcare professionals survey. BMJ Support Palliat Care. 2020;
42. Lee JS, McLaughlin S, Collard HR. Comprehensive care of the patient with idiopathic pulmonary fibrosis. Curr Opin Pulm Med. 2011;17(5):348–54.
43. Higginson IJ, Addington-Hall JM. Palliative care needs to be provided on basis of need rather than diagnosis. BMJ. 1999;318(7176):123.
44. van Manen MJ, Geelhoed JJ, Tak NC, Wijsenbeek MS. Optimizing quality of life in patients with idiopathic pulmonary fibrosis. Ther Adv Respir Dis. 2017;11(3):157–69.
45. British Thoracic Society. BTS ILD Registry; 2019. Available from: https://www.nice.org.uk/guidance/qs79/chapter/Quality-statement-5-Palliative-care.
46. Duck A, Spencer LG, Bailey S, Leonard C, Ormes J, Caress AL. Perceptions, experiences and needs of patients with idiopathic pulmonary fibrosis. J Adv Nurs. 2015;71(5):1055–65.
47. Russell AM, Ripamonti E, Vancheri C. Qualitative European survey of patients with idiopathic pulmonary fibrosis: patients' perspectives of the disease and treatment. BMC Pulm Med. 2016;16:10.

48. Schoenheit G, Becattelli I, Cohen AH. Living with idiopathic pulmonary fibrosis: an in-depth qualitative survey of European patients. Chron Respir Dis. 2011;8(4):225–31.
49. Overgaard D, Kaldan G, Marsaa K, Nielsen TL, Shaker SB, Egerod I. The lived experience with idiopathic pulmonary fibrosis: a qualitative study. Eur Respir J. 2016;47(5):1472–80.
50. Morisset J, Dube BP, Garvey C, Bourbeau J, Collard HR, Swigris JJ, et al. The unmet educational needs of patients with interstitial lung disease. Setting the stage for tailored pulmonary rehabilitation. Ann Am Thorac Soc. 2016;13(7):1026–33.
51. Ramadurai D, Corder S, Churney T, Graney B, Harshman A, Meadows S, et al. Understanding the informational needs of patients with IPF and their caregivers: 'You get diagnosed, and you ask this question right away, what does this mean?'. BMJ Open Qual. 2018;7(1):e000207.
52. Cottin V, Bourdin A, Crestani B, Prevot G, Guerin M, Bouquillon B. Healthcare pathway and patients' expectations in pulmonary fibrosis. ERJ Open Res. 2017;3(2)
53. van Manen MJ, Kreuter M, van den Blink B, Oltmanns U, Palmowski K, Brunnemer E, et al. What patients with pulmonary fibrosis and their partners think: a live, educative survey in the Netherlands and Germany. ERJ Open Res. 2017;3(1)
54. Kreuter M, Wuyts WA, Wijsenbeek M, Bajwah S, Maher TM, Stowasser S, et al. Health-related quality of life and symptoms in patients with IPF treated with nintedanib: analyses of patient-reported outcomes from the INPULSIS(R) trials. Respir Res. 2020;21(1):36.
55. Yount SE, Beaumont JL, Chen SY, Kaiser K, Wortman K, Van Brunt DL, et al. Health-related quality of life in patients with idiopathic pulmonary fibrosis. Lung. 2016;194(2):227–34.
56. Rajala K, Lehto JT, Sutinen E, Kautiainen H, Myllarniemi M, Saarto T. mMRC dyspnoea scale indicates impaired quality of life and increased pain in patients with idiopathic pulmonary fibrosis. ERJ Open Res. 2017;3(4)
57. Shah RJ, Collard HR, Morisset J. Burden, resilience and coping in caregivers of patients with interstitial lung disease. Heart Lung. 2018;47(3):264–8.
58. Belkin A, Albright K, Swigris JJ. A qualitative study of informal caregivers' perspectives on the effects of idiopathic pulmonary fibrosis. BMJ Open Respir Res. 2014;1(1):e000007.
59. Hearn J, Higginson IJ. Development and validation of a core outcome measure for palliative care: the palliative care outcome scale. Palliative Care Core Audit Project Advisory Group. Qual Health Care. 1999;8(4):219–27.
60. Highet G, Crawford D, Murray SA, Boyd K. Development and evaluation of the Supportive and Palliative Care Indicators Tool (SPICT): a mixed-methods study. BMJ Support Palliat Care. 2014;4(3):285–90.
61. Groenvold M, Petersen MA, Aaronson NK, Arraras JI, Blazeby JM, Bottomley A, et al. The development of the EORTC QLQ-C15-PAL: a shortened questionnaire for cancer patients in palliative care. Eur J Cancer. 2006;42(1):55–64.
62. Boland JW, Reigada C, Yorke J, Hart SP, Bajwah S, Ross J, et al. The adaptation, face, and content validation of a needs assessment tool: progressive disease for people with interstitial lung disease. J Palliat Med. 2016;19(5):549–55.
63. Reigada C, Papadopoulos A, Boland JW, Yorke J, Ross J, Currow DC, et al. Implementation of the Needs Assessment Tool for patients with interstitial lung disease (NAT:ILD): facilitators and barriers. Thorax. 2017;72(11):1049–51.
64. Johnson MJ, Jamali A, Ross J, Fairhurst C, Boland J, Reigada C, et al. Psychometric validation of the needs assessment tool: progressive disease in interstitial lung disease. Thorax. 2018;73(9):880–3.
65. Sharp C, Lamb H, Jordan N, Edwards A, Gunary R, Meek P, et al. Development of tools to facilitate palliative and supportive care referral for patients with idiopathic pulmonary fibrosis. BMJ Support Palliat Care. 2018;8(3):340–6.
66. Lim RK, Humphreys C, Morisset J, Holland AE, Johannson KA, Collaborators OD. Oxygen in patients with fibrotic interstitial lung disease: an international Delphi survey. Eur Respir J. 2019;54(2)
67. Du Plessis JP, Fernandes S, Jamal R, Camp P, Johannson K, Schaeffer M, et al. Exertional hypoxemia is more severe in fibrotic interstitial lung disease than in COPD. Respirology. 2018;23(4):392–8.

68. Rantala HA, Leivo-Korpela S, Lehtimaki L, Lehto JT. Predictors of impaired survival in subjects with long-term oxygen therapy. Respir Care. 2019;64(11):1401–9.
69. Wijsenbeek MS, Holland AE, Swigris JJ, Renzoni EA. Comprehensive supportive care for patients with fibrosing interstitial lung disease. Am J Respir Crit Care Med. 2019;200(2):152–9.
70. Khor YH, Goh NSL, McDonald CF, Holland AE. Oxygen therapy for interstitial lung disease. A mismatch between patient expectations and experiences. Ann Am Thorac Soc. 2017;14(6):888–95.
71. Visca D, Mori L, Tsipouri V, Fleming S, Firouzi A, Bonini M, et al. Effect of ambulatory oxygen on quality of life for patients with fibrotic lung disease (AmbOx): a prospective, open-label, mixed-method, crossover randomised controlled trial. Lancet Respir Med. 2018;6(10):759–70.
72. Khor YH, Holland AE, Goh NS, Miller BR, Vlahos R, Bozinovski S, et al. Ambulatory oxygen in fibrotic ILD: a pilot, randomised, triple-blinded, sham-controlled trial. Chest. 2020;
73. Khor YH, Smith DJF, Johannson KA, Renzoni E. Oxygen for interstitial lung diseases. Curr Opin Pulm Med. 2020;26(5):464–9.
74. Spruit MA, Singh SJ, Garvey C, ZuWallack R, Nici L, Rochester C, et al. An official American Thoracic Society/European Respiratory Society statement: key concepts and advances in pulmonary rehabilitation. Am J Respir Crit Care Med. 2013;188(8):e13–64.
75. Dowman L, Hill CJ, Holland AE. Pulmonary rehabilitation for interstitial lung disease. Cochrane Database Syst Rev. 2014;10:CD006322.
76. Dowman LM, McDonald CF, Hill CJ, Lee AL, Barker K, Boote C, et al. The evidence of benefits of exercise training in interstitial lung disease: a randomised controlled trial. Thorax. 2017;72(7):610–9.
77. Jarosch I, Schneeberger T, Gloeckl R, Kreuter M, Frankenberger M, Neurohr C, et al. Short-term effects of comprehensive pulmonary rehabilitation and its maintenance in patients with idiopathic pulmonary fibrosis: a randomized controlled trial. J Clin Med. 2020;9(5)
78. Holland AE, Hill CJ, Glaspole I, Goh N, McDonald CF. Predictors of benefit following pulmonary rehabilitation for interstitial lung disease. Respir Med. 2012;106(3):429–35.
79. Holland AE, Fiore JF Jr, Goh N, Symons K, Dowman L, Westall G, et al. Be honest and help me prepare for the future: what people with interstitial lung disease want from education in pulmonary rehabilitation. Chron Respir Dis. 2015;12(2):93–101.
80. Kolb M, Raghu G, Wells AU, Behr J, Richeldi L, Schinzel B, et al. Nintedanib plus sildenafil in patients with idiopathic pulmonary fibrosis. N Engl J Med. 2018;379(18):1722–31.
81. Bajwah S, Davies JM, Tanash H, Currow DC, Oluyase AO, Ekstrom M. Safety of benzodiazepines and opioids in interstitial lung disease: a national prospective study. Eur Respir J. 2018;52(6)
82. Kronborg-White SUAC, Hilberg O, Bendstrup E. Oral morphine is safe in symptomatic patients with fibrotic interstitial lung diseases. Eur Respir J. 2019;54:PA1351.
83. Higginson IJ, Wilcock A, Johnson MJ, Bajwah S, Lovell N, Yi D, et al. Randomised, double-blind, multicentre, mixed-methods, dose-escalation feasibility trial of mirtazapine for better treatment of severe breathlessness in advanced lung disease (BETTER-B feasibility). Thorax. 2020;75(2):176–9.
84. Higginson IJ, Bausewein C, Reilly CC, Gao W, Gysels M, Dzingina M, et al. An integrated palliative and respiratory care service for patients with advanced disease and refractory breathlessness: a randomised controlled trial. Lancet Respir Med. 2014;2(12):979–87.
85. Cheng JZ, Wilcox PG, Glaspole I, Corte TJ, Murphy D, Hague CJ, et al. Cough is less common and less severe in systemic sclerosis-associated interstitial lung disease compared to other fibrotic interstitial lung diseases. Respirology. 2017;22(8):1592–7.
86. van Manen MJG, Wijsenbeek MS. Cough, an unresolved problem in interstitial lung diseases. Curr Opin Support Palliat Care. 2019;
87. Kilduff CE, Counter MJ, Thomas GA, Harrison NK, Hope-Gill BD. Effect of acid suppression therapy on gastroesophageal reflux and cough in idiopathic pulmonary fibrosis: an intervention study. Cough. 2014;10:4.

88. Dutta P, Funston W, Mossop H, Ryan V, Jones R, Forbes R, et al. Randomised, double-blind, placebo-controlled pilot trial of omeprazole in idiopathic pulmonary fibrosis. Thorax. 2019;74(4):346–53.
89. Horton MR, Santopietro V, Mathew L, Horton KM, Polito AJ, Liu MC, et al. Thalidomide for the treatment of cough in idiopathic pulmonary fibrosis: a randomized trial. Ann Intern Med. 2012;157(6):398–406.
90. van Manen MJG, Birring SS, Vancheri C, Vindigni V, Renzoni E, Russell AM, et al. Effect of pirfenidone on cough in patients with idiopathic pulmonary fibrosis. Eur Respir J. 2017;50(4)
91. Birring SS, Wijsenbeek MS, Agrawal S, van den Berg JWK, Stone H, Maher TM, et al. A novel formulation of inhaled sodium cromoglicate (PA101) in idiopathic pulmonary fibrosis and chronic cough: a randomised, double-blind, proof-of-concept, phase 2 trial. Lancet Respir Med. 2017;5(10):806–15.
92. Tashkin DP, Volkmann ER, Tseng CH, Roth MD, Khanna D, Furst DE, et al. Improved cough and cough-specific quality of life in patients treated for scleroderma-related interstitial lung disease: results of scleroderma lung study II. Chest. 2017;151(4):813–20.
93. Chamberlain Mitchell SA, Garrod R, Clark L, Douiri A, Parker SM, Ellis J, et al. Physiotherapy, and speech and language therapy intervention for patients with refractory chronic cough: a multicentre randomised control trial. Thorax. 2017;72(2):129–36.
94. Kahlmann V, Moor CC, Wijsenbeek MS. Managing fatigue in patients with interstitial lung disease. Chest. 2020;
95. Sharpe M, Wilks D. Fatigue. BMJ. 2002;325(7362):480–3.
96. Gruet M. Fatigue in chronic respiratory diseases: theoretical framework and implications for real-life performance and rehabilitation. Front Physiol. 2018;9:1285.
97. Spruit MA, Vercoulen JH, Sprangers MAG, Wouters EFM, Consortium FA. Fatigue in COPD: an important yet ignored symptom. Lancet Respir Med. 2017;5(7):542–4.
98. Swigris JJ, Yorke J, Sprunger DB, Swearingen C, Pincus T, du Bois RM, et al. Assessing dyspnea and its impact on patients with connective tissue disease-related interstitial lung disease. Respir Med. 2010;104(9):1350–5.
99. Basta F, Afeltra A, Margiotta DPE. Fatigue in systemic sclerosis: a systematic review. Clin Exp Rheumatol. 2018;36 Suppl 113(4):150–60.
100. Mermigkis C, Bouloukaki I, Antoniou KM, Mermigkis D, Psathakis K, Giannarakis I, et al. CPAP therapy in patients with idiopathic pulmonary fibrosis and obstructive sleep apnea: does it offer a better quality of life and sleep? Sleep Breath. 2013;17(4):1137–43.
101. Mermigkis C, Bouloukaki I, Antoniou K, Papadogiannis G, Giannarakis I, Varouchakis G, et al. Obstructive sleep apnea should be treated in patients with idiopathic pulmonary fibrosis. Sleep Breath. 2015;19(1):385–91.
102. Swigris JJ, Fairclough DL, Morrison M, Make B, Kozora E, Brown KK, et al. Benefits of pulmonary rehabilitation in idiopathic pulmonary fibrosis. Respir Care. 2011;56(6):783–9.
103. Saketkoo LA, Karpinski A, Young J, Adell R, Walker M, Hennebury T, et al. Feasibility, utility and symptom impact of modified mindfulness training in sarcoidosis. ERJ Open Res. 2018;4(2)
104. Ryerson CJ, Berkeley J, Carrieri-Kohlman VL, Pantilat SZ, Landefeld CS, Collard HR. Depression and functional status are strongly associated with dyspnea in interstitial lung disease. Chest. 2011;139(3):609–16.
105. Ryerson CJ, Arean PA, Berkeley J, Carrieri-Kohlman VL, Pantilat SZ, Landefeld CS, et al. Depression is a common and chronic comorbidity in patients with interstitial lung disease. Respirology. 2012;17(3):525–32.
106. Holland AE, Fiore JF Jr, Bell EC, Goh N, Westall G, Symons K, et al. Dyspnoea and comorbidity contribute to anxiety and depression in interstitial lung disease. Respirology. 2014;19(8):1215–21.
107. Akhtar AA, Ali MA, Smith RP. Depression in patients with idiopathic pulmonary fibrosis. Chron Respir Dis. 2013;10(3):127–33.
108. van Manen MJG, van't Spijker A, Tak NC, Baars CT, Jongenotter SM, van Roon LR, et al. Patient and partner empowerment programme for idiopathic pulmonary fibrosis. Eur Respir J. 2017;49(4)

109. Bajwah S, Ross JR, Wells AU, Mohammed K, Oyebode C, Birring SS, et al. Palliative care for patients with advanced fibrotic lung disease: a randomised controlled phase II and feasibility trial of a community case conference intervention. Thorax. 2015;70(9):830–9.
110. Janssen K, Rosielle D, Wang Q, Kim HJ. The impact of palliative care on quality of life, anxiety, and depression in idiopathic pulmonary fibrosis: a randomized controlled pilot study. Respir Res. 2020;21(1):2.
111. Lindell KO, Olshansky E, Song MK, Zullo TG, Gibson KF, Kaminski N, et al. Impact of a disease-management program on symptom burden and health-related quality of life in patients with idiopathic pulmonary fibrosis and their care partners. Heart Lung. 2010;39(4):304–13.
112. Lindell KO, Nouraie M, Klesen MJ, Klein S, Gibson KF, Kass DJ, et al. Randomised clinical trial of an early palliative care intervention (SUPPORT) for patients with idiopathic pulmonary fibrosis (IPF) and their caregivers: protocol and key design considerations. BMJ Open Respir Res. 2018;5(1):e000272.
113. Wijsenbeek M, Bendstrup E, Ross J, Wells A. Cultural differences in palliative care in patients with idiopathic pulmonary fibrosis. Chest. 2015;148(2):e56.
114. Skorstengaard MH, Neergaard MA, Andreassen P, Brogaard T, Bendstrup E, Lokke A, et al. Preferred place of care and death in terminally ill patients with lung and heart disease compared to cancer patients. J Palliat Med. 2017;20(11):1217–24.
115. Kalluri M, Claveria F, Ainsley E, Haggag M, Armijo-Olivo S, Richman-Eisenstat J. Beyond idiopathic pulmonary fibrosis diagnosis: multidisciplinary care with an early integrated palliative approach is associated with a decrease in acute care utilization and hospital deaths. J Pain Symptom Manag. 2018;55(2):420–6.
116. Ahmadi Z, Wysham NG, Lundstrom S, Janson C, Currow DC, Ekstrom M. End-of-life care in oxygen-dependent ILD compared with lung cancer: a national population-based study. Thorax. 2016;71(6):510–6.

# Chapter 12
# The Role of Palliative Care in Lung Cancer

**Donald R. Sullivan**

## Symptom Burden

Patients with lung cancer experience significant disease-related symptom burden (Fig. 12.1) Although the frequency of symptoms varies widely across studies likely related to patient selection, inconsistent definitions, and reporting bias, commonly reported physical symptoms include fatigue, pain, anorexia, insomnia, cough, and dyspnea [1–4]. Traditionally, patients with lung cancer presented with one or more of these nonspecific symptoms prompting a clinical evaluation and subsequent diagnosis. Symptom burden can be a prognostic indicator of worse clinical outcome; [5, 6] however, this is likely confounded by the association between symptom severity and stage at diagnosis [7]. Symptoms will worsen in untreated disease; however, treatments can exacerbate or contribute to additional symptom burden. Additionally, about 10% of patients with lung cancer suffer from paraneoplastic syndromes which cause a host of additional systemic physical symptoms related to neurologic, endocrine, dermatologic, rheumatologic, hematologic, and ophthalmological syndromes and may include hypoglycemia, acromegaly, gynecomastia, hyperthyroidism, and hypercalcemia [8, 9].

Besides the impact of physical symptoms, patients with lung cancer suffer from considerable psychological symptom burden. A life-threatening diagnosis such as lung cancer evokes stress in many patients, and the prevalence of major depressive disorder ranges from 5% to 13%, whereas up to 44% of patients with lung cancer

D. R. Sullivan (✉)
Division of Pulmonary and Critical Care Medicine, Department of Medicine, Oregon Health & Science University, Portland, OR, USA

Center to Improve Veteran Involvement in Care, Portland VA Healthcare System, Portland, OR, USA
e-mail: sullivad@ohsu.edu


K. O. Lindell, S. K. Danoff (eds.), *Palliative Care in Lung Disease*, Respiratory Medicine, https://doi.org/10.1007/978-3-030-81788-6_12

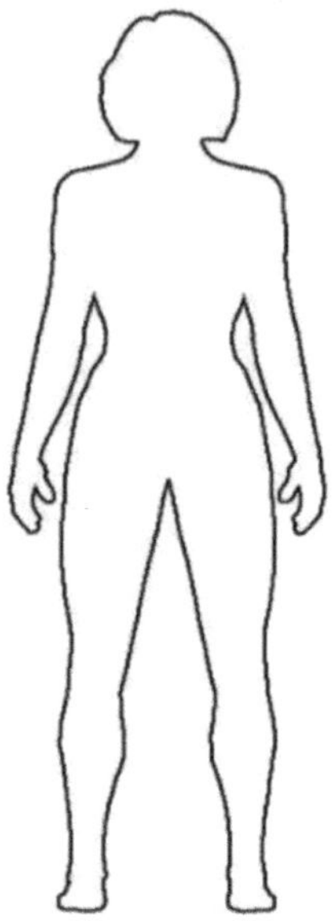


**Fig. 12.1** Constellation of physical and psychological symptom burden among patients with lung cancer

may experience depression symptoms [10–13]. Patients with lung cancer also report high levels of psychological distress and anxiety [14–17]. Estimates of psychological symptom burden are consistently higher among patients with lung cancer compared to other cancer types [12, 18]. This may be partially due to lung cancer stigma, which is a perceived health-related stigma that results from negative perceptions about the causal relationship between smoking and lung cancer [11, 19]. Unfortunately, emotional distress [20] and depression symptoms [10] are associated with worse survival in patients with lung cancer, particularly among patients with early-stage disease.

Lung cancer physical and psychological symptoms are inextricably linked, and not surprisingly, both physical and psychological symptom burdens significantly impact patients' quality of life (QOL) [3, 13, 21]. QOL is among the most important patient-reported outcome [22, 23] and is an independent prognostic factor for survival among patients with lung cancer [24]. Unfortunately, improvement in survival, which is the primary outcome for most cancer treatment trials, does not always equate to better QOL [25], and there is evidence that successful treatment does not necessarily result in improved QOL [26]. Furthermore, low QOL after treatment is not adequately explained by pre-cancer QOL, stage at diagnosis, or treatment outcomes [13].

Overall, patients with lung cancer suffer considerable physical and psychological symptom burden at diagnosis and during treatment which significantly affect patients' functional status and can reduce QOL. Among patients with lung cancer, QOL is an independent prognostic factor for survival which likely contributes to the association between symptom burden and survival. Therefore, reduction of patients' physical and psychological symptom burden is an essential component of disease management among patients with lung cancer.

## Evidence Basis

### *Randomized Controlled Trials*

Several randomized controlled trials (RCTs) of palliative care or early palliative care, several with low risk of bias [27], were conducted among more than 800 patients with advanced cancer which are summarized in Table 12.1 (randomized controlled trials of palliative care in lung cancer). Trials conducted entirely among or enrolling a sizable representation of patients with lung cancer are included. Most trials designated quality of life (QOL) as a primary outcome, and secondary outcomes included physical and psychological symptom burden, healthcare resource use including chemotherapy receipt in the last weeks of life, and survival [28–32]. Interventions are discussed in detail in Section "Models of Delivery".

Chronologically, the first RCT (ENABLE II) was conducted from November 2003 through May 2008 enrolling 322 patients with advanced cancer [30]. Patients with advanced solid tumors (36% had lung cancer) were randomized to either a multicomponent, psychoeducational intervention (ENABLE [Educate, Nurture, Advise, Before Life Ends]) conducted by advanced practice nurses consisting of four weekly educational sessions and monthly follow-up sessions until death or study completion vs. usual care. Eligible patients had a disease prognosis of approximately 1 year and were within 8–12 weeks of a new cancer diagnosis. The intervention used a case management and educational-based approach; in-person protocols were manualized to a telephone-based format to improve study access in this rural population.

The primary outcome was QOL measured by the Functional Assessment of Chronic Illness Therapy for Palliative Care (FACIT-Pal) [33]. Participants were well balanced based on baseline sociodemographics. Longitudinal intention-to-treat analyses for the total sample revealed higher QOL (mean [standard error (SE)],4.6 [2]; $p = 0.02$) (FACITPC) and lower depressed mood (mean [SE], −1.8 [0.81]; $p = 0.02$) (Center for Epidemiological Studies Depression (CES-D) scores) in the intervention compared with the usual care group. Differences in symptom intensity, hospital days, days in the intensive care unit, or emergency department visits were not significantly different between groups. Post hoc exploratory analyses demonstrated no statistically significant differences in survival between the two groups. Median survival was 14 months (95% confidence interval (CI), 10.6–18.4 months) in the intervention group and 8.5 months (95% CI, 7.0–11.1 months) for the usual care group (log-rank test, $p = 0.14$).

The next landmark trial for palliative care was conducted from June 2006 to July 2009 among 151 ambulatory patients with newly diagnosed metastatic non-small cell lung cancer (NSCLC) [28]. Eligible patients were enrolled within 8 weeks after diagnosis and had an Eastern Cooperative Oncology Group (ECOG) performance status of 0 to 2. Patients who were assigned to the intervention group met with a member of the palliative care team, within 3 weeks after enrollment and at least monthly thereafter, in the outpatient setting until death. General guidelines for the

**Table 12.1** Randomized controlled trials of palliative care in lung cancer

| Source[A] (by year) | No. of patients randomized | | Population | Setting | Primary outcome | Secondary outcomes | Notes |
|---|---|---|---|---|---|---|---|
| | Intervention | Control | | | | | |
| Bakitas M, et al., JAMA. 2009; (ENABLE II) [30] | 161 | 161 | GI (unresectable stages III–IV) (41%), lung (stages IIIB–IV NSCLC or extensive SCLC) (36%), genitourinary (stage IV) (12%), or breast (stage IV and visceral crisis, lung or liver metastasis, ER −, Her 2 neu+) (10%) cancer | Home | QOL, mean difference = 4.6 (SE = 2), $P = 0.02$; symptom intensity, mean difference = 27.8 (SE = 15), $P = 0.06$; resource utilization, hospital days (6.6 vs. 6.5, $P = 0.14$), ICU days (0.06 vs. 0.06, $P = 1$) or emergency department visits (0.86 vs. 0.63, $P = 0.53$) | Mood, mean difference = −1.8 (SE = 0.81), $P = 0.02$ | Inclusion criteria: enrolled within 8–12 weeks of cancer diagnosis Population: 64% of patients in the intervention arm had advanced solid malignancies other than lung cancer |
| Temel J, et al., N Engl J Med 2010 [28, 40]; Secondary analysis [40] | 77 | 74 | Advanced stage NSCLC | Ambulatory | QOL at 12 weeks, 98.0 vs. 91.5, $P = 0.03$; adjusted mean difference = 5.4 (SE = 2.4), 95% CI:0.7–10.0; $P = 0.03$ | Depression symptoms (16% vs. 38%, $P = 0.01$; aggressive EOL care (33% vs. 54%, $P = 0.05$); median survival (11.6 mo. vs. 8.9 mo., $P = 0.02$; QOL (adjusted difference in mean scores, 5.2 ± 1.8; 95% CI:1.6–8.9; $P = 0.005$; lung cancer symptoms (adjusted difference in mean scores, 1.0 ± 0.6; 95% CI:–0.2–2.3; $P = 0.12$) Secondary analysis: intervention group had lower odds of receiving chemotherapy within 60 days of death (OR = 0.47, 95% CI:0.23–0.99; $P = 0.05$), a longer interval between the last dose of chemotherapy and death (median, 64.0 days [range, 3–406 days] vs. 40.5 days [range, 6–287 days]; $P = 0.02$), and higher enrollment in hospice care for >1 week (60.0% [36/60 patients] vs. 33.3% [21/63 patients]; $P = 0.004$) | Inclusion criteria: enrolled within 8 weeks of cancer diagnosis and ECOG performance status 0–2 |

| | | | | | | | |
|---|---|---|---|---|---|---|---|
| Northhouse LL, et al., Psychooncology. 2013 [29] | 321 | 163 | Advanced solid tumor (stage III or IV): breast, 32%; lung, 29%; colorectal, 25%; and prostate, 13% within 6 months of diagnosis, progression, or change in treatment | Home | Group x time (3 and 6 month assessments) interactions in dyads' coping ($P = 0.013$), self-efficacy ($P = 0.024$), and social QOL ($P = 0.002$) and group x time x role interaction in caregivers' emotional QOL ($P =$ o.042) were improved in the intervention group; there were no differences in appraisal | | Population: patient and family caregiver dyads |
| Bakitas M, et al., J Clin Oncol. 2015; (ENABLE III) [31] | 104 | 103 | Advanced stage solid tumor or hematologic malignancy (lung, 44%; GI tract, 25%; breast, 10%; other solid tumors, 10%; genitourinary tract, 7%; and hematologic malignancy, 5%) | Home | QOL at 3 months, 129.9; 95% CI:126.6–133.3 vs. 127.2; 95% CI:124.1–130.3, $P = 0.34$; symptoms at 3 months, 11.4; 95% CI:10.8–12.1 vs. 12.2; 95% CI:11.6–12.8; $P = 0.09$; and depression symptoms: 11.2; 95% CI:9.7–12.7 vs. 10.8; 95% CI:9.5–12.1; $P = 0.33$ | 1-year survival rates were 63% vs. 48% (difference = 15%; $P = 0.04$); however, median survival was 18.3 months vs. 11.8 months, per log-rank test $P = 0.18$; relative rate of chemotherapy use in the last 2 weeks of life = 1.57; 95% CI:0.37–6.7, $P = 0.54$; died at home 54% vs. 47%, $P = 0.60$ | Inclusion criteria: oncologist-determined prognosis of 6–24 months and enrolled within 30–60 days of advanced cancer diagnosis, cancer recurrence, or progression |

(continued)

**Table 12.1** (continued)

| Source[A] (by year) | No. of patients randomized | | Population | Setting | Primary outcome | Secondary outcomes | Notes |
|---|---|---|---|---|---|---|---|
| | Intervention | Control | | | | | |
| Temel J, et al., J Clin Oncol. 2017 [32, 41] Secondary analysis [41] | 175 | 175 | Advanced stage lung (NSCLC, small cell, or mesothelioma) (55%) or non-colorectal GI (45%) (pancreatic, esophageal, gastric, or hepatobiliary) cancer | Ambulatory | QOL at 12 weeks, 0.39 vs. 1.13; *P* = 0.339; adjusted mean difference = 2.40 (SE = 1.41) 95% CI:-0.38–5.18, *P* = 0.091; only lung cancer patients: adjusted mean difference = 5.04 (SE = 2.21) 95% CI:0.68–9.41, *P* = 0.024 | QOL at 24 weeks 1.59 vs. 3.40; *P* = 0.010; depression symptoms at 24 weeks, (adjusted mean difference, 21.17; 95% CI: 22.33–20.01; *P* = 0.048); reported primary goal of cancer treatment was cured at 12 weeks, 28.7% vs. 34.5%, *P* = 0.289; discussed EOL wishes with their oncologist, 30.2% vs. 14.5%; *P* = 0.004<br>Secondary analysis: caregivers of 350 patients participated (intervention = 137) Caregivers' distress at 12 weeks (HADS-total adjusted mean difference = −1.45, 95% CI: −2.76 to −0.15; *p* = 0.029) and depression subscale (HADS depression adjusted mean difference = −0.71, 95% CI: −1.38 to −0.05; *p* = 0.036) improved. QOL and HADS anxiety subscale was not different at or 12 weeks. No differences in caregivers' outcomes were noted at 24 weeks | Inclusion criteria: enrolled within 8 weeks after cancer diagnosis and ECOG performance status 0–2<br>Population: 46% in the intervention arm had advanced GI cancer |

[a]Randomized controlled trials with <29% lung cancer patient enrollment were excluded

Abbreviations: *ENABLE* Educate, Nurture, Advise Before Life Ends, *GI* gastrointestinal, *QOL* quality of life, *MO* months, *ECOG* Eastern Cooperative Oncology Group, *CI* confidence interval. *SE* standard error, and *NSCLC* non-small cell lung cancer

palliative care visits were adapted from the National Consensus Project for Quality Palliative Care [34].

The primary outcome was QOL measured by the Functional Assessment of Cancer Therapy–Lung (FACT-L) Trial Outcome Index (TOI), and patients in the intervention group had a 2.3-point increase in mean TOI score from baseline to 12 weeks, as compared with a 2.3-point decrease in the usual care group ($p = 0.04$). After controlling for baseline QOL values, the group assignment significantly predicted scores at 12 weeks on the total FACT-L scale (adjusted difference in mean [±SE] scores, 5.4 ± 2.4; 95% CI, 0.7–10.0; $p = 0.03$) and the TOI (adjusted difference in mean scores, 5.2 ± 1.8; 95% CI, 1.6–8.9; $p = 0.005$). The percentage of patients with depression at 12 weeks, as measured by the Hospital Anxiety and Depression Scale (HADS) and 9-Item Patient Health Questionnaire (PHQ-9), was significantly lower in the palliative care group than in the usual care group. Among the 70% of patients who died at the time of study publication, a greater percentage of usual care patients compared to intervention patients received aggressive end-of-life care (i.e., chemotherapy within 14 days before death, no hospice care, or late admission to hospice 3 days or less before death) (54% [30 of 56 patients] vs. 33% [16 of 49 patients], $p = 0.05$). In addition, more patients in the intervention than in the usual care group had resuscitation preferences documented in the outpatient electronic medical record (53% vs. 28%, $p = 0.05$). Median estimates of survival were as follows: 9.8 months (95% CI, 7.9–11.7) in the entire sample (151 patients), 11.6 months (95% CI, 6.4–16.9) in the intervention group, and 8.9 months (95% CI, 6.3–11.4) in the standard care group (log-rank test, $p = 0.02$).

In an innovative study design, 484 dyads (advanced cancer patients [29% with lung cancer] and their caregivers) were randomized to a home-based intervention that provided information and support to cancer patients and their caregivers [29]. Eligible participants were diagnosed with advanced breast, colorectal, lung, or prostate cancer (i.e., stage III or IV) and were within 6 months of a new diagnosis, progression of their disease, or recent change in treatment with a life expectancy ≥6 months and had a family caregiver willing to participate. The primary outcome was QOL measured with the general Functional Assessment of Cancer Therapy-General (FACT-G) that assesses QOL in four domains: social, emotional, functional, and physical well-being. There were no significant differences in the emotional, functional, or physical well-being domains. There was a significant group by time effect for social QOL ($F = 4.28$, $p = 0.002$). Control dyads had a significant decline in their social QOL at 3 months, while intervention dyads maintained their social QOL at 3-month or 6-month follow-up. There were also significant group by time effects on coping variables ($F = 2.15$, $p = 0.013$) and self-efficacy ($F = 2.84$, $p = 0.024$) measured via the Brief Cope Scale and the Lewis Cancer Self-efficacy Scale, respectively.

ENABLE III was conducted between October 2010 and March 2013 among 207 patients with advanced cancer (42.5% were diagnosed with lung cancer) [31]. Participants were randomly assigned to receive early (within 30–60 days of being informed of an advanced cancer diagnosis, cancer recurrence, or progression, with, in the opinion of the oncologist, prognosis between 6 and 24 months) or delayed (within 3 months or later of the above criteria). The intervention consisted of an in-person palliative care consultation, structured palliative care telehealth nurse coaching sessions (1/week for six sessions), and monthly follow-ups that used the same multicomponent intervention as ENABLE II. There were no significant differences in QOL via the FACIT-Pal, symptom impact via the quality of life at the end of life (QUAL-E) symptom impact subscale, or mood via the CES-D. There was a 15% difference in survival at 1 year (early group, 63%, vs. delayed group, 48%; $p = 0.038$), and the median overall survival was 18.3 months for the early group and 11.8 months for the delayed group. However, the overall log-rank test was not significant ($p = 0.18$), suggesting no difference in survival after 12 months. There were no significant differences in resource use (hospital, ICU days, ED visits, and chemotherapy receipt in the last 2 weeks of life) and location of death between groups.

The most recent RCT was conducted between May 2011 and July 2015 among 350 patients with incurable lung (55%) or non-colorectal GI cancer [32]. Eligible patients were within 8 weeks of cancer diagnosis and had an ECOG performance status of 0 to 2, and patients who were already receiving palliative care services were excluded. Intervention group patients met with a palliative care clinician at least once per month until death, whereas those who received usual care could consult a palliative care clinician upon request. The primary end point was change in QOL via the FACT-G from baseline. At 24 weeks, intervention patients reported a 1.59-point increase in FACT-G scores, and usual care patients reported a 3.40-point decrease from baseline ($p = 0.010$; Cohen's d, 0.33). Patient PHQ-9, HADS Depression, and HADS Anxiety scores did not differ significantly between groups from baseline to weeks 12 or 24. However, after controlling for baseline variables, significant differences that favored the intervention for PHQ-9 scores at 24 weeks (mean difference = −1.1.7 (SE 0.59), $p = 0.048$) were seen among patients with lung cancer. At 24 weeks, more intervention patients reported that they had discussed their end-of-life wishes with their oncologist compared with usual care patients (30.2% vs. 14.5%; $p = 0.004$).

Overall, in randomized controlled trials, palliative care significantly improved QOL among patients with advanced lung cancer including some effects on family caregivers in a single trial. Palliative care was associated with either improved or no difference in survival compared to usual oncology care. Palliative care also demonstrated some beneficial effects on psychological symptom burden such as mood and depression symptoms. Results were mixed regarding the effects of palliative care on healthcare resource utilization such as emergency department visits, ICU admission, and chemotherapy receipt in the final weeks of life. Thus, there is a growing body of literature that demonstrates that palliative care improves patient outcomes without significantly shortening survival.

## *Cohort Studies*

While randomized controlled trials yield the highest level of evidence for causality, cohort studies may represent an important contribution toward understanding the potential impact of palliative care as these studies occur in uncontrolled or real-world settings. While not an exhaustive list, this is a sampling of cohort studies that examined palliative care use among patients with lung cancer in both Europe and the United States.

Among NSCLC lung cancer patients in Norway, early (3 months prior to death) or late (within 3 months of death) receipt of palliative care was compared to nonreceipt of palliative care [35]. The likelihood of active anticancer treatment (e.g., chemotherapy) in the last month of life was lowest in the early palliative care group. Patients who received early or late palliative care were significantly more likely to have a documented resuscitation preference or to become hospitalized in the last 3 months of life compared to patients who did not receive palliative care.

Using SEER-Medicare data from the United States from 2001 to 2015 among a cohort of metastatic NSCLC patients, palliative care use was associated with significantly lower healthcare costs compared with those who did not receive palliative care, from US$3180 less in 2011 to $1285 less in 2015 [36]. Outpatient palliative care was also associated with improved survival compared with patients who received palliative care in other settings [36].

Among a population of advanced stage lung cancer patients in the Veterans Health Administration (VA) diagnosed between 2007 and 2013, palliative care was associated with improved survival if it was received 31–365 days after a cancer diagnosis compared to patients who did not receive palliative care [37]. Patients who received palliative care were also less likely to die in acute care settings. In this same cohort, palliative care was associated with reduced admission to the intensive care in the last 30 days of life, while outpatient palliative care was associated with reduced emergency department visits any time after diagnosis and hospitalizations in the last 30 days of life [38]. Early palliative care in this study (i.e., received within 90 days of cancer diagnosis) was associated with reduced receipt of any chemotherapy and high-intensity chemotherapy [39].

Overall, trial and observational research demonstrates palliative care significantly improves QOL and survival, reduces healthcare use (particularly in the last weeks of life), and improves psychological symptom burden especially mood and depression symptoms among patients with advanced lung cancer. Thus, there is a considerable body of evidence suggesting palliative care should be considered a complementary approach among patients with lung cancer as it significantly improves patient outcomes.

## Models of Delivery

Traditionally, palliative is delivered in inpatient settings by consult teams when patients with lung cancer are hospitalized [42]. The development of these models is largely influenced by fee-for-service bundled payment systems as palliative care can reduce overall hospital costs [43]. The two dominant models in inpatient settings are specialist consultation services and inpatient palliative care units, where the palliative care team may function as the primary service caring for the patient. As a likely result of this foundation, palliative services are concentrated in inpatient settings in the United States [44–46].

Today, newer models of palliative care delivery enjoy widespread adoption including multidisciplinary clinics [28, 32, 41, 47, 48], home- or community-based care [29, 49], alternative delivery models including those that use telephone and telehealth methods [30, 50, 51], and outpatient palliative care specialty clinics [52–54]. These newer models of delivery are preferable as the focus is on upstream integration of palliative care in ambulatory settings where the mechanisms of care coordination and follow-up are better established compared to inpatient delivery models [55]. Several of these newer or upstream models of palliative care delivery are discussed in more detail below.

### *Multidisciplinary Clinics*

The optimal timing of palliative care integration is based on patients' perceived needs, however, other suggested assessments include patients' prognosis, interval from diagnosis to median survival based on stage, treament trajectory (i.e., first or second line of treatment etc.), and performance status [56]. Integration of palliative care among patients with lung cancer in ambulatory settings alongside their lung cancer treatment team in thoracic oncology clinics is an established model of delivery associated with improved patient outcomes [28, 32]. Similarly, breathlessness clinics have been developed which are a multi-professional integrated service that in some instances combine respiratory, physiotherapy, occupational therapy, and palliative care assessments and management in a one-stop shopping treatment model. Although not exclusive to patients with lung cancer, this model of delivery improved breathlessness mastery (i.e., patients feeling of control over their respiratory disease and its effects on QOL and function) compared to a control group by 16% [48]. A systematic review of breathlessness services including 37 articles, representing 18 different services mostly among patients with thoracic cancer, noted significant reductions in distress due to breathlessness and depression scores comparing breathlessness services to control groups [57]. In this systematic review, no differences in health status or QOL were noted. Integration of palliative care in ambulatory multidisciplinary settings may be the best-suited model among patients with lung cancer to help coordinate care with the lung cancer treatment team, especially among patients also receiving disease-directed therapy such as chemotherapy or radiation. However, significant potential barriers to widespread implementation are identified including a shortage of palliative care clinicians and lack of capacity in ambulatory cancer settings [44, 58–60].

## *Community-Based Care*

The origins of this model may derive from the interdisciplinary community-based care provided through certified home health or hospice agencies outside of the Medicare Hospice Benefit [61]. Some of the earlier studies of this model among patients with serious illness, including about 61% with advanced cancer, showed increased satisfaction, less care in the emergency department, fewer hospital days, and fewer skilled nursing facility days compared with patients in usual care [62]. The decreased use of healthcare resources also led to a 45% decrease in healthcare costs. Community-based palliative care is expected to play an increasingly significant role in the delivery of palliative care; [49] however, in the fee-for-service world of the United States healthcare system, community-based palliative care programs cannot offset the costs of fee-for-service billing alone. Therefore, if the evolution of palliative care is expected to include community-based programs in the United States, a transition to value-based care as proposed by the Affordable Care Act is needed [63]. Currently, the evidence supporting community-based palliative care among patients with lung cancer is somewhat limited.

## *Alternative*

Delivery models including telephone and telehealth methods have been suggested to reduce travel demands on patients and their families, especially those residing in rural settings. Project ENABLE incorporated telephone-based assessments to help deliver palliative care as they enrolled a rural population of patients with advanced cancer demonstrating improved QOL [30, 64]. The feasibility of a nurse-led entirely telephone-based palliative care intervention among lung cancer patients is also established [51]. While alternative palliative care delivery models will likely include combinations of approaches including telehealth methods, currently evidence is limited to observational, noncontrolled studies and a few quasi-experimental studies [65]. A more recent review of systematic reviews also concluded there is still limited evidence regarding telehealth approaches in palliative care [66].

A significant criticism of telehealth approaches are technology complaints, especially with live video platforms. Commonly cited complaints include connectivity, loss of connection, slow video feed, or issues with understanding how to employ the technology particularly among older patients [67]. Patients from lower socioeconomic groups, people of color, and those residing in rural settings are most affected by these issues, raising important disparity questions. Additionally, among a group of patients receiving palliative lung cancer radiation, clinicians felt the sickest patients had the least amount of benefit from telehealth options for symptom management [68]. There remain important research opportunities to explore the intersection of palliative care and telehealth.

There are several established and many more innovative models of palliative care delivery among patients with lung cancer. Patients' significant symptom burden and their frequent inpatient clinical encounters make inpatient delivery models reasonable; however, ambulatory models allow for earlier integration and improved patient outcomes based on available evidence. Ultimately, combinations of delivery methods based on available resources and context are often necessary to deliver timely palliative care in accordance with the American Society of Clinical Oncologists (ASCO) guidelines, which suggest palliative care is initiated within 8 weeks of an advanced lung cancer diagnosis [69].

## Palliative Therapies in Lung Cancer

According to ASCO's Choosing Wisely guidelines, cancer-directed therapy for solid tumors should not be used for patients with low performance status, no benefit from prior evidence-based interventions, not eligible for a clinical trial, and no strong evidence supporting the clinical value of further anticancer treatment [70]. Additionally, palliative chemotherapy may not change QOL among patient with poor baseline performance status and may actually worsen QOL among patients with good baseline performance status [71]. Studies demonstrate early palliative care integration may reduce receipt of cancer-directed therapy among patients with advanced lung cancer, especially at the end of life [28, 39]. However, advances in lung cancer therapies have resulted in patients living longer with advanced stage lung cancer [72, 73]. Therefore, a greater number of patients are likely to receive or be offered cancer-directed therapies (e.g., chemotherapy) or treatment for lung cancer complications (e.g., malignant pleural effusion). If the goal of this therapy is to alleviate symptoms and improve QOL, then the following therapies may be considered.

### *Chemotherapy*

Palliative chemotherapy may improve QOL and survival [74, 75]. However, in some advanced stage disease patients with poor performance status, the side effects of chemotherapy in reducing QOL may outweigh the benefits of receiving it [71].

Unfortunately, almost 70% of patients receiving chemotherapy for incurable lung cancer may not understand that chemotherapy is unlikely to be curative, which may compromise their ability to make informed treatment decisions [76]. Therefore, initiation of palliative chemotherapy should be preceded by a thorough discussion of risks, benefits, and goals and expectations of this therapy among patients and their clinicians to ensure therapy is consistent with patients' values and preferences.

## *Radiation*

Palliative radiation can be effective at relieving respiratory symptoms and is generally well-tolerated [77]. It may be particularly effective in treating symptomatic metastases to the central nervous system and bone, and the most common treatment sites are the brain, thorax, and bone [78]. Endobronchial brachytherapy (EBB) utilizes the placement of a radioactive source (usually iridium-192) within the airway to treat a local tumor, and external beam radiation therapy (EBRT) involves external radiation application to a tumor. EBB can be used as a sole modality or in combination with EBRT. For EBRT, patients often receive multiple treatments over the course of several days to weeks which may limit use in practice among the sickest patients. As radiation must pass through nonmalignant tissues in EBRT, the potential for rib fractures, pneumonitis, esophagitis, and chest wall pain exists [79, 80].

The 2011 American Society for Radiation Oncology (ASTRO) evidence-based clinical practice guidelines suggest EBB is not recommended as either sole or adjunctive therapy for palliation of airway obstruction based on randomized trials evaluating EBB and EBRT [81]. Current ASTRO guidelines suggest among patients with stage III NSCLC deemed unsuitable for curative therapy, but who are candidates for chemotherapy based on performance status and have a minimum life expectancy of 3 months, administration of chemotherapy concurrently with EBRT is recommended over treatment with either modality alone. Guidelines further state that in the palliative management of patients with stage IV NSCLC, the use of concurrent thoracic chemotherapy and EBRT is not recommended, and this practice should be reserved for clinical trials [82].

Advances in radiation techniques such as stereotactic ablative radiotherapy (SABR) or stereotactic body radiation therapy (SBRT) may increase the role of palliative radiation among patients with advanced lung cancer as therapy is delivered with increasing accuracy limiting potential toxicity to surrounding tissues [83]. While evidence suggests some symptomatic patients with advanced lung cancer may benefit from palliative radiation therapy, trends in the provision of palliative radiation therapy have demonstrated decreased use from 2011 to 2018 among patients enrolled in hospice [84]. Potential barriers to receipt of palliative radiation therapy include costs, transportation, life expectancy, and knowledge of potential benefits among referring clinicians. As with any palliative treatment, it is important to ensure patients and families understand the intent and expectations of such therapy to ensure treatment is consistent with patients' goals, values, and priorities.

## *Surgery and Invasive Procedures*

### Malignant Pleural Effusion

Malignant pleural effusions (MPEs) occur when pleural fluid production overwhelms absorption due to increased production or impaired absorption (e.g., impaired lymphatic drainage from tumor cells or tumor compression) [85]. Patient symptoms include cough, shortness of breath, chest pain, and inability to lay flat among others. Common interventions to treat symptomatic a MPE may include thoracentesis, placement of an indwelling pleural catheter (Fig. 12.2), and/or pleurodesis. In patients with known or suspected MPE who are asymptomatic, guidelines suggest therapeutic pleural interventions should not be performed, [86] although it is expected that the majority of patients with MPEs will eventually develop shortness of breath leading to consideration of potential interventions.

Thoracentesis involves inserting a needle and sometimes a catheter into the pleural space and evacuating the fluid which is commonly done during lung cancer staging procedures when a sizable pleural effusion is present. However, if the MPE recurs and patients are expected to live longer than 1 month, society guidelines suggest consideration of longer-term therapies such as indwelling pleural catheter placement and/or pleurodesis [87]. Drainage of MPEs can serve two important

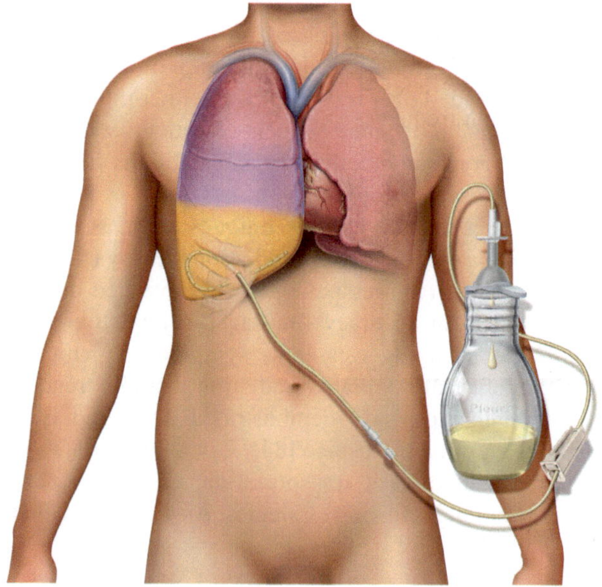

**Fig. 12.2** Indwelling pleural catheters are a longer-term therapy to help manage recurrent MPEs that are symptomatic. (Courtesy and © Becton, Dickinson and Company)

functions: (1) relieve patient symptoms and (2) allow lung re-expansion. However, nonexpendable lung occurs in about 30% of patients with MPEs [88] and is a contraindication to pleurodesis [89].

Either indwelling pleural catheter placement or pleurodesis may be used among patients with symptomatic MPEs. Guidelines do not recommend one approach over another; however, indwelling pleural catheter placement may be favored as this approach is expected to result in fewer days spent in the hospital, but is associated with higher rates of cellulitis compared to pleurodesis [86]. Although retrospective data from 11 centers in North America, Europe, and Australia revealed only 4.9% of patients developed catheter-associated infections and overall morality from these infections was very low (0.3%) [90], a recent randomized trial (IPC-Plus study) comparing indwelling pleural catheter with talc slurry infused into the catheter versus saline infusion resulted in higher pleurodesis rates and improved QOL in the talc slurry group [91].

## *Central Airway Obstruction and Massive Hemoptysis*

Obstruction of the central airways is a significant and common cause of patient distress in advanced lung cancer affecting an estimated of 20–30% of all patients [92]. These patients may develop distressing symptoms such as cough, dyspnea, or chest pain and are at risk for post-obstructive atelectasis and pneumonia [93, 94]. Traditionally, oxygen, opiates, glucocorticoids, and heliox were suggested palliative adjuncts for these patients; however [95, 96], newer interventional pulmonary therapies may be useful for palliation.

Bronchoscopic interventions may include argon plasma coagulation, laser, electrocautery, photodynamic therapy, cryoablation, balloon bronchoplasty, and airway stenting [97]. These interventions can be performed in the operating room under general anesthesia using a rigid bronchoscope or in an endoscopy suite with sedating medications using a flexible bronchoscope. Using these methods, clinicians may relieve intrinsic or extrinsic compression of the airway lumen resulting in airway recannulation and possible destruction of a portion of the tumor. Often one or more of these interventions may be used in a single procedure. While in the right setting these interventions may improve QOL for some patients [97], evidence demonstrating the effectiveness of bronchoscopic interventions in randomized controlled trials is nonexistent [92, 97]. However, invasive interventions may be indicated in specific circumstances as urgent therapeutic bronchoscopy allowed a majority of patients (52%) to be liberated from the ventilator caused by malignant central airway obstruction [98].

Another indication for invasive palliative interventions in lung cancer could include bronchoscopic therapies to treat massive hemoptysis, defined as more than 100 mL/24 hr. [99] Massive hemoptysis can be particularly distressing to patients, families, and clinicians [100]. Therapeutic bronchoscopic techniques may include balloon tamponade and infusion of vasoactive agents such as epinephrine, or if the area of bleeding can be visualized, laser coagulation or electrocautery can be considered with reasonable response rates [101–106].

Overall, studies have demonstrated potential roles for palliative therapies or interventions providing benefits to some patients with advanced stage lung cancer to alleviate distressing physical symptoms. However, careful patient selection is a critical aspect of initiation of these types of therapies to reduce potential complications and to avoid worsening of patients' QOL. Therefore, these therapies should be reserved for patients with high performance status. Additionally, some of these therapies should only be offered in the setting of a clinical trial. Most importantly, the use of these therapies needs to include a thorough discussion of the goals of therapy with patients and their families to ensure there is an accurate understanding of expectations.

## Emerging Therapies

Lung cancer is not a singular entity, and major histologic subtypes have traditionally included non-small cell lung cancer (NSCLC) and small cell lung cancer (SCLC). However, these traditional histological distinctions are oversimplified, and advances in molecular pathology have identified driver genetic mutations in NSCLC tumors [107]. These genetic mutations include epidermal growth factor receptor (EGFR) and anaplastic lymphoma kinase (ALK) among others. Identification of these tumor mutations have led to the development of targeted therapies and a major paradigm shift in the treatment and staging of advanced NSCLC [107, 108]. However, traditional platinum-based doublet therapy remains the standard regimen among most patients with advanced NSCLC, as identified driver mutations only account for a minority of NSCLC tumors [109].

Targeted therapies and the incorporation of immunotherapy have improved survival and provided expanded treatment options for some patients with advanced stage disease. However, the introduction of novel therapies is not expected to reduce the need for integrated palliative care. Instead, these therapies are expected to increase palliative care needs as some patients with advanced disease are living longer with serious illness and these therapies can contribute to serious side effects including cardiomyopathy and hypersensitivity pneumonitis [110–113]. Overall, as lung cancer treatments advance over time, we expect the role of integrated palliative care to be ever more important.

## Summary

Patients with lung cancer experience significant symptom burden during and after treatment that can worsen QOL and survival. The evidence base for palliative care integration among patients with lung cancer is robust and includes several innovative models of care delivery. Palliative therapies are suggested to alleviate pain and suffering and improve QOL; however, most treatments lack sufficient evidence to be considered part of usual care. Finally, advances in care and the ever-changing treatment paradigm are unlikely to diminish the critical role of palliative care in the treatment of patients with lung cancer and their families.

**Acknowledgments** I dedicate this work to my loving family MCR, NKS, EGS, and EDS who inspire me each and every day.

The Department of Veterans Affairs did not have a role in the preparation of this work. The views expressed are those of the author and do not necessarily reflect the position or policy of the Department of Veterans Affairs or the US Government.

## References

1. Cooley ME. Symptoms in adults with lung cancer. A systematic research review. J Pain Symptom Manag. 2000;19(2):137–53.
2. Krech R, Davis J, Walsh D, Curtis E. Symptoms of lung cancer. Palliat Med. 1992;6(4):309–15.
3. Tanaka K, Akechi T, Okuyama T, Nishiwaki Y, Uchitomi Y. Impact of dyspnea, pain, and fatigue on daily life activities in ambulatory patients with advanced lung cancer. J Pain Symptom Manag. 2002;23(5):417–23.
4. Vainio A, Auvinen A. Prevalence of symptoms among patients with advanced cancer: An international collaborative study. Symptom prevalence group. J Pain Symptom Manag. 1996;12(1):3–10.
5. Barney BJ, Wang XS, Lu C, et al. Prognostic value of patient-reported symptom interference in patients with late-stage lung cancer. Qual Life Res. 2013;22(8):2143–50.
6. Cheville AL, Novotny PJ, Sloan JA, et al. The value of a symptom cluster of fatigue, dyspnea, and cough in predicting clinical outcomes in lung cancer survivors. J Pain Symptom Manag. 2011;42(2):213–21.
7. Mendoza TR, Kehl KL, Bamidele O, et al. Assessment of baseline symptom burden in treatment-naïve patients with lung cancer: an observational study. Support Care Cancer. 2019;27(9):3439–47.
8. Pelosof LC, Gerber DE. Paraneoplastic syndromes: an approach to diagnosis and treatment. Mayo Clin Proc. 2010;85(9):838–54.
9. Spiro SG, Gould MK, Colice GL. American College of Chest Physicians. Initial evaluation of the patient with lung cancer: symptoms, signs, laboratory tests, and paraneoplastic syndromes: ACCP evidenced-based clinical practice guidelines (2nd edition). Chest. 2007;132(3 Suppl):149S–60S.
10. Sullivan DR, Forsberg CW, Ganzini L, et al. Longitudinal changes in depression symptoms and survival among patients with lung cancer: a national cohort assessment. J Clin Oncol. 2016;34(33):3984–91.
11. Cataldo JK, Jahan TM, Pongquan VL. Lung cancer stigma, depression, and quality of life among ever and never smokers. Eur J Oncol Nurs. 2012;16(3):264–9.
12. Linden W, Vodermaier A, Mackenzie R, Greig D. Anxiety and depression after cancer diagnosis: prevalence rates by cancer type, gender, and age. J Affect Disord. 2012;141(2–3):343–51.
13. Brown Johnson CG, Brodsky JL, Cataldo JK. Lung cancer stigma, anxiety, depression, and quality of life. J Psychosoc Oncol. 2014;32(1):59–73.
14. Arrieta O, Angulo LP, Núñez-Valencia C, et al. Association of depression and anxiety on quality of life, treatment adherence, and prognosis in patients with advanced non-small cell lung cancer. Ann Surg Oncol. 2013;20(6):1941–8.

15. Graves KD, Arnold SM, Love CL, Kirsh KL, Moore PG, Passik SD. Distress screening in a multidisciplinary lung cancer clinic: prevalence and predictors of clinically significant distress. Lung Cancer. 2007;55(2):215–24.
16. Jung JY, Lee JM, Kim MS, Shim YM, Zo JI, Yun YH. Comparison of fatigue, depression, and anxiety as factors affecting posttreatment health-related quality of life in lung cancer survivors. Psychooncology. 2018;27(2):465–70.
17. Zabora J, BrintzenhofeSzoc K, Curbow B, Hooker C, Piantadosi S. The prevalence of psychological distress by cancer site. Psychooncology. 2001;10(1):19–28.
18. Massie MJ. Prevalence of depression in patients with cancer. J Natl Cancer Inst Monogr. 2004;32:57–71. doi(32):57–71.
19. Cataldo JK, Slaughter R, Jahan TM, Pongquan VL, Hwang WJ. Measuring stigma in people with lung cancer: psychometric testing of the cataldo lung cancer stigma scale. Oncol Nurs Forum. 2011;38(1):E46–54.
20. Faller H, Bülzebruck H, Drings P, Lang H. Coping, distress, and survival among patients with lung cancer. Arch Gen Psychiatry. 1999;56(8):756–62.
21. Smith EL, Hann DM, Ahles TA, et al. Dyspnea, anxiety, body consciousness, and quality of life in patients with lung cancer. J Pain Symptom Manag. 2001;21(4):323–9.
22. Gralla RJ, Hollen PJ, Msaouel P, Davis BV, Petersen J. An evidence-based determination of issues affecting quality of life and patient-reported outcomes in lung cancer: results of a survey of 660 patients. J Thorac Oncol. 2014;9(9):1243–8.
23. Sullivan DR, Eden KB, Dieckmann NF, et al. Understanding patients' values and preferences regarding early stage lung cancer treatment decision making. Lung Cancer. 2019;131:47–57.
24. Sloan JA, Zhao X, Novotny PJ, et al. Relationship between deficits in overall quality of life and non-small-cell lung cancer survival. J Clin Oncol. 2012;30(13):1498–504.
25. Kovic B, Jin X, Kennedy SA, et al. Evaluating progression-free survival as a surrogate outcome for health-related quality of life in oncology: a systematic review and quantitative analysis. JAMA Intern Med. 2018;178(12):1586–96.
26. Sarna L, Cooley ME, Brown JK, et al. Women with lung cancer: quality of life after thoracotomy: a 6-month prospective study. Cancer Nurs. 2010;33(2):85–92.
27. Kavalieratos D, Corbelli J, Zhang D, Dionne-Odom JN, Ernecoff NC, Hanmer J, Hoydich ZP, Ikejiani DZ, Klein-Fedyshin M, Zimmermann C, Morton SC, Arnold RM, Heller L, Schenker Y. Association between palliative care and patient and caregiver outcomes: A systematic review and meta-analysis. [PMID: 27893131; PMCID: PMC5226373.]. 2016;22;316(20):2104–2104-211.
28. Temel JS, Greer JA, Muzikansky A, et al. Early palliative care for patients with metastatic non-small-cell lung cancer. N Engl J Med. 2010;363(8):733–42.
29. Northouse LL, Mood DW, Schafenacker A, et al. Randomized clinical trial of a brief and extensive dyadic intervention for advanced cancer patients and their family caregivers. Psychooncology. 2013;22(3):555–63.
30. Bakitas M, Lyons KD, Hegel MT, et al. Effects of a palliative care intervention on clinical outcomes in patients with advanced cancer: the project ENABLE II randomized controlled trial. JAMA. 2009;302(7):741–9.
31. Bakitas MA, Tosteson TD, Li Z, et al. Early versus delayed initiation of concurrent palliative oncology care: patient outcomes in the ENABLE III randomized controlled trial. J Clin Oncol. 2015;33(13):1438–45.
32. Temel JS, Greer JA, El-Jawahri A, et al. Effects of early integrated palliative care in patients with lung and GI cancer: a randomized clinical trial. J Clin Oncol. 2017;35(8):834–41.
33. Lyons KD, Bakitas M, Hegel MT, Hanscom B, Hull J, Ahles TA. Reliability and validity of the functional assessment of chronic illness therapy-palliative care (FACIT-pal) scale. J Pain Symptom Manag. 2009;37(1):23–32.
34. Clinical practice guidelines for quality palliative care. Pediatrics. 2019;143(1):e20183310. https://doi.org/10.1542/peds.2018-3310.

35. Nieder C, Tollåli T, Haukland E, Reigstad A, Flatøy LR, Engljähringer K. Impact of early palliative interventions on the outcomes of care for patients with non-small cell lung cancer. Support Care Cancer. 2016;24(10):4385–91.
36. Huo J, Hong YR, Turner K, et al. Timing, costs, and survival outcome of specialty palliative care in medicare beneficiaries with metastatic non-small-cell lung cancer. JCO Oncol Pract. 2020:OP2000298.
37. Sullivan DR, Chan B, Lapidus JA, et al. Association of early palliative care use with survival and place of death among patients with advanced lung cancer receiving care in the veterans health administration. JAMA Oncol. 2019;5(12):1702–9.
38. Vranas KC, Lapidus JA, Ganzini L, Slatore CG, Sullivan DR. Association of palliative care use and setting with health-care utilization and quality of care at the end of life among patients with advanced lung cancer. Chest. 2020;158(6):2667–74.
39. Lammers A, Slatore CG, Fromme EK, Vranas KC, Sullivan DR. Association of early palliative care with chemotherapy intensity in patients with advanced stage lung cancer: a national cohort study. J Thorac Oncol. 2019;14(2):176–83.
40. Greer JA, Pirl WF, Jackson VA, et al. Effect of early palliative care on chemotherapy use and end-of-life care in patients with metastatic non-small-cell lung cancer. J Clin Oncol. 2012;30(4):394–400.
41. El-Jawahri A, Greer JA, Pirl WF, et al. Effects of early integrated palliative care on caregivers of patients with lung and gastrointestinal cancer: a randomized clinical trial. Oncologist. 2017;22(12):1528–34.
42. Dumanovsky T, Augustin R, Rogers M, Lettang K, Meier DE, Morrison RS. The growth of palliative care in U.S. hospitals: a status report. J Palliat Med. 2016;19(1):8–15.
43. Smith TJ, Coyne P, Cassel B, Penberthy L, Hopson A, Hager MA. A high-volume specialist palliative care unit and team may reduce in-hospital end-of-life care costs. J Palliat Med. 2003;6(5):699–705.
44. Hui D, Elsayem A, De la Cruz M, et al. Availability and integration of palliative care at US cancer centers. JAMA. 2010;303(11):1054–61.
45. Morrison RS, Augustin R, Souvanna P, Meier DE. America's care of serious illness: a state-by-state report card on access to palliative care in our nation's hospitals. J Palliat Med. 2011;14(10):1094–6.
46. Center to Advance Palliative Care. America's care of serious illness: A state-by-state report card on access to palliative care in our nation's hospitals. Available at: https://reportcard.capc.org/ (Accessed on August 08, 2020).
47. Rabow MW, Dibble SL, Pantilat SZ, McPhee SJ. The comprehensive care team: a controlled trial of outpatient palliative medicine consultation. Arch Intern Med. 2004;164(1):83–91.
48. Higginson IJ, Bausewein C, Reilly CC, et al. An integrated palliative and respiratory care service for patients with advanced disease and refractory breathlessness: a randomised controlled trial. Lancet Respir Med. 2014;2(12):979–87.
49. Kamal AH, Currow DC, Ritchie CS, Bull J, Abernethy AP. Community-based palliative care: the natural evolution for palliative care delivery in the U.S. J Pain Symptom Manag. 2013;46(2):254–64.
50. Chua IS, Zachariah F, Dale W, et al. Early integrated telehealth versus in-person palliative care for patients with advanced lung cancer: a study protocol. J Palliat Med. 2019;22(S1):7–19.
51. Reinke LF, Vig EK, Tartaglione EV, Backhus LM, Gunnink E, Au DH. Protocol and pilot testing: the feasibility and acceptability of a nurse-led telephone-based palliative care intervention for patients newly diagnosed with lung cancer. Contemp Clin Trials. 2018;64:30–4.
52. Meier DE, Beresford L. Outpatient clinics are a new frontier for palliative care. J Palliat Med. 2008;11(6):823–8.
53. Rabow MW, Dahlin C, Calton B, Bischoff K, Ritchie C. New frontiers in outpatient palliative care for patients with cancer. Cancer Control. 2015;22(4):465–74.
54. Rabow M, Kvale E, Barbour L, et al. Moving upstream: a review of the evidence of the impact of outpatient palliative care. J Palliat Med. 2013;16(12):1540–9.

55. Pantilat SZ, Kerr KM, Billings JA, Bruno KA, O'Riordan DL. Palliative care services in California hospitals: program prevalence and hospital characteristics. J Pain Symptom Manag. 2012;43(1):39–46.
56. David Hui, Breffni Hannon, Camilla Zimmermann, and Eduardo Bruera. CA Cancer J Clin. 2018;68(5):356–76 https://doi.org/10.3322/caac.21490.
57. Brighton LJ, Miller S, Farquhar M, Booth S, Yi D, Gao W, Bajwah S, Man WD-C, Higginson IJ, Maddocks M. Holistic services for people with advanced disease and chronic breathlessness: a systematic review and meta-analysis. Thorax. 2019;74(3):270–81.
58. Lupu D, American Academy of Hospice and Palliative Medicine Workforce Task Force. Estimate of current hospice and palliative medicine physician workforce shortage. J Pain Symptom Manag. 2010;40(6):899–911.
59. Kamal AH, Bull JH, Swetz KM, Wolf SP, Shanafelt TD, Myers ER. Future of the palliative care workforce: preview to an impending crisis. Am J Med. 2017;130(2):113–4.
60. Spetz J, Dudley N, Trupin L, Rogers M, Meier DE, Dumanovsky T. Few hospital palliative care programs meet national staffing recommendations. Health Aff (Millwood). 2016;35(9):1690–7.
61. Center to Advance Palliative Care. Hospital hospice partnerships in palliative care: creating a continuum of service. 2001.
62. Brumley RD, Enguidanos S, Cherin DA. Effectiveness of a home-based palliative care program for end-of-life. J Palliat Med. 2003;6(5):715–24.
63. The Patient Protection and Affordable Care Act, 42 U.S.C. &18031; PUBLIC LAW 111–148, (2010).
64. Bakitas M, Stevens M, Ahles T, et al. Project ENABLE: a palliative care demonstration project for advanced cancer patients in three settings. J Palliat Med. 2004;7(2):363–72.
65. Capurro D, Cole K, Echavarría MI, Joe J, Neogi T, Turner AM. The use of social networking sites for public health practice and research: a systematic review. J Med Internet Res. 2014;16(3):e79.
66. Rogante M, Giacomozzi C, Grigioni M, Kairy D. Telemedicine in palliative care: a review of systematic reviews. Ann Ist Super Sanita. 2016;52(3):434–42.
67. Katalinic O, Young A, Doolan D. Case study: the interact home telehealth project. J Telemed Telecare. 2013;19(7):418–24.
68. Cox A, Illsley M, Knibb W, et al. The acceptability of e-technology to monitor and assess patient symptoms following palliative radiotherapy for lung cancer. Palliat Med. 2011;25(7):675–81.
69. Ferrell BR, Temel JS, Temin S, et al. Integration of palliative care into standard oncology care: American society of clinical oncology clinical practice guideline update. J Clin Oncol. 2017;35(1):96–112.
70. American Society of Clinical Oncology. Ten things physicians and patients should question. Updated 2019 2012, 2013.
71. Prigerson HG, Bao Y, Shah MA, et al. Chemotherapy use, performance status, and quality of life at the end of life. JAMA Oncol. 2015;1(6):778–84.
72. National Comprehensive Cancer Network. CCN clinical practice guidelines in oncology: palliative care. https://www.nccn.org/professionals/physician_gls/f_guidelines.asp#palliative. Accessed Dec 2016.
73. Planchard D, Popat S, Kerr K, et al. Metastatic non-small cell lung cancer: ESMO clinical practice guidelines for diagnosis, treatment and follow-up. Ann Oncol. 2018;29(Suppl 4):iv192–237.
74. Macbeth F, Stephens R. Palliative treatment for advanced non-small cell lung cancer. Hematol Oncol Clin North Am. 2004;18(1):115–30.
75. Non-Small Cell Lung Cancer Collaborative Group. Chemotherapy and supportive care versus supportive care alone for advanced non-small cell lung cancer. Cochrane Database Syst Rev. 2010;(5):CD007309. doi(5):CD007309.
76. Weeks JC, Catalano PJ, Cronin A, et al. Patients' expectations about effects of chemotherapy for advanced cancer. N Engl J Med. 2012;367(17):1616–1625. Accessed 20121025. doi: https://doi.org/10.1056/NEJMoa1204410.

77. Reinfuss M, Mucha-Małecka A, Walasek T, et al. Palliative thoracic radiotherapy in non-small cell lung cancer. An analysis of 1250 patients. Palliation of symptoms, tolerance and toxicity. Lung Cancer. 2011;71(3):344–9.
78. Chen AB, Cronin A, Weeks JC, et al. Palliative radiation therapy practice in patients with metastatic non-small-cell lung cancer: a cancer care outcomes research and surveillance consortium (CanCORS) study. J Clin Oncol. 2013;31(5):558–64.
79. Andolino DL, Forquer JA, Henderson MA, et al. Chest wall toxicity after stereotactic body radiotherapy for malignant lesions of the lung and liver. Int J Radiat Oncol Biol Phys. 2011;80(3):692–7.
80. Timmerman R, McGarry R, Yiannoutsos C, et al. Excessive toxicity when treating central tumors in a phase II study of stereotactic body radiation therapy for medically inoperable early-stage lung cancer. J Clin Oncol. 2006;24(30):4833–9.
81. Rodrigues G, Videtic GM, Sur R, et al. Palliative thoracic radiotherapy in lung cancer: an american society for radiation oncology evidence-based clinical practice guideline. Pract Radiat Oncol. 2011;1(2):60–71.
82. Moeller B, Balagamwala EH, Chen A, et al. Palliative thoracic radiation therapy for non-small cell lung cancer: 2018 update of an american society for radiation oncology (ASTRO) evidence-based guideline. Pract Radiat Oncol. 2018;8(4):245–50.
83. Jumeau R, Vilotte F, Durham AD, Ozsahin EM. Current landscape of palliative radiotherapy for non-small-cell lung cancer. Transl Lung Cancer Res. 2019;8(Suppl 2):S192–201.
84. Hsu SH, Wang SY. Trends in provision of palliative radiotherapy and chemotherapy among hospices in the United States, 2011–2018. JAMA Oncol. 2020;6(7):1106–8.
85. Stathopoulos GT, Kalomenidis I. Malignant pleural effusion: tumor-host interactions unleashed. Am J Respir Crit Care Med. 2012;186(6):487–92.
86. Feller-Kopman DJ, Reddy CB, DeCamp MM, et al. Management of malignant pleural effusions. An official ATS/STS/STR clinical practice guideline. Am J Respir Crit Care Med. 2018;198(7):839–49.
87. Roberts ME, Neville E, Berrisford RG, Antunes G, Ali NJ, BTS Pleural Disease Guideline Group. Management of a malignant pleural effusion: British thoracic society pleural disease guideline 2010. Thorax. 2010;65 Suppl 2:ii32–40.
88. Dresler CM, Olak J, Herndon JE 2nd, et al. Phase III intergroup study of talc poudrage vs talc slurry sclerosis for malignant pleural effusion. Chest. 2005;127(3):909–15.
89. Scarci M, Caruana E, Bertolaccini L, et al. Current practices in the management of malignant pleural effusions: a survey among members of the european society of thoracic surgeons. Interact Cardiovasc Thorac Surg. 2017;24(3):414–7.
90. Fysh ETH, Tremblay A, Feller-Kopman D, et al. Clinical outcomes of indwelling pleural catheter-related pleural infections: an international multicenter study. Chest. 2013;144(5):1597–602.
91. Bhatnagar R, Keenan EK, Morley AJ, et al. Outpatient talc administration by indwelling pleural catheter for malignant effusion. N Engl J Med. 2018;378(14):1313–22.
92. Ernst A, Feller-Kopman D, Becker HD, Mehta AC. Central airway obstruction. Am J Respir Crit Care Med. 2004;169(12):1278–97.
93. Beamis JF Jr. Interventional pulmonology techniques for treating malignant large airway obstruction: an update. Curr Opin Pulm Med. 2005;11(4):292–5.
94. Ginsberg RJ, Vokes EE, Ruben A. Non–small cell lung cancer. In: DeVita VT, Hellman S, Rosenberg SA, editors. Cancer: principles and practice of oncology. 5th ed. Philadelphia: Lippincott-Raven; 1997. p. 858–911.
95. Kamal AH, Maguire JM, Wheeler JL, Currow DC, Abernethy AP. Dyspnea review for the palliative care professional: treatment goals and therapeutic options. J Palliat Med. 2012;15(1):106–14.
96. Curtis JL, Mahlmeister M, Fink JB, Lampe G, Matthay MA, Stulbarg MS. Helium-oxygen gas therapy. Use and availability for the emergency treatment of inoperable airway obstruction. Chest. 1986;90(3):455–7.
97. Mallow C, Hayes M, Semaan R, et al. Minimally invasive palliative interventions in advanced lung cancer. Expert Rev Respir Med. 2018;12(7):605–14.

98. Colt HG, Harrell JH. Therapeutic rigid bronchoscopy allows level of care changes in patients with acute respiratory failure from central airways obstruction. Chest. 1997;112(1):202–6.
99. Radchenko C, Alraiyes AH, Shojaee S. A systematic approach to the management of massive hemoptysis. J Thorac Dis. 2017;9(Suppl 10):S1069–86.
100. Corner J, Hopkinson J, Fitzsimmons D, Barclay S, Muers M. Is late diagnosis of lung cancer inevitable? Interview study of patients' recollections of symptoms before diagnosis. Thorax. 2005;60(4):314–9.
101. Gottlieb LS, Hillberg R. Endobronchial tamponade therapy for intractable hemoptysis. Chest. 1975;67(4):482–3.
102. Swersky RB, Chang JB, Wisoff BG, Gorvoy J. Endobronchial balloon tamponade of hemoptysis in patients with cystic fibrosis. Ann Thorac Surg. 1979;27(3):262–4.
103. Valipour A, Kreuzer A, Koller H, Koessler W, Burghuber OC. Bronchoscopy-guided topical hemostatic tamponade therapy for the management of life-threatening hemoptysis. Chest. 2005;127(6):2113–8.
104. Hetzel MR, Smith SG. Endoscopic palliation of tracheobronchial malignancies. Thorax. 1991;46(5):325–33.
105. Morice RC, Ece T, Ece F, Keus L. Endobronchial argon plasma coagulation for treatment of hemoptysis and neoplastic airway obstruction. Chest. 2001;119(3):781–7.
106. Jain PR, Dedhia HV, Lapp NL, Thompson AB, Frich JC Jr. Nd:YAG laser followed by radiation for treatment of malignant airway lesions. Lasers Surg Med. 1985;5(1):47–53.
107. Chan BA, Hughes BG. Targeted therapy for non-small cell lung cancer: current standards and the promise of the future. Transl Lung Cancer Res. 2015;4(1):36–54.
108. Alamgeer M, Ganju V, Watkins DN. Novel therapeutic targets in non-small cell lung cancer. Curr Opin Pharmacol. 2013;13(3):394–401.
109. Yuan M, Huang LL, Chen JH, Wu J, Xu Q. The emerging treatment landscape of targeted therapy in non-small-cell lung cancer. Signal Transduct Target Ther. 2019;4:61–019–0099-9. eCollection 2019.
110. Zaborowska-Szmit M, Krzakowski M, Kowalski DM, Szmit S. Cardiovascular complications of systemic therapy in non-small-cell lung cancer. J Clin Med. 2020;9(5):1268. https://doi.org/10.3390/jcm9051268.
111. Mackintosh JA, Marshall HM, Fong KM. A targeted approach to the complications of targeted therapy. J Thorac Oncol. 2019;14(4):577–9.
112. Fujimoto D, Kato R, Morimoto T, et al. Characteristics and prognostic impact of pneumonitis during systemic anti-cancer therapy in patients with advanced non-small-cell lung cancer. PLoS One. 2016;11(12):e0168465.
113. Ricciardi S, Tomao S, de Marinis F. Toxicity of targeted therapy in non-small-cell lung cancer management. Clin Lung Cancer. 2009;10(1):28–35.

# Chapter 13
# Palliative Care in Patients with Neuromuscular Diseases

**Marianne de Visser**

Palliative care started in the 1960s as hospice care for patients who suffered from unbearable pain due to advanced cancer [1]. For a long time, palliative care was only administered to patients with malignancies. Over the last decades, there has been increasing awareness of the role palliative care could play in the care of people with progressive neurological disease, initially focused on amyotrophic lateral sclerosis/motor neuron disease (ALS/MND), to increase quality of life and promote patient autonomy [2]. The importance of providing palliative care early in the disease trajectory of patients suffering from a life-limiting illness as recommended by the WHO was underlined by the European Academy of Neurology [3, 4].

Advance care planning (ACP) is a substantial part of palliative care and is an iterative process "whereby a patient, in consultation with health care providers, family members and important others, makes decisions about his or her future health care, should he or she become incapable of participating in medical treatment decisions"[5]. In chronic progressive neurological, often life-limiting disorders, ACP conversations usually start after the patient has been informed about the diagnosis, albeit there is often uncertainty about timing and content (e.g., focused on preferences for future care) in which cultural factors may play an important role [6]. In ALS in which the mean life expectancy is 3 years after onset of the symptoms and for which no curative treatment exists, ACP should start right after diagnosis.

ACP is about listening to the patient and the significant others, understanding their values, beliefs, and goals of care and identifying their wishes about treatment options which might also include discontinuation or withholding interventions.

---

The author is based at a center which is part of the European Reference Network EURO-NMD.

---

M. de Visser (✉)
Department of Neurology, Amsterdam University Medical Centers, University of Amsterdam, Amsterdam Neuroscience, Amsterdam, Netherlands
e-mail: m.devisser@amsterdamumc.nl



K. O. Lindell, S. K. Danoff (eds.), *Palliative Care in Lung Disease*, Respiratory Medicine, https://doi.org/10.1007/978-3-030-81788-6_13

Although ALS is often considered the paradigmatic disease of palliative care [7], there are many more neuromuscular diseases which are associated with a severe burden both for the patient and his carer and which have a reduced life expectancy. Neuromuscular diseases (NMD) include genetic and acquired conditions originating in the lower motor neuron, i.e., the anterior horn cell, peripheral nerve, neuromuscular junction, and skeletal muscle. Onset ranges from the neonatal period to late adulthood, and there is considerable variability as regards the severity, ranging from death in infancy and early childhood (e.g., Pompe's disease or spinal muscular atrophy) to mild signs and symptoms in the sixth or seventh decade (e.g., late-onset myotonic dystrophy type 1). Most NMD in which palliative care may be offered at some point during the disease course are hereditary by nature, including muscular dystrophy, congenital myopathy/muscular dystrophy, mitochondrial myopathies, myotonic dystrophy type 1, and spinal muscular atrophy, albeit this list is not comprehensive. These diseases are not only characterized by progressive muscle weakness of the limbs; there is often also cardiac and respiratory involvement which may be associated with premature death. In some of these diseases, treatment has become possible changing the perspective of life expectancy and disabilities which makes ACP even more challenging. Among acquired NMD, inclusion body myositis and those myositis subtypes associated with rapidly progressive interstitial lung disease or progressive dysphagia leading to aspiration pneumonia may cause severe incapacities and not seldom an increased mortality.

However, literature and research on palliative care in neuromuscular disorders other than ALS are conspicuously absent or sparse. Nevertheless, there is a tendency to establish standards of care in various NMD in which palliative care gets a place. What could be the cause of underutilization of palliative care in neuromuscular disease? First, palliative care is often considered to be synonymous with hospice care or end-of-life care, both by health-care professionals and patients [8, 9]. Second, illness trajectories of progressive neurological diseases vary from rapidly progressive (infantile Pompe's disease, spinal muscular atrophy (SMA), ALS) to chronic progressive (among others, muscular dystrophies, myotonic dystrophy type 1, mitochondrial myopathies, myofibrillar myopathy, inclusion body myositis) and sometimes fluctuating (myositis). Patients with neuromuscular diseases have different symptom profiles, needs, preferences, and psychosocial issues. Third, knowledge about palliative care needs in NMD other than ALS is just emerging. Fourth, health-care professionals in general are found to be less familiar with communication skills needed to deliver bad news and to discuss advance care planning [9].

In this chapter, the most recent literature on palliative care in patients with the following NMD will be discussed: ALS, SMA, Duchenne muscular dystrophy and other muscular dystrophies (limb-girdle, congenital), Pompe's disease, and myotonic dystrophy type 1. We will also discuss which chronic, incurable, autonomy-impairing, and often life-shortening NMD, where patients have unmet physical and psychological needs, could be candidates for palliative care.

# Amyotrophic Lateral Sclerosis/Motor Neuron Disease

## *Epidemiology, Clinical Picture, and Diagnosis*

Amyotrophic lateral sclerosis (ALS) is a relentlessly progressive disease with an incidence of 2/100,000 persons-years. Progressive muscular atrophy (PMA) and primary lateral sclerosis (PLS) together with ALS belong to the motor neuron disease (MND) spectrum. ALS is the most common form in which degeneration of both the upper and in particular the lower motor neurons leads to progressive weakness of muscles innervated by the motor neurons in the spinal cord and the brain stem. The most common presentation is limb-onset muscle weakness, bulbar-onset accounting for 25–30% of cases [10]. Limb-onset ALS presents with asymmetrical clumsiness of the hands or weakness of the proximal arm muscles, or gait difficulty due to a drop foot, and bulbar-onset ALS is characterized by progressive swallowing difficulty or speech impairment often associated with forced laughter, crying, or yawning (pseudobulbar affect). A variable degree of spasticity can be observed [10]. Roughly 8% of the patients suffer from the behavioral variant of frontotemporal dementia, and in 20–50% of the patients cognitive impairment, behavioral disturbances or both can be demonstrated which have a negative impact on survival [10, 11]. About 90–95% of the patients are sporadic cases. In PMA, only lower motor neuron features are present, albeit in a proportion of the patients in due course upper motor neuron signs may occur. PLS is characterized by upper motor neuron signs only. Diagnosis is made on the history and clinical picture supported by electrophysiology and after excluding mimics. In ALS, 50% of patients die within 30 months of symptom onset and in PMA within 48 months [12, 13]. PLS has a more protracted course. In ALS and PMA, death is usually caused by respiratory failure as a result of progressive muscle weakness.

## *Management*

Riluzole is the first FDA-approved drug which prolongs life by 3 months. Edaravone has a beneficial effect on progression in a highly selected cohort of patients with early onset and rapidly progressive disease. It has been licensed by the FDA but not by the European Medicines Agency [10]. The mainstay of management consists mainly of supportive interventions, such as feeding via gastrostomy tube and noninvasive ventilation (NIV). These interventions are associated with a somewhat prolonged survival and improved health-related quality of life and therefore recommended to be offered to patients with MND, in a timely manner. A multidisciplinary evidence-based guideline on the care and management of MND commissioned by the National Institute for Health and Care Excellence provided recommendations on recognition and referral, information and support at diagnosis, coordination of (multidisciplinary) care, planning for end-of-life care, and symptom management, including dysphagia, respiratory dysfunction, and cognitive and behavioral impairment [14]. ACP plays an important role during the whole disease course.

As mentioned above, in ALS communication of the diagnosis is the start of palliative care. If not done properly with great adherence to effective communication techniques, particularly displaying empathy, it may lead to dissatisfaction and compromise the relationship between the patient and carers and the treating physician [15]. An Australian survey among neurologists showed that nearly 70% of neurologists reported finding it "somewhat to very difficult" communicating the MND diagnosis, and 65% reported feeling moderate to high stress and anxiety at the delivery of diagnosis [16]. Family carers' experiences of receiving the news of diagnosis showed that not only the duration of the consultation was of importance but also the physician's knowledge and skills on the (progression of) symptoms [17]. Follow-up assessment and care with an ACP approach should be offered shortly after breaking of the bad news and provided by a multidisciplinary team including at least a physician (neurologist, rehabilitation physician, or palliative care specialist), nurse, social worker, and psychologist/counselor [14, 18]. Since the disease follows a progressive course, preferences of the patients may change accordingly, and therefore, regular assessment of physical symptoms and psychosocial issues should be performed. End-of-life care includes recognition of deterioration over the last months and weeks in order to allow appropriate management in the dying phase. In addition to motor symptoms (difficulty with breathing and swallowing and loss of mobility), there are also extra-motor symptoms (cognitive and behavioral disturbances, depression) and – often underrecognized – pain which have to be taken into account [19]. Open discussion about the dying process and about the wish for hastened death should be encouraged, even if there are legal, religious, or cultural barriers for euthanasia, physician-assisted suicide, or palliative sedation as is the case in most countries.

Withdrawal of NIV is legal, but patients are often not aware of this option, and health-care professionals might find it ethically and legally challenging [20]. A gastrostomy tube may be withdrawn at the request of the patient when the burden of the intervention outweighs the patient's quality of life. In 2016, the ESPEN Guideline on Ethical Aspects of Artificial Nutrition and Hydration discussed the indications for artificial nutrition and also the ethical issues with regard to withdrawal or withholding this treatment [21]. The decision to discontinue enteral feeding is a unique journey for every patient and their families and should be communicated properly. It is the duty of the health-care professionals to adequately manage the symptoms of dysphagia when the tube has been removed.

Support should be extended to the carers not only during the disease course but also for bereavement, albeit an Australian study of ALS family carers reported that half of them did not recall receiving offers of bereavement support [22]. It is also important to reduce emotional exhaustion and avoid burnout in health-care professionals by preventive strategies at personal level aiming at improving the physical well-being and professional and organizational level [23].

## Spinal Muscular Atrophy

### *Epidemiology, Clinical Picture, and Diagnosis*

Spinal muscular atrophy (SMA) is the second most common autosomal recessive disease, with an incidence of 1 in every 6000–10,000 live births. SMA is caused by mutations of the survival of motor neuron 1 gene (SMN1), resulting in SMN protein deficiency. The almost identical SMN2 gene produces a small amount of functional SMN protein, and SMN2 copy number is recognized as a major modulator of the SMA phenotype. SMA exhibits a variable progression of muscle weakness. Based on age at presentation and severity, SMA is classified into four categories. SMA type I presents during the first 6 months of life. These patients show an arrest in the development of their motor skills and are never able to walk or even sit. In 50%, death occurs by 7 months, in 95% by 17 months. Patients with SMA type II have a better prognosis than those with type I disease, with 93% surviving to 25 years. These children never learn to walk unaided. SMA type III causes symptoms after 18 months of age, and the life expectancy is generally in line with that of the general population. SMA type IV, finally, presents in the third decade of life, and walking ability is retained during adult years. The diagnosis of SMA is based on molecular genetic testing. Genetic testing of SMN1/SMN2 is highly reliable, and it is first-line investigation when the condition is suspected in a typical case [24].

### *Management*

Supportive care is the cornerstone in the treatment of severe SMA, focusing on preventing complications of weakness and maintaining quality of life following the updated consensus statement for standards of care. Key issues here include respiratory and nutritional support [24, 25], albeit marked variability in the implementation of the standards of care, particularly in the use of ventilation, nutritional support, and scoliosis surgery, has been observed [26].

Most of the therapeutic strategies are aimed at increasing the expression of the SMN2 protein. Nusinersen – the first drug approved for treating SMA – is an antisense oligonucleotide that promotes the production of full-length SMN protein and is administered intrathecally. A systematic review showed that nusinersen improved both survival without permanent respiratory support and motor development; improvements were strongest in younger children. Treatment of presymptomatic children led to a near-normal motor development [27]. However, not all treated patients benefit as the authors of a double-blind sham-controlled randomized clinical trial stated at the end of their paper "Several of the infants who received nusinersen died, none achieved normal motor development, and some needed continued feeding and ventilatory support; these findings indicate that nusinersen is not a cure in symptomatic patients" [28]. As long-term efficacy is as yet unknown, palliative care is still much needed. Gene replacement therapy is an alternative strategy. There are now other drugs on or about to come on the market: onasemnogene abeparvovec (Zolgensma®), an adeno-associated viral vector-based gene therapy designed to deliver a functional copy of the SMN1 gene to the motor neurons through a single intravenous infusion, and another splicing modifier (risdiplam), a small molecule that is administered orally.

Given the lack of hard evidence on palliative care, the updated standards of care for SMA defined key areas for future analysis: (1) the concept of palliative care as applied to SMA, (2) patient management and decision-making, and (3) managing expectations [25]. Research has been performed to obtain data on parents' experiences with receiving the diagnosis and discussion of treatment decisions. A nationwide survey in Sweden conducted among bereaved parents of children with SMA and parents of children who were still alive showed that the majority of parents were satisfied with the manner the diagnosis was discussed. Ninety percent was told that their child would have a short life, but up to almost a third reported that a health-care professional had told, in the child's last days, that he or she would pass away shortly. The vast majority reported feeling confident about the treatment decisions. However, a quarter of the parents reported that they were not given information about respiratory support, which indicates that the parents did not sufficiently understand the available treatment options and that their child thereby may not receive the kind of care recommended in guidelines [29]. A recent study from France including both retrospective and prospective data showed that over time, palliative management occurred more frequently at home with increased levels of technical supportive care and that dedicated pediatric palliative care teams were increasingly involved in the management of SMA type 1 patients. Usually long-term ventilation was not administered, and that reflects the explicit choice that has been made by the French pediatricians involved in the management of neuromuscular patients. The authors stressed the importance of active collaboration and coordination between the different actors involved to ensure the child and family's best quality of life as well as the importance of parents' input about their wishes for their child's treatments and end-of-life conditions. Although only few nusinersen-treated patients were included in the study, the authors noted a far more invasive supportive care, which calls for a revisit of standards of care [30].

## Duchenne Muscular Dystrophy

### *Epidemiology, Clinical Picture, and Diagnosis*

Duchenne muscular dystrophy (DMD) is an X-linked recessively inherited muscular dystrophy. DMD manifests with progressive muscle weakness and wasting which first affects the pelvic girdle and lower limbs and subsequently the shoulder girdle, upper limbs, and respiratory muscles. The estimated worldwide prevalence of DMD among males is 4.78 per 100,000 males [31]. DMD is caused by a mutation in the *DMD* gene encoding for the protein dystrophin. In DMD, dystrophin is virtually absent [32]. Diagnosis can be established by showing absence of dystrophin in the muscle tissue, but mostly diagnosis is based on molecular genetic testing. Because approximately 70% of individuals with DMD have a single-exon or multi-exon deletion or duplication in the dystrophin gene, deletion and duplication testing is usually the first test. If this test is negative, (next-generation) sequencing should take place [33].

The accurate and early diagnosis of DMD plays a crucial role in the effective management of patients because it ends the diagnostic odyssey and has the potential to lead to earlier intervention and appropriate genetic counseling [34]. However, reports indicate that there are significant delays in diagnosis of DMD. The median age of diagnosis is 5 years [35]. The mean age at which first symptoms of DMD are noticed by the parents is approximately 2.5 years. The boys often have a waddling gait with tiptoe walking. Following a plateau phase, which is usually reached at age 4–8 years, muscle weakness progresses relentlessly, not only in the proximal leg muscles but also in the lower legs, and subsequently the proximal arm and neck muscles become also affected. By the age of 13, boys with DMD have generally lost the ability to walk independently. At a later stage, respiratory muscles become weak. Patients who undergo spinal surgery and nocturnal ventilation have a mean survival of 30 years [36]. Although all DMD patients above age 18 will show evidence of cardiac muscle disease (rhythm disturbances and dilated cardiomyopathy), only slightly more than half will complain of any symptoms. Approximately 30% of the boys with DMD have mental retardation with an IQ < 70. In addition, learning problems and behavioral disorders occur more frequently.

## Management

Although there is currently no cure for DMD, improvements in multidisciplinary care have slowed disease progression and thereby prolonged the life expectancy of affected individuals. Standards of care are proposed for rehabilitation and neuromuscular, respiratory, cardiac, orthopedic, nutritional, and psychosocial aspects of care [33, 37, 38]. Corticosteroids are used by the majority of patients to extend the ambulant phase in DMD by 1–2 years. Palliative care consultation at various times throughout the lifespan of a person with DMD is recommended in these care considerations.

There are currently targeted treatments such as antisense oligonucleotides (AONs) used for exon skipping which aim to restore dystrophin production in DMD. There are now three AONs approved. The clinical efficacy of the first one, eteplirsen, is somewhat disappointing and showed delay of disease progression, rather than a significant improvement in symptoms. For other AONs, clinical studies are underway [39]. Another treatment (ataluren) - applicable to a small proportion of DMD patients with a specific nonsense mutation resulting in a premature stop in the production of normal dystrophin - repairs the effect of premature stop codons and leads to dystrophin expression in DMD boys. Recently, it was shown that ataluren treatment was well tolerated and was associated with clinical benefit – delaying loss of ambulation and worsening motor performance, when compared with patients who only received the standard of care [40].

There is sparse solid evidence on palliative care in DMD. A systematic review on conversations of patients, parents, and health-care professionals about end-of-life care in neuromuscular diseases yielded only three papers on DMD or SMA [41]. The authors report that none of the papers showed evidence of conversations taking place between the patient and health-care professionals. One paper reported that parents found it difficult to initiate conversations about end-of-life care. Of note, the patient's view on participating in these conversations had not been addressed. Few parents were familiar with the term palliative care or with the concept of ACP. No paper considered the preferences of patients or health-care professionals (HCPs) about timing and content of conversations about end-of-life care. The papers did not provide much insight into the barriers to end-of-life conversations other than the wait-and-see policy of the HCPs who were found to be reluctant to initiate these conversations.

A qualitative study among DMD patients, aged 20–45 years, revealed that none of them could recall that any of their medical professionals had discussed end-of-life care and most patients assumed that the clinicians had been too anxious to address this issue. There was a clear need to be given proactive messages and cues that the topic of end of life could be raised. They also voiced the desire to know more about the possible causes of death and the management of end of life in terms of support and pain control. The DMD patients also expressed their wish to discuss the last stages of life and the options of hastened death. The study also showed that wills or formal written information about their wishes about place of death and funeral arrangements were not present and that was a concern to most of the patients. Conspicuously, effective emotional and psychological support seemed to be absent [42]. Patients and carers' lack of awareness of palliative care and the misconception about palliative care only being end-of-life care may play a role. An older survey among DMD families in the USA showed that only 15% of the respondents were familiar with the term palliative care [43]. There was no association with education, income, or ethnicity suggesting that there may simply be a lack of knowledge about palliative care services. Respiratory care was received by a majority of the young men with DMD, and skilled nursing services were received by half of the males. Attendant care and case manager services were received by somewhat less than half of the individuals, whereas services such as respite care, transportation assistance, pain management, and hospice services were received by <20%. Less than 25% of respondents reported having any type of directive document (living will, advance directive) in place. Also from the USA was a survey among a large cohort of 233 primary caregivers for an equal number of patients with Duchenne and Becker muscular dystrophy older than 12 years [44]. The data were collected over a period of 2007–2012. Although palliative care use had increased as compared to a previous survey, there was still an underutilization. The authors also noted a huge variation in use of services with high percentages for case management and a low percentage for pain management which is remarkable since this is a common complaint among these patients.

One might argue that these papers date back to the first decade of 2000 and that by now HCPs are more knowledgeable about the benefits of palliative care and thus proactively anticipate and facilitate patient and family decision-making as the disease progresses. However, recent research showed that HCPs (experienced physicians, nurses, and social workers) often feel uncomfortable with discussing (pediatric) advance care planning (ACP) despite the perceived benefits [45]. Perceived barriers include unrealistic expectations by parents, differences between physicians and patients/parents' understanding of prognosis, and parents not being ready for pediatric discussions [46].

Only fairly recently there is increasing awareness of the importance of palliative care in patients with DMD which may be provided through a joint neuromuscular/ palliative care clinic [47]. The adult DMD patients do express the desire to talk about their wishes and needs regarding treatment but also about end-of-life care [42]. Even in parts of the world where talking about the latter is considered taboo [48].

## Limb-Girdle Muscular Dystrophies

### *Epidemiology, Clinical Picture, and Diagnosis*

During an international workshop under the auspices of the European Neuromuscular Centre, consensus was achieved on the definition of limb-girdle muscular dystrophy (LGMD): "……. a genetically inherited condition that primarily affects skeletal muscle leading to progressive, predominantly proximal muscle weakness at presentation caused by a loss of muscle fibres. To be considered a form of limb girdle muscular dystrophy the condition must be described in [.....] families with affected individuals achieving independent walking, must have an elevated serum creatine kinase activity, must demonstrate degenerative changes on muscle imaging over the course of the disease, and have dystrophic changes on muscle histology, ultimately leading to end-stage pathology for the most affected muscles " [49]. In accordance with this definition, the historical classification was replaced by a nomenclature including the mode of inheritance (D for dominant and R for recessive), the affected protein, and a number based upon the order of discovery of the affected protein. Still, LGMDs are a heterogeneous group of myopathies. The age at onset is usually from adolescence to early adulthood, ranging from early childhood to late adult life. Most LGMDs are rare, with a pooled prevalence of limb-girdle muscular dystrophy of 1.63 per 100,000 [31]. Patients suffering from LGMD typically present with slowly progressing symmetrical weakness affecting proximal muscles of the arms and legs. Cases presenting in early childhood resemble DMD with wheelchair dependency before adolescence and respiratory and cardiac involvement, and therefore the patients have the same care needs and preferences as DMD patients. However, there is a lack of studies investigating the benefits of palliative care in LGMD.

### *Management*

An evidence-based guideline from the USA on the diagnosis and treatment of limb-girdle muscular dystrophies (LGMD) guideline touches upon the topic of shared decision-making with respect for the autonomy of the patient in a paragraph on rehabilitative management: "While respecting and protecting patient autonomy, clinicians should proactively anticipate and facilitate patient and family decision-making as the disease progresses, including decisions regarding loss of mobility, need for assistance with activities of daily living, medical complications, and end-of-life care" [50]. The American Academy of Neurology (AAN) formed a multidisciplinary work group to identify and define quality measures toward improving outcomes for patients with a muscular dystrophy. The work group recommended multidisciplinary care with at least a palliative care specialist in the team and discussed many desired outcomes for the care of patients diagnosed with a muscular dystrophy. One of the outcome measures was "increase patient and family engagement," i.e., participation in advanced decision-making in order to facilitate patients, parents, and caregivers to make informed choices that are consistent with their own values. Quality measures were also formulated. All patients with a diagnosis of a muscular dystrophy or their caregivers should be counseled about advanced health-care decision-making, palliative care, or end-of-life issues at least once annually. The multidimensional approach of palliative care should be integrated with curative interventions. Active palliative care anticipates important events such as loss of ambulation, respiratory insufficiency, or cardiac failure which call for flexible re-evaluation of goals of care in line with prognosis.

## Congenital Muscular Dystrophies (CMDs)

### *Epidemiology, Clinical Picture, and Diagnosis*

CMDs are a group of rare genetic neuromuscular disorders with muscle weakness presenting at birth or early infancy. In addition to muscle weakness, the heart, brain, and eye may be affected [51]. The pooled prevalence of congenital muscular dystrophy in all age groups was 0.99 per 100,000 and 0.82 per 100,000 in children only [31]. Patients with CMD experience a broad spectrum of respiratory, musculoskeletal, nutritional, cognitive, and cardiac complications.

### *Management*

In 2010, a CMD care guideline aimed at improving quality of life was published [52]. The guideline was established by bringing together experts in the field but was also fed by the results of an online survey of families and affected individuals with CMD. The guideline addressed how to establish and deliver the diagnosis and discussed management of respiratory, cardiac, orthopedic, nutritional, and speech issues. Palliative care was specifically dealt with. As in the other muscular dystrophies, the guidelines stress that incorporating palliative care from diagnosis can benefit the patient, family, and medical team as they anticipate and make decisions regarding interventions that affect both the duration and quality of these patients' lives [52].

The survey among CMD patients showed that there is wide variability as regards the introduction of palliative care to the patient and family as well as in the availability and composition of palliative care. The guideline recommends to start individualized end-of-life discussions, especially for the more severe life-limiting CMD diagnoses (e.g., Walker-Warburg syndrome), ideally before the first life-threatening event. Educating the parents about the potentially life-limiting character of the disease which can be associated with life-threatening episodes is crucial [52].

## Other Neuromuscular Diseases Which Are Associated with a Reduced Life Expectancy Pompe Disease (Glycogen Storage Disease Type II (GSD2))

### *Epidemiology, Clinical Picture, and Diagnosis*

Pompe disease is a rare autosomal recessively inherited lysosomal disorder caused by mutation in the GAA gene leading to acid α-glucosidase deficiency. Depending largely on how much enzyme activity is preserved, it can present at different ages, from soon after birth to late adulthood. Incidence including all GSD2 forms varies according to ethnicity and region and ranges between 1:40,000 and 1:14,000 [53]. Patients with the classic infantile form (IOPD) present in the first months of life with generalized muscle weakness, hypertrophic cardiomyopathy, respiratory problems, and feeding difficulties. If untreated, they usually die before age two due to cardiorespiratory insufficiency. Late-onset Pompe disease (LOPD) typically shows greater heterogeneity in symptoms with a variable progression and is usually characterized by proximal and axial muscle weakness leading to respiratory insufficiency and ambulatory problems, without cardiac involvement in the majority of patients. Longer disease duration tends to lead to a more severe and more rapidly progressive disease, increasing the likelihood for ventilation support and wheelchair dependency [53].

The diagnosis of Pompe disease is usually based on typical clinical presentation followed by the demonstration of deficiency of GAA enzyme activity in muscle, skin fibroblasts, or dried blood spots as well as *GAA* mutation analysis.

### *Management*

Since 2006, enzyme replacement therapy (ERT) is available to which about half of the infants respond. In adults, ERT has a significant effect on mortality and a short-lasting (2–3 years) beneficial effect on ventilation (forced vital capacity) and mobility (6-minute walk test) [54].

Given the suboptimal clinical response in patients with LOPD and a proportion of patients with IOPD, palliative care is appropriate to discuss treatment options if respiratory or nutritional issues occur or if ERT is no longer beneficial and thus should be discontinued [55, 56]. In an evidence-based guideline on diagnosis and management, palliative care is specifically mentioned in more or less general terms [56]. To the best of our knowledge, there are no studies on palliative care in Pompe disease. A systematic review on the impact of the disease on health-related quality in LOPD (there were no studies on IOPD) showed that LOPD patients have a significantly lower health-related quality of life as compared to the normal population despite treatment with ERT [57].

## Myotonic Dystrophy Type 1 (DM1)

### *Epidemiology, Clinical Picture, and Diagnosis*

DM1 is the most common hereditary (autosomal dominant inheritance) myopathy in adults with an estimated prevalence of 1/8000 in most American and European populations and caused by an expansion of an unstable CTG trinucleotide repeat in the 3'untranslated region of the *myotonic dystrophy protein kinase* (*DMPK*) gene. DM1 is a multisystem disorder affecting not just the skeletal muscles but also the heart, respiratory system, endocrine system, central nervous system, gastrointestinal system, skin, and eyes, and it may cause psychiatric issues. Patients with DM1 can be divided into four main categories determined by the number of repeat expansions, each presenting specific clinical features: congenital, childhood-onset, adult-onset, and late-onset/asymptomatic. Congenital myotonic dystrophy (CDM) occurs in 25% of offspring of mothers with DM1 and is characterized by profound hypotonia, facial weakness, difficulties in sucking and swallowing, and often severe respiratory distress. Survivors may have delayed motor and speech development and mental retardation [58]. Patients with the childhood-onset form of DM1 have cognitive deficits and learning abnormalities [58]. The core features in classic adult-onset

DM1 are distal muscle weakness, leading to difficulty with performing tasks requiring fine dexterity of the hands and foot drop, dysphagia (often unnoticed), and facial weakness. Diagnosis relies on showing expansion of the trinucleotide repeat; the size of the abnormal expansion in affected individuals has a positive association with the severity of symptoms. Disease progression is slow, with gradual involvement of the proximal limb and truncal muscles. The heart is involved in the majority of patients, and sudden death caused by complete AV block is the worst cardiac complication. Diaphragmatic and intercostal muscle weakness may result in alveolar hypoventilation and chronic bronchitis [58]. Acute respiratory failure and pneumonia are the main causes of death in DM1, and the life expectancy is greatly reduced with a mean age at death of 53 years [59, 60]. Central nervous system involvement includes cognitive-behavioral impairment of frontal type which leads slowly but progressively to intellectual and social deterioration. More than half of the patients are disease-unaware which makes patient-centered care challenging [61]. However, a study on the impact of the disease assessed by using the Individualized Neuromuscular Quality of Life, a patient-reported outcome tool, showed that the disease burden is substantial [62]. In particular symptoms as muscle weakness and fatigue were relevant to the patients [62]. A study among patients with congenital or childhood-onset DM and their parents on the relevant symptoms impacting health-related quality of life revealed that communication difficulties, cognitive impairment, and social role limitations were the most important themes [63].

## *Management*

Currently, there are no disease-modifying therapies for patients with DM1 and management aims at handling motor symptoms and hypersomnia, and monitoring cardiac and pulmonary function. A qualitative study among physicians treating patients with complex disorders such as myotonic dystrophy and Huntington's disease conducted in Canada suggested that physicians perceived that they were qualified to treat symptoms, but were less comfortable addressing patients' and caregivers' social and quality-of-life issues. The authors concluded that traditional physician-led clinical models may not be sufficient, that there is a need for greater involvement from allied health professionals, and that it may also be necessary to modify current medical education curricula and resident training programs to ensure that clinicians are better equipped to holistically integrate the complex needs of patients living with chronic disease into collaborative practices [64]. Recently consensus-based care recommendations have been published including a section on palliative care. The first recommendation stressed that palliative care should be introduced at the time of diagnosis and at regular intervals thereafter and that palliative care should be considered as a therapeutic option in the pathway of care to control symptoms, when necessary and not only during the end-of-life stages of disease [65].

## Mitochondrial Diseases

### *Epidemiology, Clinical Picture, and Diagnosis*

Mitochondrial diseases are genetic disorders that impair oxidative phosphorylation and mitochondrial ATP synthesis. Together, they affect about 1 in 5000 adults and children. They are a clinically, biochemically, and genetically heterogeneous group of disorders with a variable age of onset and rate of disease progression and may lead to a range of well-defined, but overlapping, clinical syndromes, including LHON (Leber's hereditary optic neuropathy, adolescents and adults), MELAS (mitochondrial encephalomyopathy with lactic acidosis and stroke-like episodes, children, adults, and adolescents), MERRF (myoclonic epilepsy with ragged red fibers, children and adults), Kearns-Sayre syndrome (children and adolescents), Pearson syndrome (infants), Leigh syndrome (infants), MNGIE (mitochondrial neuro-gastrointestinal encephalopathy, children), benign reversible myopathy (infants), and Alpers-Huttenlocher syndrome (children) [66]. Mitochondrial disease may affect almost every single organ and often results in multisystemic disorders, both in children and adults. Symptoms and signs are muscular (muscle weakness, myalgia, chronic progressive ophthalmoplegia with ptosis, exercise intolerance, or motor developmental delay) or neurological (developmental delay, intellectual deficit, migraine, dystonia, ataxia, spasticity, neuropathy, seizures, encephalopathy) or have a multisystem character (gastrointestinal tract disease, growth delay or failure to thrive, endocrine abnormalities (diabetes mellitus, hypothyroidism), bone marrow failure, visual deficit (optic atrophy, retinitis pigmentosa, cataracts), sensorineural hearing loss, renal tubular acidosis, cardiac involvement) [67].

Numerous nuclear genes are known to cause mitochondrial disease, with autosomal recessive, autosomal dominant, and X-linked inheritance patterns, affecting both children and adults. In adult patients, mitochondrial disease is mainly caused by mutations in the mitochondrial genome and shows exclusive maternal inheritance. Diagnosis is based on molecular genetics. If no molecular genetic diagnosis is available and there is a high clinical suspicion of mitochondrial disease, biochemical or histological studies may be helpful. Still, the diagnostic odyssey of patients with mitochondrial disease is complex and burdensome.

More than half of the patients first receive one or more non-mitochondrial diagnoses before the final mitochondrial diagnosis [68].

### *Management*

There is no curative treatment for mitochondrial diseases, and therefore management is supportive, and it is crucial to prevent acute illness related to deterioration of chronic conditions or to febrile infections, surgery and anesthesia, dietary changes, long periods of fasting, or specific medications. Life expectancy is reduced in most infancy/childhood-onset clinical syndromes and in mitochondrial diseases which are associated with cardiomyopathy (MELAS), arrhythmia (Kearns-Sayre syndrome), or severe muscle weakness and dysphagia leading to respiratory failure/aspiration pneumonia. In a retrospective study from the UK, the life expectancy and causes of death of 30 adults with a mitochondrial disease were evaluated [69]. The causes of death were predominantly respiratory or cardiac. The authors were struck by the fact that most patients died at home where palliative care was delivered by the general practitioner without awareness of the involved tertiary specialists. Thus, they recommend that the primary care physician should coordinate the patient care and the specialist center should provide a point of contact for the patient. They also stress that this communication is equally important in relation to end-of-life issues where effective management may avoid unnecessary intervention in the terminal phase of an illness and allow early initiation of palliative care. The authors mention that timing of when to have "end-of-life discussions" with patients and family will depend on a number of factors including the particular form of mitochondrial disease, the patient's willingness to engage, and the rate of disease progression which may be difficult to determine in patients who experience gradual deterioration [69]. In 2017, consensus-based recommendations for standardized treatment and preventive health care of patients with primary mitochondrial disease were published which also include the usefulness of palliative care consultation, albeit without further details [70].

## Idiopathic Inflammatory Myopathies (IIM)

### *Epidemiology, Clinical Picture, and Diagnosis*

The current classification includes dermatomyositis (DM), immune-mediated necrotizing myopathy (IMNM), overlap myositis (OM) including anti-synthetase syndrome (ASS), and inclusion body myositis (IBM) [71]. Based on the presence of myositis-associated or myositis-specific antibodies (MAA/MSA), there are numerous subtypes, but this is beyond the scope of this chapter. Diagnosis is based on clinicoseropathological findings [72]. IIMs are rare (estimated incidence of 6–10 per million persons per year and a prevalence of 12 per 100,000 persons). IBM is the most common acquired muscle disease in patients older than 50 years, with an estimated incidence of 1–3 per million persons per year and a prevalence of 2–5 per 100,000 persons [73].

Classic DM is characterized by specific skin features. Muscle weakness is usually preceded by skin rash but may never develop, i.e., amyopathic dermatomyositis. The association with cancer is another important feature of adult-onset DM and associated with specific MSAs [74]. Histopathology (skin, muscle) shows characteristic changes [72]. IMNM is generally characterized by severe muscle weakness.

Two autoantibodies are associated specifically with IMNM: anti-SRP and anti-HMGCR autoantibodies. In approximately half of patients with the latter, a history of statin use is found. Seronegative and anti-HMGCR-positive adult-onset IMNM are associated with cancer. Histopathology of IMNM is characterized by extensive muscle fiber necrosis and the absence of (significant) lymphocytic infiltrates in the muscles as seen in other myositis subgroups [75, 76]. Overlap myositis (OM) forms a category without distinctive clinical, pathological, and/or serological features. OM is frequently associated with MAAs, other connective tissue disorders, and extramuscular disease activity [77, 78]. Anti-synthetase syndrome (ASS) can be considered an overlap myositis since it is characterized by a combination of myositis, Raynaud phenomenon, "mechanic hands," nonerosive polyarthritis, and interstitial lung disease (ILD) [79]. Not all symptoms may be present, and ASS may present with ILD which may cause a diagnostic delay [74]. Distinction from DM is sometimes cumbersome since in about 25% characteristic DM features can be found in ASS. Serology is of diagnostic value; anti-Jo1 autoantibodies are the ones most commonly found [79]. IBM is the outlier of the IIMs since it is as yet an incurable disease and characterized by both proximal and distal muscle weaknesses (the quadriceps femoris and deep finger flexor muscles) [80].

Extramuscular disease activity (ILD in particular) and cancer significantly contribute to myositis-related morbidity and determine myositis-related mortality. Hence, screening for extramuscular disease activity and cancer is of cardinal importance. Screening for ILD should be based on the clinicoserological profile of a patient with myositis. An example is the East Asian patient with anti-MDA5 autoantibodies who should be monitored closely for the development of rapidly progressive ILD [81]. Screening for cancer in subtypes of DM and IMNM (see above) should be performed for 3–5 years after diagnosis of myositis. Probably there is also cardiac involvement – in particular potentially reversible (peri)myocarditis that may lead to arrhythmias and/or cardiomyopathy – however, this has not yet been sufficiently studied in a systematic manner.

Dysphagia occurs in all myositis subtypes. A recently published systematic review and meta-analysis comprising 109 studies including 10,382 subjects showed an overall estimate of dysphagia prevalence of 36% in IIM [82]. In IBM patients, a prevalence of 56% was estimated.

## *Management*

There are manifold therapeutic regimes, including numerous immunosuppressants or immunomodulation modalities, aimed at ameliorating muscle weakness including dysphagia in IIM [83]. As IBM does not respond to these pharmacological interventions, dysphagia management remains of major concern as this condition progresses [84]. Botulinum toxin, cricopharyngeal dilatation, or myotomy may be beneficial dependent on the mechanism of dysphagia. All three abovementioned interventions have been performed in IIM with varying results as regards improvement of the swallowing function and the duration of the symptom relief, which perhaps is not surprising since most interventions take place without thorough evaluation of the cause of dysphagia. Even more concerning is the fact that there are no interventional trials with meaningful clinical endpoints.

In the literature on management of IIM and IBM in particular, no mention is made of palliative care whereas dysphagia negatively affects quality of life but is also associated with increased morbidity (i.e., dehydration, malnutrition, and aspiration pneumonia) and increased mortality, probably due to aspiration pneumonia which is significantly more prevalent in dysphagic as compared to non-dysphagic IIM patients, and especially in IBM [82, 84]. In literature on ILD caused by pulmonary fibrosis which causes considerable symptom burden and reduced quality of life, early integrated palliative care and regular counseling of the patient and caregiver are recommended [85]. However, a retrospective study published in 2018 on the use of palliative care in the terminal stage in which the patients suffered from severe dyspnea showed that referral to palliative care and use of palliative medications occurred just prior to death [86]. As mentioned before in this chapter, misconception about palliative care being synonymous with end-of-life care and the stigma of prescribing opioids and benzodiazepines contributes to the unnecessarily suffering of the patients [85]. In an excellent review, the structured approach to comprehensive care, including palliative care throughout the disease course in ILD, has been described, including the barriers to provide optimal palliative care which may be ILD-, patient-, or HCP-related. The authors also take cultural factors and religious beliefs into consideration [85].

## Conclusion

Disease burden in most neuromuscular diseases is considerable due to incapacitating disability and reduced life expectancy. ALS is exemplary, but the same holds for SMA, DMD, and congenital muscular dystrophies. In these disorders, the significance of integrated palliative care as part of standard of care is gradually recognized. There are only few studies evaluating the provision of palliative care. The studies are mostly qualitative and show appreciation by the patients and their caregivers if advance care planning is provided, e.g., in ALS. At the same time, there are apparently also obstacles which hamper the initiation of palliative care, such as lack of awareness of health-care professionals, patients, and parents and reluctance to participate in discussions on advance care planning and in particular on end-of-life issues. Cultural and religious factors may play a role in this. Therefore, palliative care is underutilized, as was shown in studies on DMD and myositis-related ILD. There is, however, increasing awareness about the role palliative care can play in chronic progressive, life-limiting neuromuscular diseases, in particular in SMA and DMD. In both diseases, palliative care is explicitly included in consensus statements on standards of care, and in DMD, reports are emerging on joint clinics of neuromuscular and palliative care. In other diseases, in which palliative care would be appropriate given the unmet needs of patients and caregivers, such as Pompe disease, myotonic dystrophy type 1, and inflammatory myopathies, a palliative care approach is not considered or in very general terms. However, every disease is unique, and that also holds for the needs, wishes, and preferences of the patients and carers. This calls for more condition-specific research and also for the development of evidence-based valid instruments, like patient-related outcome measures, which could accurately measure the impact of a specific disease on the patient's quality of life and that of the caregiver [85, 87].

Optimal palliation requires various skills, provided by a multidisciplinary team of health-care professionals. Education of these health-care professionals, directed toward improving communication strategies, is crucial in this respect.

## References

1. Saunders C. The evolution of palliative care. J R Soc Med. 2001;94:430–2. https://doi.org/10.1177/014107680109400904.
2. Borasio GD. The role of palliative care in patients with neurological diseases. Nat Rev Neurol. 2013;9:292–5. https://doi.org/10.1038/nrneurol.2013.49.
3. Gaertner J, Wolf J, Ostgathe C, Toepelt K, Glossmann JP, Hallek M, et al. Specifying WHO recommendation: moving toward disease-specific guidelines. J Palliat Med. 2010; 13:1273-6. https://doi.org/10.1089/jpm.2010.0016.
4. Oliver DJ, Borasio GD, Caraceni A, de Visser M, Grisold W, Lorenzl S, et al. A consensus review on the development of palliative care for patients with chronic and progressive neurological disease. Eur J Neurol. 2016;23:30-8. https://doi.org/10.1111/ene.12889.
5. Singer PA, Robertson G, Roy DJ. Bioethics for clinicians: 6. Advance care planning. CMAJ. 1996;155:1689–92.
6. Miyashita J, Kohno A, Cheng SY, Hsu SH, Yamamoto Y, Shimizu S, et al. Patients' preferences and factors influencing initial advance care planning discussions' timing: a cross-cultural mixed-methods study. Palliat Med. 2020;34:906–16. https://doi.org/10.1177/0269216320914791.
7. Borasio GD, Shaw PJ, Hardiman O, Ludolph AC, Sales Luis ML, Silani V. Standards of palliative care for patients with amyotrophic lateral sclerosis: results of a European survey. Amyotroph Lateral Scler Other Mot Neuron Disord. 2001;2:159-64. https://doi.org/10.1080/146608201753275517.
8. van Vliet LM, Gao W, DiFrancesco D, Crosby V, Wilcock A, Byrne A, et al. How integrated are neurology and palliative care services? Results of a multicentre mapping exercise. BMC Neurol. 2016;16:63. https://doi.org/10.1186/s12883-016-0583-6.
9. Walter HAW, Seeber AA, Willems DL, De Visser M. The role of palliative care in chronic progressive neurological diseases-a survey amongst neurologists in the Netherlands. Front Neurol. 2019;10:1157. https://doi.org/10.3389/fneur.2018.01157.
10. Hardiman O, Al-Chalabi A, Chio A, Corr EM, Logroscino G, Robberecht W, et al. Amyotrophic lateral sclerosis. Nat Rev Dis Prim. 2017;3:17071. https://doi.org/10.1038/nrdp.2017.71.
11. Beeldman E, Govaarts R, De Visser M, Klein Twennaar M, Van Der Kooi AJ, Van Den Berg LH, et al. Progression of cognitive and behavioural impairment in early amyotrophic lateral sclerosis. J Neurol Neurosurg Psychiatry. 2020;91:779-80. https://doi.org/10.1136/jnnp-2020-322992.
12. Visser J, Van Den Berg-Vos RM, Franssen H, Van Den Berg LH, Wokke JH, De Jong JMV, et al. Disease course and prognostic factors of progressive muscular atrophy. Arch Neurol. 2007;64:522-8. https://doi.org/10.1001/archneur.64.4.522.

13. Talbot K. Motor neuron disease. Pract Neurol. 2009;9:303–9. https://doi.org/10.1136/jnnp.2009.188151.
14. Oliver D, Radunovic A, Allen A, McDermott C. The development of the UK National Institute of Health and Care Excellence evidence-based clinical guidelines on motor neurone disease. Amyotroph Lateral Scler Frontotemporal Degener. 2017;18(5-6):313-23.
15. Seeber AA, Pols AJ, Hijdra A, Grupstra HF, Willems DL, de Visser M. Experiences and reflections of patients with motor neuron disease on breaking the news in a two-tiered appointment: a qualitative study. BMJ Support Palliat Care. 2019:9:e8. https://doi.org/10.1136/bmjspcare-2015-000977.
16. Aoun SM, Breen LJ, Edis R, Henderson RD, Oliver D, Harris R, et al. Breaking the news of a diagnosis of motor neurone disease: a national survey of neurologists' perspectives. J Neurol Sci. 2016;367:368–74. https://doi.org/10.1016/j.jns.2016.06.033.
17. Aoun SM, Breen LJ, Oliver D, Henderson RD, Edis R, O'Connor M, et al. Family carers' experiences of receiving the news of a diagnosis of motor neurone disease: a national survey. J Neurol Sci. 2017;372:144–51. https://doi.org/10.1016/j.jns.2016.11.043.
18. Seeber AA, Pols AJ, Hijdra A, Grupstra HF, Willems DL, De Visser M. Advance care planning in progressive neurological diseases: lessons from ALS. BMC Palliat Care. 2019;18:50. https://doi.org/10.1186/s12904-019-0433-6.
19. Chiò A, Mora G, Lauria G. Pain in amyotrophic lateral sclerosis. Lancet Neurol. 2017;16:144–57. https://doi.org/10.1016/S1474-4422(16)30358-1.
20. Faull C, Haynes CR, Oliver D. Issues for palliative medicine doctors surrounding the withdrawal of non-invasive ventilation at the request of a patient with motor neurone disease: a scoping study. BMJ Support Palliat Care. 2014;4:43–9. https://doi.org/10.1136/bmjspcare-2013-000470.
21. Druml C, Ballmer PE, Druml W, Oehmichen F, Shenkin A, Singer P, et al. ESPEN guideline on ethical aspects of artificial nutrition and hydration. Clin Nutr. 2016;35:545-56. https://doi.org/10.1016/j.clnu.2016.02.006.
22. O'Brien MR, Whitehead B, Jack BA, Mitchell JD. From symptom onset to a diagnosis of amyotrophic lateral sclerosis/motor neuron disease (ALS/MND): experiences of people with ALS/MND and family carers – a qualitative study. Amyotroph Lateral Scler. 2011;12:97–104. https://doi.org/10.3109/17482968.2010.546414.
23. Dobre C, Duceac L, Grierosu C, Mihai D, Zaharia A, Stafie L, et al. Efficient measures for burnout prevention in palliative care. Int J Med Dent. 2017;21:81–4.
24. Mercuri E, Finkel RS, Muntoni F, Wirth B, Montes J, Main M, et al. Diagnosis and management of spinal muscular atrophy: part 1: recommendations for diagnosis, rehabilitation, orthopedic and nutritional care. Neuromuscul Disord. 2018;28:103–15. https://doi.org/10.1016/j.nmd.2017.11.005.
25. Finkel RS, Mercuri E, Meyer OH, Simonds AK, Schroth MK, Graham RJ, et al. Diagnosis and management of spinal muscular atrophy: part 2: pulmonary and acute care; medications, supplements and immunizations; other organ systems; and ethics. Neuromuscul Disord. 2018;28:197–207. https://doi.org/10.1016/j.nmd.2017.11.004.
26. Oskoui M, Ng P, Liben S, Zielinski D. Physician driven variation in the care of children with spinal muscular atrophy type 1. Pediatr Pulmonol. 2017;52:662–8. https://doi.org/10.1002/ppul.23616.
27. Albrechtsen SS, Born AP, Boesen MS. Nusinersen treatment of spinal muscular atrophy – a systematic review. Dan Med J. 2020;67:1–12.
28. Finkel RS, Mercuri E, Darras BT, Connolly AM, Kuntz NL, Kirschner J, et al. Nusinersen versus sham control in infantile-onset spinal muscular atrophy. N Engl J Med. 2017;377:1723–32. https://doi.org/10.1056/nejmoa1702752.
29. Lövgren M, Sejersen T, Kreicbergs U. Parents' experiences and wishes at end of life in children with spinal muscular atrophy types I and II. J Pediatr. 2016;175:201–5. https://doi.org/10.1016/j.jpeds.2016.04.062.

30. Hully M, Barnerias C, Chabalier D, Le Guen S, Germa V, Deladriere E, et al. Palliative care in SMA type 1: a prospective multicenter French study based on parents' reports. Front Pediatr. 2020;8:4. https://doi.org/10.3389/fped.2020.00004.
31. Mah JK, Korngut L, Fiest KM, Dykeman J, Day LJ, Pringsheim T, et al. A systematic review and meta-analysis on the epidemiology of the muscular dystrophies. Can J Neurol Sci. 2015;43:163–77. https://doi.org/10.1017/cjn.2015.311.
32. Hoffman EP, Brown RH, Kunkel LM. Dystrophin: the protein product of the duchenne muscular dystrophy locus. Cell. 1987;51:919–28. https://doi.org/10.1016/0092-8674(87)90579-4.
33. Birnkrant DJ, Bushby K, Bann CM, Apkon SD, Blackwell A, Brumbaugh D, et al. Diagnosis and management of Duchenne muscular dystrophy, part 1: diagnosis, and neuromuscular, rehabilitation, endocrine, and gastrointestinal and nutritional management. Lancet Neurol. 2018;17:251–67. https://doi.org/10.1016/S1474-4422(18)30024-3.
34. Aartsma-Rus A, Hegde M, Ben-Omran T, Buccella F, Ferlini A, Gallano P, et al. Evidence-based consensus and systematic review on reducing the time to diagnosis of Duchenne muscular dystrophy. J Pediatr. 2019;204:305–313.e14. https://doi.org/10.1016/j.jpeds.2018.10.043.
35. Wong SH, McClaren BJ, Archibald AD, Weeks A, Langmaid T, Ryan MM, et al. A mixed methods study of age at diagnosis and diagnostic odyssey for Duchenne muscular dystrophy. Eur J Hum Genet. 2015;23:1294–300. https://doi.org/10.1038/ejhg.2014.301.
36. Eagle M, Bourke J, Bullock R, Gibson M, Mehta J, Giddings D, et al. Managing Duchenne muscular dystrophy – the additive effect of spinal surgery and home nocturnal ventilation in improving survival. Neuromuscul Disord. 2007;17:470–5. https://doi.org/10.1016/j.nmd.2007.03.002.
37. Birnkrant DJ, Bushby K, Bann CM, Alman BA, Apkon SD, Blackwell A, et al. Diagnosis and management of Duchenne muscular dystrophy, part 2: respiratory, cardiac, bone health, and orthopaedic management. Lancet Neurol. 2018;17:347–61. https://doi.org/10.1016/S1474-4422(18)30025-5.
38. Birnkrant DJ, Bushby K, Bann CM, Apkon SD, Blackwell A, Colvin MK, et al. Diagnosis and management of Duchenne muscular dystrophy, part 3: primary care, emergency management, psychosocial care, and transitions of care across the lifespan. Lancet Neurol. 2018;17:445–55. https://doi.org/10.1016/S1474-4422(18)30026-7.
39. Dzierlega K, Yokota T. Optimization of antisense-mediated exon skipping for Duchenne muscular dystrophy. Gene Ther. 2020;27:407–16. https://doi.org/10.1038/s41434-020-0156-6.
40. Mercuri E, Muntoni F, Osorio AN, Tulinius M, Buccella F, Morgenroth LP, et al. Safety and effectiveness of ataluren: comparison of results from the STRIDE Registry and CINRG DMD Natural History Study. J Comp Eff Res. 2020;9:341–60. https://doi.org/10.2217/cer-2019-0171.
41. Hiscock A, Kuhn I, Barclay S. Advance care discussions with young people affected by life-limiting neuromuscular diseases: a systematic literature review and narrative synthesis. Neuromuscul Disord. 2017;27:115–9. https://doi.org/10.1016/j.nmd.2016.11.011.
42. Abbott D, Prescott H, Forbes K, Fraser J, Majumdar A. Men with Duchenne muscular dystrophy and end of life planning. Neuromuscul Disord. 2017;27:38–44. https://doi.org/10.1016/j.nmd.2016.09.022.
43. Arias R, Andrews J, Pandya S, Pettit K, Trout C, Apkon S, et al. Palliative care services in families of males with Duchenne muscular dystrophy. Muscle Nerve. 2011;44:93–101. https://doi.org/10.1002/mus.22005.
44. Andrews JG, Pandya S, Trout C, Jaff T, Matthews D, Cunniff C, et al. Palliative care services in families of males with muscular dystrophy: data from MD STARnet. SAGE Open Med. 2019;7:205031211984051. https://doi.org/10.1177/2050312119840518.
45. Lotz JD, Jox RJ, Borasio GD, Führer M. Pediatric advance care planning from the perspective of health care professionals: a qualitative interview study. Palliat Med. 2015;29:212–22. https://doi.org/10.1177/0269216314552091.
46. Durall A, Zurakowski D, Wolfe J. Barriers to conducting advance care discussions for children with life-threatening conditions. Pediatrics. 2012;129:e975-82 https://doi.org/10.1542/peds.2011-2695.

47. Macfarlane M, Willis TA, Easthope-Mowatt Y, Bassie C, Willis D. Adult neuromuscular disorders: a joint palliative/neuromuscular clinic. BMJ Support Palliat Care. 2019:1–2. https://doi.org/10.1136/bmjspcare-2019-001821.
48. Tapawan SJC, Wang FS, Lee MW, Chua AQ, Lin JB, Han V, et al. Perspectives on palliative care among Duchenne muscular dystrophy patients and their families in Singapore. Ann Acad Med Singap. 2020;49:72–7.
49. Straub V, Murphy A, Udd B. 229th ENMC international workshop: limb girdle muscular dystrophies – nomenclature and reformed classification Naarden, the Netherlands, 17–19; 2017. Neuromuscul Disord. 2018;28:702-10. https://doi.org/10.1016/j.nmd.2018.05.007.
50. Narayanaswami P, Weiss M, Selcen D, David W, Raynor E, Carter G, et al. Evidence-based guideline summary: diagnosis and treatment of limb-girdle and distal dystrophies: report of the Guideline Development Subcommittee of the American Academy of Neurology and the Practice Issues Review Panel of the American Association of Neuromuscular & Electrodiagnostic Medicine. Neurology. 2014;83:1453–63. https://doi.org/10.1212/WNL.0000000000000892.
51. Schorling DC, Kirschner J, Bönnemann CG. Congenital muscular dystrophies and myopathies: an overview and update. Neuropediatrics. 2017;48:247–61. https://doi.org/10.1055/s-0037-1604154.
52. Wang CH, Bonnemann CG, Rutkowski A, Sejersen T, Bellini J, Battista V, et al. Consensus statement on standard of care for congenital muscular dystrophies. J Child Neurol. 2010;25:1559–81. https://doi.org/10.1177/0883073810381924.
53. Dasouki M, Jawdat O, Almadhoun O, Pasnoor M, McVey AL, Abuzinadah A, et al. Pompe disease: literature review and case series. Neurol Clin. 2014;32:751–76. https://doi.org/10.1016/j.ncl.2014.04.010.
54. Schoser B, Stewart A, Kanters S, Hamed A, Jansen J, Chan K, et al. Survival and long-term outcomes in late-onset Pompe disease following alglucosidase alfa treatment: a systematic review and meta-analysis. J Neurol. 2017;264:621–30. https://doi.org/10.1007/s00415-016-8219-8.
55. van der Ploeg AT, Kruijshaar ME, Toscano A, Laforêt P, Angelini C, Lachmann RH, et al. European consensus for starting and stopping enzyme replacement therapy in adult patients with Pompe disease: a 10-year experience. Eur J Neurol. 2017;24:768–e31. https://doi.org/10.1111/ene.13285.
56. Tarnopolsky M, Katzberg H, Petrof BJ, Sirrs S, Sarnat HB, Myers K, et al. Pompe disease: diagnosis and management. Evidence-based guidelines from a Canadian Expert Panel. Can J Neurol Sci. 2016;43:472–85. https://doi.org/10.1017/cjn.2016.37.
57. Schoser B, Bilder DA, Dimmock D, Gupta D, James ES, Prasad S. The humanistic burden of Pompe disease: are there still unmet needs? A systematic review. BMC Neurol. 2017;17:202. https://doi.org/10.1186/s12883-017-0983-2.
58. Meola G, Cardani R. Myotonic dystrophies: an update on clinical aspects, genetic, pathology, and molecular pathomechanisms. Biochim Biophys Acta Mol basis Dis. 1852;2015:594–606. https://doi.org/10.1016/j.bbadis.2014.05.019.
59. De Die-Smulders CEM, Höweler CJ, Thijs C, Mirandolle JF, Anten HB, Smeets HJM, et al. Age and causes of death in adult-onset myotonic dystrophy. Brain. 1998;121:1557–63. https://doi.org/10.1093/brain/121.8.1557.
60. Mathieu J, Allard P, Potvin L, Prévost C, Begin P. A 10-year study of mortality in a cohort of patients with myotonic dystrophy. Neurology. 1999;52:1658–62. https://doi.org/10.1212/wnl.52.8.1658.
61. Baldanzi S, Bevilacqua F, Lorio R, Volpi L, Simoncini C, Petrucci A, et al. Disease awareness in myotonic dystrophy type 1: an observational cross-sectional study. Orphanet J Rare Dis. 2016;11:34. https://doi.org/10.1186/s13023-016-0417-z.
62. Landfeldt E, Nikolenko N, Jimenez-Moreno C, Cumming S, Monckton DG, Gorman G, et al. Disease burden of myotonic dystrophy type 1. J Neurol. 2019;266:998–1006.
63. Johnson NE, Luebbe E, Eastwood E, Chin N, Moxley RT, Heatwole CR. The impact of congenital and childhood myotonic dystrophy on quality of life: a qualitative study of associated symptoms. J Child Neurol. 2014;29:983–6. https://doi.org/10.1177/0883073813484804.

64. Ladonna KA, Watling CJ, Ray SL, Piechowicz C, Venance SL. Myotonic dystrophy and Huntington's disease care: we like to think we're making a difference. Can J Neurol Sci. 2016;43:678–86. https://doi.org/10.1017/cjn.2016.257.
65. Ashizawa T, Gagnon C, Groh WJ, Gutmann L, Johnson NE, Meola G, et al. Consensus-based care recommendations for adults with myotonic dystrophy type 1. Neurol Clin Pract. 2018;8:507–20. https://doi.org/10.1212/CPJ.0000000000000531.
66. Gorman GS, Schaefer AM, Ng Y, Gomez N, Blakely EL, Alston CL, et al. Prevalence of nuclear and mitochondrial DNA mutations related to adult mitochondrial disease. Ann Neurol. 2015;77:753–9. https://doi.org/10.1002/ana.24362.
67. Kanungo S, Morton J, Neelakantan M, Ching K, Saeedian JGA. Mitochondrial disorders. Ann Transl Med. 2018;6:475–92.
68. Grier J, Hirano M, Karaa A, Shepard E, Thompson JLP. Diagnostic odyssey of patients with mitochondrial disease results of a survey. Neurol Genet. 2018;4:e230. https://doi.org/10.1212/NXG.0000000000000230.
69. Barends M, Verschuren L, Morava E, Nesbitt V, Turnbull D, McFarland R. Causes of death in adults with mitochondrial disease. JIMD Rep. 2016;26:103–13. https://doi.org/10.1007/8904_2015_449.
70. Parikh S, Goldstein A, Karaa A, Koenig MK, Anselm I, Brunel-Guitton C, et al. Patient care standards for primary mitochondrial disease: a consensus statement from the mitochondrial medicine society. Genet Med. 2017;19:1–18. https://doi.org/10.1038/gim.2017.107.
71. Hoogendijk JE, Amato AA, Lecky BR, Choy EH, Lundberg IE, Rose MR, et al. 119th ENMC international workshop: trial design in adult idiopathic inflammatory myopathies, with the exception of inclusion body myositis, 10–12 October 2003, Naarden, The Netherlands. Neuromuscul Disord. 2004;14:337-45. https://doi.org/10.1016/j.nmd.2004.02.006.
72. Tanboon J, Nishino I. Classification of idiopathic inflammatory myopathies: pathology perspectives. Curr Opin Neurol. 2019;32:704–14. https://doi.org/10.1097/WCO.0000000000000740.
73. Meyer A, Meyer N, Schaeffer M, Gottenberg JE, Geny B, Sibilia J. Incidence and prevalence of inflammatory myopathies: a systematic review. Rheumatol (UK). 2014;54:50–63. https://doi.org/10.1093/rheumatology/keu289.
74. Lundberg IE, De Visser M, Werth VP. Classification of myositis. Nat Rev Rheumatol. 2018;14:269-78. https://doi.org/10.1038/nrrheum.2018.41.
75. Allenbach Y, Mammen AL, Benveniste O, Stenzel W, Allenbach Y, Amato A, et al. 224th ENMC International Workshop:: Clinico-sero-pathological classification of immune-mediated necrotizing myopathies Zandvoort, The Netherlands, 14–16 October 2016. Neuromuscul Disord. 2018;28:87-99. https://doi.org/10.1016/j.nmd.2017.09.016.
76. Allenbach Y, Benveniste O, Goebel HH, Stenzel W. Integrated classification of inflammatory myopathies. Neuropathol Appl Neurobiol. 2017;43:62–81. https://doi.org/10.1111/nan.12380.
77. Van der Meulen MFG, Bronner IM, Hoogendijk JE, Burger H, Van Venrooij WJ, Voskuyl AE, et al. Polymyositis: an overdiagnosed entity. Neurology. 2003;61:316-21. https://doi.org/10.1212/WNL.61.3.316.
78. van de Vlekkert J, Hoogendijk JE, de Haan RJ, Algra A, van der Tweel I, van der Pol WL, et al. Oral dexamethasone pulse therapy versus daily prednisolone in sub-acute onset myositis, a randomised clinical trial. Neuromuscul Disord. 2010;20:382-9. https://doi.org/10.1016/j.nmd.2010.03.011.
79. Noguchi E, Uruha A, Suzuki S, Hamanaka K, Ohnuki Y, Tsugawa J, et al. Skeletal muscle involvement in antisynthetase syndrome. JAMA Neurol. 2017;74:992–9. https://doi.org/10.1001/jamaneurol.2017.0934.
80. Lloyd TE, Mammen AL, Amato AA, Weiss MD, Needham M, Greenberg SA. Evaluation and construction of diagnostic criteria for inclusion body myositis. Neurology. 2014;83:426-33. https://doi.org/10.1212/WNL.0000000000000642.
81. Li L, Wang Q, Yang F, Wu C, Chen S, Wen X, et al. Anti-MDA5 antibody as a potential diagnostic and prognostic biomarker in patients with dermatomyositis. Oncotarget. 2017;8:26552–64. https://doi.org/10.18632/oncotarget.15716.

82. Labeit B, Pawlitzki M, Ruck T, Muhle P, Claus I, Suntrup-Krueger S, et al. The impact of dysphagia in myositis: a systematic review and meta-analysis. J Clin Med. 2020 8;9:2150.
83. Gordon PA, Winer JB, Hoogendijk JE, Choy EH. Immunosuppressant and immunomodulatory treatment for dermatomyositis and polymyositis. Cochrane Database Syst Rev. 2012; 2012:CD003643. https://doi.org/10.1002/14651858.cd003643.pub4.
84. Price MA, Barghout V, Benveniste O, Christopher-Stine L, Corbett A, De Visser M, et al. Mortality and causes of death in patients with sporadic inclusion body myositis: survey study based on the clinical experience of specialists in Australia, Europe and the USA. J Neuromuscul Dis. 2016; 3:67-75. https://doi.org/10.3233/JND-150138.
85. Kreuter M, Bendstrup E, Russell AM, Bajwah S, Lindell K, Adir Y, et al. Palliative care in interstitial lung disease: living well. Lancet Respir Med. 2017;5:968–80. https://doi.org/10.1016/S2213-2600(17)30383-1.
86. Mann J, Guo H, Goh N, Smallwood N. Palliative and symptomatic care of patients with fibrotic interstitial lung disease; Eur Resp J 2018: Suppl. 62, PA4788. https://doi.org/10.1183/13993003.congress-2018.pa4788.
87. Powell PA, Carlton J, Woods HB, Mazzone P. Measuring quality of life in Duchenne muscular dystrophy: a systematic review of the content and structural validity of commonly used instruments. Health Qual Life Outcomes. 2020;18:263. https://doi.org/10.1186/s12955-020-01511-z.

# Chapter 14
# Palliative Care in Pulmonary Arterial Hypertension

**David Christiansen, Jason Weatherald, and Evan Orlikow**

## Section 1: Pathophysiology and Physical Symptoms of PAH

### *PAH Pathophysiology*

Under normal circumstances, the right ventricle (RV) ejects blood into the low resistance pulmonary circulation. PAH is characterized by a progressive increase in pulmonary vascular resistance (PVR), ultimately resulting in RV failure. This increase in PVR is caused by changes in the small pulmonary arterioles, including vasoconstriction, proliferation and remodeling of the vessel wall, and in situ thrombosis [1]. Together, these changes result in a significant decrease in the cross-sectional area of the pulmonary circulation as well as impaired recruitment and distension of the pulmonary vasculature [2].

Increased pulmonary arterial pressure and RV afterload eventually result in RV enlargement and dysfunction (Fig. 14.1). RV enlargement results in functional tricuspid regurgitation, which further impairs forward flow. Subsequently, RV end diastolic pressure and volumes increase, which result in impaired left ventricular filling via ventricular interdependence, causing further impairment in cardiac output [4]. Low cardiac output results in lower systemic blood pressures. This, in combination with higher RV intracavitary pressures, results in hypoperfusion of RV myocardium, further impairing RV function [5]. As RV dysfunction progresses, central venous pressure rises resulting in hepatic, splanchnic, and renal congestion.

D. Christiansen (✉) · E. Orlikow
Section of Respiratory Medicine, Department of Medicine, University of Manitoba, Winnipeg, MB, Canada
e-mail: dchristiansen@sbgh.mb.ca; eorlikow@manitoba-physicians.ca

J. Weatherald
Section of Respirology, Department of Medicine, University of Calgary, Calgary, AB, Canada



K. O. Lindell, S. K. Danoff (eds.), *Palliative Care in Lung Disease*, Respiratory Medicine, https://doi.org/10.1007/978-3-030-81788-6_14

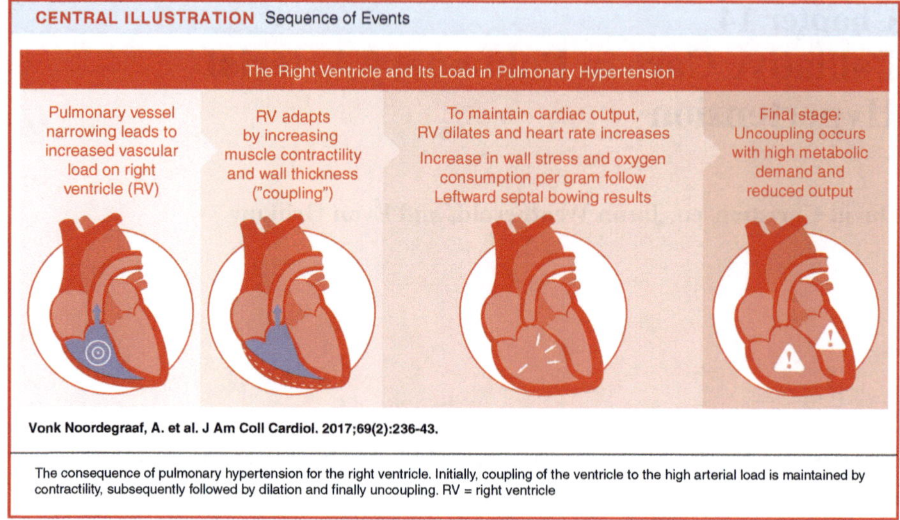


**Fig. 14.1** Features of progressive right ventricular failure that occurs in PAH. (With permission from Ref. [3])

This complex pathophysiologic cascade results in the common symptoms of PAH including shortness of breath on exertion, fatigue, presyncope, chest pain, and peripheral edema [6]. Moreover, as PAH may be secondary to another disease (e.g., systemic sclerosis, human immunodeficiency virus, cirrhosis, etc.), patients may also experience symptoms related to the specific underlying disease or symptoms related to increasingly prevalent comorbidities [7].

## *Physical Symptoms of PAH: Pathogenesis and Management*

### Dyspnea

Dyspnea arises in PAH due to a complex interplay of factors. Impaired cardiac output and skeletal muscle function result in early anaerobiosis which coupled with inefficient gas exchange and heightened chemosensitivity increases ventilatory drive and the sensation of dyspnea [8]. Dyspnea is also promoted by hypoxemia, which often occurs with exercise due to low mixed-venous oxygen saturation, ventilation-perfusion mismatch, and occasionally right-to-left shunting via a patent foramen ovale [9].

Most PAH-targeted therapies improve dyspnea when measured using a variety of clinical scores as outlined in Table 14.1. Beyond treatment of the underlying PAH, management of dyspnea should encompass rehabilitation, oxygen therapy where necessary, and pharmacologic therapy such as opioids, when needed.

**Table 14.1** PAH-targeted therapies and their effects on symptoms, exercise capacity, functional class, and HRQoL in key clinical trials, as well as important side effects

| Medication | Symptom burden (dyspnea) | Exercise capacity (6MWT) | WHO FC | HRQoL | Common or important side effects | Reference |
|---|---|---|---|---|---|---|
| Calcium channel blockers | | | | | | |
| Nifedipine, amlodipine, verapamil | NR | NR | + | NR | Systemic hypotension, RV failure | [10–12] |
| Prostacyclin pathway agonists | | | | | | |
| Epoprostenol (intravenous) | + | + | + | + | Systemic hypotension, headache, jaw pain, diarrhea, flushing, arthralgias, nausea, vomiting | [13, 14] |
| Treprostinil (subcutaneous) | + | + | NR | + | | [15] |
| Iloprost (inhaled) | + | + | + | + | | [16] |
| Selexipag (oral) | NR | + | – | + | | [17] |
| Endothelin receptor antagonists | | | | | | |
| Bosentan | + | + | + | – | Hepatotoxicity, anemia, edema | [18–20] |
| Macitentan | + | + | + | + | | [21, 22] |
| Ambrisentan | + | + | – | – | | [23] |
| PDE5 inhibitors | | | | | | |
| Sildenafil | – | + | + | + | Headache, flushing, dyspepsia. Rare hearing/vision loss | [24–26], [27] |
| Tadalafil | – | + | – | + | | [28] |
| Guanylate cyclase stimulators | | | | | | |
| Riociguat | + | + | + | + | Systemic hypotension, syncope | [29] |

Reproduced from Ref. [30]

*PAH* pulmonary arterial hypertension, *6MWT* 6-minute walk test, *WHO* World Health Organization. *FC* functional class. *HRQoL* health-related quality of life, *CCBs* calcium channel blockers, *NR* not reported, + significant improvement (in most or all studies), – no significant change or inconsistent effect across studies, *RV* right ventricular, *PDE5* phosphodiesterase type 5. Symptom and HRQoL tools included the following: Borg Dyspnea Score [15, 18–20, 23, 24, 28, 29, 31], Dyspnea-Fatigue Score [14, 15, 32], Mahler Dyspnea Index Score [16], Chronic Heart Failure Questionnaire [14, 25], Nottingham Health Profile [14], Medical Outcomes Study 36-Item Short Form [21, 23, 27, 28], Minnesota Living with Heart Failure Questionnaire [15], EuroQol Visual Analogue Scale Form [16, 27–29], and Living with Pulmonary Hypertension Questionnaire [29]

Physical inactivity is common in PAH due to cardiopulmonary limitation and as a maladaptive coping mechanism. Reduced daytime activity (<15 h/day) is associated with death or need for lung transplantation, whereas greater daytime activity is associated with increased quality of life [33]. Supervised rehabilitation programs for patients with PAH improve exercise capacity [34] and several domains of quality of life [35]. Even patients in functional class IV appear to derive a significant benefit without complications; however, attention to the safety of the prescribed exercise regime is paramount [36, 37]. Supplemental oxygen is often required in PAH with the recommendation that resting saturations be maintained above 90% and exercise saturations above 85% to reduce dyspnea and hypoxic pulmonary vasoconstriction [37, 38]. The impact of oxygen on symptoms and QoL is discussed below.

For refractory or severe dyspnea, the use of opioids is recommended by the PC guidelines of major respiratory societies [39, 40]. Evidence of efficacy is inferred from other diseases such as COPD and lung cancer [41] although there is minimal direct evidence of efficacy in PAH-related dyspnea. In a double-blinded, crossover trial of 23 patients with PAH, participants were randomized to receive morphine extended release 20 mg by mouth daily or placebo for 7 days with crossover after a 7-day washout period [42]. Four subjects withdrew while taking morphine because of dizziness, drowsiness, nausea, vomiting, and lethargy. Despite morphine producing the anticipated physiologic effects of lower respiratory rates (19.7 vs. 21.4 breaths/min) and higher end-tidal $CO_2$ levels (30.8 vs. 28.2 mmHg), scores for breathlessness "right now" were actually higher with morphine than placebo during the last 3 days of the treatment. Results were not statistically significant owing to sample size. Additionally, scores on two dyspnea scales were similar between the two interventions. For activity-provoked dyspnea, an unblinded crossover study of morphine 5 mg prior to a 6WMT in carefully selected patients with PAH found that morphine did not improve peak Borg dyspnea scores versus control, but also did not affect vital signs or demonstrate any important safety signals [43]. Given the unique physiology of PAH and potential for harm, opioids should be titrated carefully and merit further study.

## Chest Pain

Chest pain is a frequent and distressing symptom of advanced PAH [6, 44]. Pain may be anginal or non-anginal in character. Increased RV wall stress coupled with decreased RV coronary perfusion may result in angina. Occasionally, compression of the left main coronary artery by an enlarged pulmonary artery, detectable by CT coronary angiography, may respond to percutaneous coronary intervention [45]. Pharmacologic analgesic strategies include acetaminophen and opioids. Nonsteroidal anti-inflammatories and nitrates are generally contraindicated. Pericardial effusions are common in advanced PAH particularly when related to connective tissue disease [46]. Effusions are driven by high right atrial pressure and rarely signify pericarditis nor respond to anti-inflammatory therapy. Drainage is recommended only if there is hemodynamic compromise and with utmost caution owing to a risk of precipitating RV decompensation and death [47, 48].

## Syncope

RV dysfunction and reduced cardiac output contribute to fatigue and may lead to exertional presyncope. Overt syncope occurs in advanced PAH in about 10% of patients and may be associated with significant trauma [44]. Typical causes are abrupt changes in RV afterload (hypoxemia, Valsalva during coughing or defecation) or in systemic vascular resistance or preload (change in posture, exercise, hot bathing/shower). Careful attention should be paid to gait supports, sensible activity, management of constipation and cough, and adherence to supplemental oxygen.

### *Right Heart Failure*

Fluid retention is nearly universal in advanced PAH, and patients benefit from diuretics to diminish breathlessness, anorexia related to hepatic congestion, and peripheral edema. There are scant data to guide diuretic therapy, but as right heart failure progresses, often a combination of loop (e.g., furosemide 20–160 mg orally or intravenously once or twice daily), thiazide (e.g., metolazone 2.5–5 mg once weekly to twice daily), and potassium-sparing diuretics (e.g., spironolactone 25–50 mg daily) may be required to maintain euvolemia [49]. A subcutaneous form of furosemide has been developed that may improve diuresis and reduce hospitalization [50]. Frequent monitoring of blood pressure, body weight, electrolytes, and renal function may be required, depending on patient goals.

## Section 2: PAH-Targeted Therapies and Prognosis

### *PAH-Targeted Therapies*

The therapeutic landscape in PAH has evolved to include several oral, inhaled, subcutaneous, and intravenous medications. Current guidelines suggest a risk-based approach to therapy such that patients with advanced disease typically receive three PAH-targeted therapies [51]. Here we review the pharmacology and side effects of available therapies with a discussion of their effects on health-related quality of life (HRQoL) in the following section.

About 10% of patients with PAH demonstrate a favorable response to acute vasodilators at right heart catheterization. These patients enjoy a substantial and long-term positive response to oral calcium channel blockers [10–12] including amlodipine, nifedipine, or diltiazem [38]. Patients without documented vasoreactivity should not receive calcium channel blockers as these agents may depress ventricular contractility and/or systemic blood pressure.

Endothelin-1 is a potent vasoconstrictor and induces proliferation and fibrosis of pulmonary artery smooth muscle cells via its interaction with endothelin receptors A and B. Certain endothelin receptor antagonists (macitentan and bosentan) are nonselective and target both receptors, while ambrisentan is selective for $ET_A$. This class of oral medications improves exercise capacity, dyspnea, and time to clinical worsening [52]. However, these agents may cause nasopharyngitis, headache, liver enzyme abnormalities, and peripheral edema [22].

The nitric oxide pathway is augmented by two groups of oral medications, phosphodiesterase type 5 (PDE5) inhibitors such as sildenafil and tadalafil and soluble guanylate cyclase stimulators such as riociguat. Nitric oxide binds to soluble guanylate cyclase and results in production of cyclic guanosine monophosphate (cGMP), which causes vasodilation. PDE5 breaks down cGMP, and therefore PDE5 inhibitors cause vasodilation via inhibition of cGMP breakdown. Soluble guanylate cyclase stimulators increase guanylate cyclase activity leading to increased production of cGMP. The benefits of PDE5 inhibitors include improved exercise capacity and time to clinical worsening [24, 28, 53]. Riociguat also results in improvement in these domains [29]. Side effects of these agents may include systemic hypotension, headache, flushing, dyspepsia, gastroesophageal reflux, and myalgias [24, 29].

Prostacyclin is a potent pulmonary vasodilator and platelet inhibitor. There are several prostacyclin analogues available that improve exercise capacity, symptoms, and time to clinical worsening [13, 14, 54–56]. This class of medications is associated with hot flashes, gastrointestinal upset, headache, jaw pain, and myalgias. Readers are directed toward a review of the management of prostanoid side effects [32].

Epoprostenol is a synthetic prostacyclin that requires administration by continuous i.v. infusion via an implanted central venous catheter and portable pump due to its short half-life of 6 minutes. The use of epoprostenol requires considerable experience by the clinician as well as significant involvement by the patient and patient's support network. Epoprostenol is supplied as a dry powder which patients must reconstitute while maintaining sterility. Epoprostenol has been shown to reduce mortality within the confines of a single clinical trial [14]. In addition to usual prostacyclin side effects, epoprostenol may cause adverse events related to the central venous catheter and/or pump including line infections, thrombosis, or pump malfunction [57].

Treprostinil is a tricyclic benzidine analogue of prostacyclin that can be administered i.v. or via subcutaneous infusion as a result of its significantly longer half-life of 4.5 hours [15]. Subcutaneous administration has the benefits of avoiding a central line and its attendant risks as well as less frequent drug reconstitution. However, subcutaneous administration can be associated with significant pain at the injection site which may require drug discontinuation in some patients [58].

Other prostacyclin pathway agonists include iloprost which is administered via inhalation, roughly six to nine times daily [59]. Selexipag, an oral prostacyclin IP receptor agonist, is titrated similarly to parenteral prostanoids and reduces rates of clinical worsening [17]. Oral treprostinil improves symptoms and clinical outcomes when added to patients on oral monotherapy but was not effective in improving symptoms or exercise capacity in patients on an ERA and PDE5i [60, 61].

The effects of PAH-targeted therapies on symptoms and exercise capacity as well as their important side effects are summarized in Table 14.1.

## *Prognosis of PAH*

The prognosis of PAH prior to currently available treatment was unfortunately very poor with a median survival in the range of 2–3 years [62]. More recent data suggest median survival has improved to roughly 7 years [63]. There are numerous clinical, lab, hemodynamic, and imaging characteristics that inform a patient's expected prognosis, including 6-minute walk test (6MWT) distance, WHO functional class, serum B-type natriuretic peptide, hemodynamic parameters (particularly right atrial pressure and cardiac index), as well as the presence of a pericardial effusion or clinical right heart failure. Cumulatively, these variables help classify patients into low-, intermediate-, or high-risk groups, with estimated 1-year mortality rates of <5%, 5–10%, and >10%, respectively (see Table 14.2) [38]. This risk assessment plays a significant role in initial treatment selection and subsequent treatment modification. Furthermore, certain PAH patient populations (such as systemic sclerosis or portal hypertension) are known to respond less well to treatment and to have a worse prognosis [63].

Despite the significant advances in medical management of PAH, it remains a progressive disease that often results in or contributes to a patient's death. Death in patients with PAH is often due to progressive right heart failure; however, other causes include cardiac arrest or death due to an intercurrent illness [64]. Intercurrent illnesses or common conditions that are normally survivable unfortunately may result in clinical deterioration and death due to a patient's preexisting PAH. Examples of these poorly tolerated conditions include infections, pulmonary emboli, respiratory failure, arrhythmias, anemia, or pregnancy.

**Table 14.2** European Respiratory Society/European Society of Cardiology risk assessment table for PAH

| Determinants of prognosis[a] (estimated 1-year mortality) | Low risk <5% | Intermediate risk <5–10% | High risk >10% |
| --- | --- | --- | --- |
| Clinical signs of right heart failure | Absent | Absent | Present |
| Progression of symptoms | No | Slow | Rapid |
| Syncope | No | Occasional syncope[b] | Repeated syncope[c] |
| WHO functional class | I, II | III | IV |
| 6MWD | >440m | 165-440 m | <165 m |
| Cardiopulmonary exercise testing | Peak $VO_2$ > 15ml/min/kg (>65% pred.) $VE/VCO_2$ slope<36 | Peak $VO_2$ > 11-15ml/min/kg (35-65% pred.) $VE/VCO_2$ slope 36-44.9 | Peak $VO_2$ <11ml/min/kg (<35% pred.) $VE/VCO_2$ slope ≥45 |
| NT-proBNP plasma levels | BNP <50 ng/l NT-proBNP <300 ng/l | BNP 50-300 ng/l NT-proBNP 300-1400 ng/l | BNP >300 ng/l NT-proBNP >1400 ng/l |
| Imaging (echocardiography, CMR imaging) | RA area <18 $cm^2$ No pericardial effusion | RA area 18-26 $cm^2$ No or minimal, pericardial effusion | RA area >26 $cm^2$ pericardial effusion |
| Haemodynamics | RAP <8 mmHg CI ≥2.5 l/min/$m^2$ $SvO_2$ >65% | RAP 8-14 mmHg CI 2.0-2.4 l/min/$m^2$ $SvO_2$ 60-65% | RAP >14 mmHg CI <2.0 l/min/$m^2$ $SvO_2$ <60% |

6MWD: 6-minute walking distance; BNP: brain natriuretic peptide; CI: cardiac index; CMR: cardiac magnetic resonance; NT-proBNP: N-terminal pro-brain natriuretic peptide; pred.: predicted; RA: right atrium; RAP: right atrial pressure; $SvO_2$: mixed venous oxygen saturation; $VE/VCO_2$ ventitlatory equivalents for carbon dioxide; $VO_2$: oxygen consumption; WHO: World Health Organization. [a]Most of the proposed variables and cut-off values are based on expert opinion. They may provide prognostic infromation and may be used to guide therapeutic decisions, but applications to individual patients must be done carefully. One must also note that most of these variables have been validated mostly for IPAH and the cut-off levels used above may not necessarlily apply to other forms of PAH. Futhermore, the use of approved therapies and their influence on the variables should be considered in the evaluation of the risk. [b]Occasional syncope during brisk or heavy exercise, or occasional orthostatic syncope in an otherwise stable patient. [c]Repeated episodes of syncope, even with little or regular physical activity.

The trajectory toward death is inherently variable due to the different potential causes of death. The majority of PAH patients die in hospital [64, 65]. Many of these deaths occur in intensive care, often as a result of institutional policies restricting the use of prostanoid therapy to a monitored bed [65]. Patients with PAH can develop progressive right heart failure over the course of weeks to months, hypothetically allowing enough time for discussions regarding treatment escalation, consideration of lung transplant, or end-of-life care with institution of appropriate palliative care resources and treatments. In this scenario, if a palliative treatment strategy is chosen, end-of-life could occur in hospital, hospice, or at home, depending on a patient's wishes, needs, and available support. Importantly, in some jurisdictions, hospice care may preclude the use of expensive PAH-targeted therapies, and patients may decline this, viewing it as suicide [65].

On the other hand, if a patient becomes ill abruptly and is hospitalized, there may be inadequate time to fully explore the various potential locations for end-of-life care. The use of PC in this context appears to be infrequent although a study examining temporal trends from the US National Inpatient Sample did find an increased use of specialist PC consultative services in PAH over time, from 0.5% of admissions in 2001 to 7.6% in 2017, albeit with significant differences based on race, insurance status, income, and hospital size [66]. Several other studies have demonstrated that palliative treatments and resources are significantly underutilized in PAH [6, 64, 65]. In one single-center study of patients who died of PAH, the minority of patients had an advanced directive, and a significant portion of patients underwent aggressive end-of-life care including cardiopulmonary resuscitation (CPR) and/or mechanical ventilation [64]. Based on the very poor outcomes with CPR in PAH [67], it is paramount that advanced care planning reflect an informed patient decision.

## Section 3: Health-Related Quality of Life in PAH

HRQoL is a complex concept that encompasses symptoms and patient perceptions of physical, social, and psychological well-being [68]. The subjective experience of a patient with PAH extends beyond just breathlessness and the other cardinal symptoms. Although powerful, one-dimensional scales that grade the severity of physical symptoms, such as the World Health Organization (WHO) or New York Heart Association (NYHA) functional classification, do not adequately capture the spectrum of symptoms, nor the impact of symptoms on daily functioning or quality of life. In addition to the classic PAH symptoms of dyspnea, fatigue, chest pain, and presyncope, many patients endorse emotional consequences such as anxiety or depression, difficulty sleeping, and impaired sexual health [44, 69, 70]. PAH also has a life-changing effect on social well-being and greatly affects patients' families and caregivers. In an international survey of over 300 PAH patients and more than 120 caregivers, 57% of caregivers felt that PAH had a profound effect on daily life with 43% reporting exhaustion due to the additional responsibilities [71]. Nearly three quarters of partners reported that the disease negatively affected their sexual relationships. There is also a significant financial burden when facing a progressive, chronic disease like PAH. In a survey from the United Kingdom, monthly income decreased by 13–33% after the diagnosis of PAH [72]. Only 28% of patients could continue their employment without any change after their PAH diagnosis, while 22% had to reduce work hours, 23% were on long-term disability leave, and 28% gave up working completely [72]. Similarly, 29% of caregivers report that their work is affected by the demands of caring for someone with PAH [71]. As such, there has been increasing emphasis on the importance of incorporating patient perspectives in routine care of the PAH patient, including the use of patient-reported measures of HRQoL [73].

## *HRQoL Measurement Tools*

There are several generic and disease-specific instruments to measure HRQoL, which can be of value in PAH research and in routine clinical practice (Table 14.3) [73]. Generic HRQoL measurement tools, such as the Short Form-36 (SF-36) questionnaire, have been validated in PAH populations [68, 74], which allows comparison of HRQoL to the normal values in the population and to other disease states. It is clear that HRQoL is severely impaired in PAH, to a similar extent as end-stage kidney disease or cancer (Fig. 14.2) [75].

Generic HRQoL tools have important limitations, as they do not always correlate with standard measures of disease severity and may not capture the full spectrum of symptoms in PAH. Therefore, several PAH-specific HRQoL instruments have been derived and validated, which may better describe symptoms and disability in PAH. The Cambridge Pulmonary Hypertension Outcome Review (CAMPHOR) questionnaire was derived in the United Kingdom and captures symptoms, functioning, and quality of life [76, 77]. CAMPHOR has been widely validated in multiple languages, as well as in North American PAH populations [78, 79], but is considerably longer than other instruments and has an associated fee for its use. Other disease-specific questionnaires include the Minnesota Living with Heart Failure Questionnaire (MLHFQ) and Living with Pulmonary Hypertension (LPH) questionnaire. The Pulmonary Arterial Hypertension-Symptoms and Impact (PAH-SYMPACT) Questionnaire® was more recently developed to meet regulatory guidance by the Food and Drug Administration (FDA) for a patient-reported outcome (PRO) for use as an efficacy endpoint in pharmaceutical trials [80]. The PAH-SYMPACT® captures respiratory, cardiovascular, tiredness, and other related symptoms, as well as

**Table 14.3** Features of generic and PAH-specific quality-of-life scores

| Measure | Domains | Items (n) | Recall period |
|---|---|---|---|
| *Generic* | | | |
| SF-36 | Physical functioning, role limitations physical, bodily pain, general health, vitality, social functioning, role limitations emotional, mental health | 36 | Now to previous 4 weeks |
| EQ-5D | Health state description: mobility, self-care, usual activities, pain/discomfort, anxiety/depression, overall health status (Visual Analogue Scale) | 52 | Today |
| NHP | Mobility, pain, social isolation, emotional reactions, energy level, sleep | 38 | At the moment |
| HADS | Anxiety, depression | 24 | At the moment |
| *PH-specific* | | | |
| CAMPHOR | Overall symptoms (energy, breathlessness, mood), functioning, quality of life | 65 | Today |
| MLHFQ | Physical, emotional | 32 | 4 weeks |
| LPH | Physical, emotional | 32 | 1 week |
| CHFQ | Dyspnea, fatigue, emotional function, mastery | 30 | 2 weeks |
| EmPHasis-10 | Unidimensional | 10 | At the moment |
| PAH-SYMPACT | Respiratory symptoms, tiredness, cardiovascular symptoms, other symptoms, physical activities, daily activities, social impact, cognition, emotional impact | 41 | 24 h for symptoms, 7 days for impacts |

Reproduced from Ref. [73]

*SF-36* Medical Outcomes Study 36-item short form, *EQ-5D* EuroQol Group 5-Dimension Self-Report Questionnaire, *NHP* Nottingham Health Profile, *HADS* Hospital Anxiety and Depression Scale, *CAMPHOR* Cambridge Pulmonary Hypertension Outcome Review, *MLHFQ* Minnesota Living with Heart Failure Questionnaire, *LPH* Living with Pulmonary Hypertension questionnaire, *CHFQ* Chronic Heart Failure Questionnaire, *EmPHasis-10* 10-question survey proposed by the UK Pulmonary Hypertension Association

their impacts on physical activities, daily activities, social activities and relationships, cognition, and emotions [80]. The PAH-SYMPACT® correlated with HRQoL using the generic SF-36 questionnaire and the disease-specific CAMPHOR, differentiated well between varying levels of disease severity, and was sensitive to treatment-induced changes in clinician- and patient-reported HRQoL [81]. The EmPHasis-10 score is another useful disease-specific HRQoL tool, as it contains only ten items, with each scored on a scale of 0–5 (higher scores being worse), which can be easily administered in routine clinical practice [82]. It captures the key symptoms of PAH (breathlessness, fatigue, exhaustion, low energy) as well as patient perceptions of independence, being a burden, and confidence with being out in public. Although developed in the United Kingdom, the EmPHasis-10 has recently been validated in the US Pulmonary Hypertension Association Registry [83].

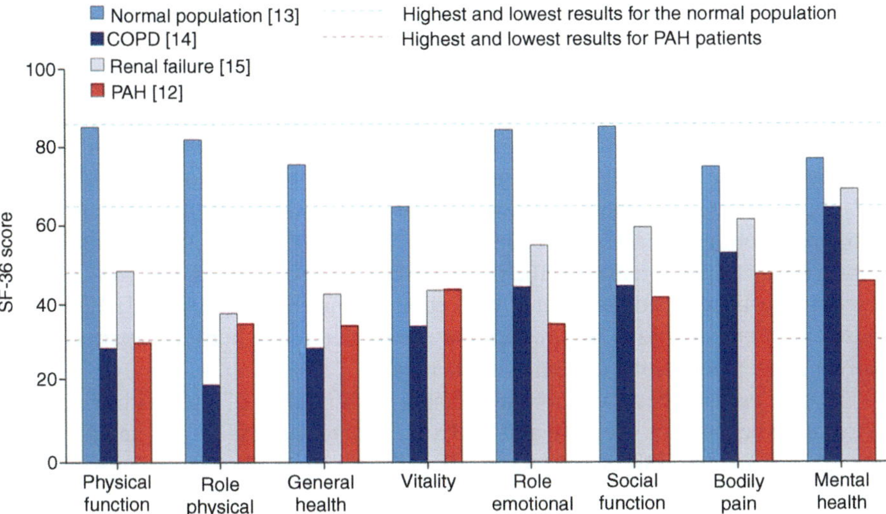


**Fig. 14.2** Effect of pulmonary arterial hypertension (PAH) on SF-36-measured health-related quality of life (HRQoL) measures versus the normal population and other disease conditions. *COPD* chronic obstructive pulmonary disease, *SF-36* Medical Outcomes Study 36-item short form. (Reproduced with permission of the © ERS 2020: European Respiratory Review 24 (138) 621–629; DOI: https://doi.org/10.1183/16000617.0063-2015 Published 30 November 2015 [75])

## *Impact of Treatment on HRQoL*

A meta-analysis of randomized trials in PAH found consistent statistical improvements in HRQoL scores with the initiation of PAH-targeted therapies [84]. However, the vast majority of clinical trials in PAH have used generic tools, such as the SF-36 or EQ-5D, and the effect sizes are frequently below the minimal clinically important difference, suggesting that that PAH treatment might not improve HRQoL in a meaningful way. While physical domains on generic HRQoL often improve with PAH therapies, the psychological or emotional domains often do not improve [74, 84]. The psychological burden of PAH is an important consideration for future PAH studies since approximate 50% of patients experience anxiety, depression, and stress and no existing PAH therapies or other interventions have been shown to improve these symptoms [85]. It is possible that generic HRQoL tools do not completely or accurately detect the effects of PAH treatments on emotional aspects of the disease or that PAH therapies truly do not improve psychological or emotional symptoms. However, based on an analysis of the Study with an Endothelin Receptor Antagonist in Pulmonary Arterial Hypertension to Improve Clinical Outcome (SERAPHIN) randomized trial, the mental component score on the SF-36 significantly worsened in the placebo group as compared to small improvements in the macitentan treatment groups [21]. Therefore, PAH therapies seem to help prevent emotional/mental symptoms from worsening at the natural rate.

The standard therapeutic strategy for newly diagnosed patients with low- or intermediate-risk PAH is initial combination therapy with two oral agents based on the Ambrisentan and Tadalafil in Patients with Pulmonary Arterial Hypertension (AMBITION) trial [51]. While initial combination therapy significantly improved clinical outcomes in AMBITION by 50% [86], there were no differences in HRQoL on the SF-36 or CAMPHOR between the combination and monotherapy groups [87]. In the pivotal clinical trial, epoprostenol improved the dyspnea, fatigue, emotional function, and mastery domains on the Chronic Heart Failure Questionnaire, improving multiple domains on the generic Nottingham Health Profile [88]. Despite its clinical efficacy, patients treated with epoprostenol reported worse HRQoL than those on oral medications [89], which may be related to the burden imparted by the daily management of this complicated therapy.

Oxygen use has been variably associated with quality of life, with a negative association between oxygen use and HRQoL in some studies [74, 90] and neutral or beneficial association in others [81, 89, 91]. In one study showing a negative association between oxygen and HRQoL, patients reported adapting to oxygen therapy but that it restricted or interfered with their daily living [90]. Oxygen use was also associated with worse physical component scores on the SF-36, but there was no difference in the mental component score between those using oxygen and those not in another observational study [74]. However, in a prospective randomized crossover trial, the use of oxygen in patients with mild or exertional hypoxemia was associated with improvements in exercise capacity and better physical component scores on the SF-36 [91]. Therefore, the best available data suggest a beneficial effect of domiciliary oxygen on HRQoL.

## *Prognostic Relevance of HRQoL in PAH*

HRQoL instruments capture the physical and emotional experience of PAH, but quality of life also has prognostic importance. Fernandes et al. found that a baseline SF-36 physical component score of <32 points was associated with worse survival and that patients with a physical component score <38 units after 16 weeks of treatment also had a worse prognosis [92]. In the SERAPHIN trial, which compared the effect of macitentan to placebo, a baseline SF-36 physical component score of >35.5 was associated with a 39% (95% CI 22–52%) lower risk of future morbidity or mortality events [21]. There was a less marked but still significant association between baseline SF-36 mental component scores and future clinical events. An SF-36 mental component score ≥42.7 portended a 22% (95% CI 1–38%) lower risk of future morbidity or mortality events. Although developed for left heart failure patients, the MLHFQ questionnaire is also linked future outcomes in PAH [93].

Disease-specific tools such as CAMPHOR and EmPHasis-10 also have prognostic utility. All three CAMPHOR domains (symptoms, activity, and quality of life) were associated with the risk of clinical deterioration in univariate analysis, but only the quality-of-life domain score predicted clinical deterioration after adjustment for

NYHA functional class and 6-minute walk distance [94]. The EmPHasis-10 tool has important advantages of being considerably shorter to administer than SF-36 and CAMPHOR. One study found that a 10-point increase in EmPHasis-10 score was associated with a 59% increased risk of death in PAH patients, with a threshold of >32 points being optimal for predicting outcomes [95]. A large study of 1745 PAH patients found that EmPHasis-10 was associated with survival, independent of other important prognostic factors such as age, sex, type of PAH, hemodynamics, and walking distance [96].

### *When to Measure HRQoL*

Assessment of HRQoL is an important component in the care of PAH patients. As discussed above, HRQoL tools better capture patient experience than individual symptoms or functional classification. Just as clinicians routinely monitor functional classification, exercise capacity, and right ventricular function after any therapeutic changes, it is essential to measure HRQoL regularly to understand the impact of clinical decisions or disease worsening on patient well-being. There are a variety of validated tools for measuring HRQoL in PAH, and simple convenient tools, such as the EmPHasis-10, can be routinely collected in clinical practice. Just as HRQoL measurement may inform assessment of treatment response and prognosis, it could also conceivably identify individuals most likely to benefit from palliative care.

## Section 4: Palliative Care Implementation in PAH

### *Primary Versus Specialist Palliative Care for PAH*

PAH care is often provided in comprehensive care centers. These use multidisciplinary teams that often include a physician, nurse, and social worker [97]. Centers are accustomed to caring for a high number of PAH patients, many of whom will unfortunately die each year. Given the long-term relationships many patients establish with their team, it is most practical that the multidisciplinary team become familiar with providing PC, termed "primary" palliative care [98]. Team members who may be unfamiliar or uncomfortable with PC provision can be directed to available resources to improve their skills.[1]

Specialist PC refers to PC provided by specialty trained clinicians. Specialist PC consultation should be requested for refractory symptoms and existential distress or to help resolve difficult situations around treatment expectations, goals of care,

[1] VitalTalk (https://vitaltalk.org), Robert Wood Johnson Foundation Promoting Excellence Initiative (http://www.promotingexcellence.org)

family dynamics, or futility [99]. Specialist PC may also allow access to community PC resources that provide an additional network of support to patients and families [100].

## *Efficacy of Palliative Care*

PC efficacy can be assessed by a variety of outcomes including symptom scores, HRQoL, patient satisfaction, and, occasionally, rates of health-care utilization and survival. A landmark study in patients with advanced lung cancer who received PC in addition to usual oncologic care demonstrated that PC significantly improved depression and HRQoL scores as well as median survival by around 3 months [101]. While there are no randomized trials of PC in PAH, studies have shown an improvement in HRQoL with PC in other respiratory diseases [102] as well as in larger populations of patients predominantly with cancer [103]. PC may also result in cost savings [104] and a reduction in health-care utilization toward death [105].

## *Barriers to Palliative Care in PAH*

As discussed above, the use of specialized PC appears to be uncommon in PAH. In a survey of 276 patients with PAH, despite 40% reporting significant impairment of HRQoL, only 1.4% reported receiving specialized PC services [6]. Interestingly, 63% did not report being "sick enough" to warrant PC involvement, suggesting that patients may not recognize poor HRQoL is potentially remediable. Another study demonstrated that patients with greater cardiopulmonary symptoms and cognitive/emotional impact of PAH (as measured by PAH-SYMPACT) displayed stronger negative emotional reactions toward PC as measured by the Perceptions of Palliative Care Instrument [106]. This suggests that stigma around PC, driven by the perception it is only for end-of-life care, may be part of the reason for low utilization. Awareness may also be a barrier. In a survey of 36 families of patients who had recently died of PAH, only 11% reported PC had been involved in the care of the decedent, and 30% had been unaware of palliative services [65].

PAH clinicians vary in terms of comfort with PC provision. In a survey, 76 physicians caring for patients with PAH reported high levels of confidence in symptom management (87% of respondents) and in discussing end-of-life care plans with patients and their families (88%) [107]. However, comfort with managing QoL issues (33%) and pain (14%) was low. PC referral was more commonly requested for hospice and end-of-life care than for symptom management or impaired QoL, despite the physicians' lack of comfort managing these issues. Barriers to PC referral cited by physicians included non-approval by patient/family (53%) or concern that PC referral is perceived by the patient as "giving up hope" (43%). Based on the studies above, these appear to correctly mirror the concerns of patients. Thus, in order to increase acceptance of PC, physicians must be mindful of how a discussion of PC is framed and of the stigma surrounding PC [106]. It should be emphasized to the patient that PC can continue in parallel with aggressive, goal-oriented care [108] and that the patient will not be abandoned.

## *Triggers for Palliative Care in PAH*

PAH treatment guidelines recommend PC for PAH but provide only vague guidance on the timing of PC initiation [109]. Referral to specialist PC services is recommended "when appropriate" and in those "approaching the end of life" [110]. In reality, PAH is a chronic health condition with high morbidity, and PC should be integrated earlier in the disease course for more symptomatic patients. As discussed above, regular assessment of prognosis and HRQoL may assist in identifying those more likely to benefit from PC. Importantly, hospitalizations have been identified to be a powerful indicator of prognosis and should prompt the reassessment of HRQoL and disease trajectory [111]. It may also be reasonable to empower any team member to raise the need for PC including respiratory therapists supervising 6MWTs or pulmonary rehabilitation since they directly observe the symptoms provoked by activities of daily living.

## *Key Elements of Palliative Care in PAH*

### Symptom Control

Elements of comprehensive PC for PAH are outlined in Fig. 14.3. Physical symptoms increase as PAH progresses and correlate with HRQoL. Symptoms may be due to the disease itself or may also be caused by side effects of PAH-targeted therapies, the underlying disease causing PAH (e.g., scleroderma), or by comorbidities (e.g., ischemic heart disease). As discussed above, knowledge of PAH pathophysiology, targeted therapies, and interaction with other conditions are required to appropriately address each symptom that arises.

### Psychological, Emotional, and Spiritual Support

Feelings of isolation, loss, frustration, anger, and "enforced dependency" are common in PAH [75, 112, 113]. Patients desire more information on the emotional consequences of PAH [71]. The primary PAH team should practice supportive listening and narrative competence, described as the ability to "acknowledge, absorb, interpret, and act on the stories and plights of others" [73]. Social workers should be engaged to help the patient navigate the emotional, financial, and relationship aspects of the disease. Pastoral care may be desired by patients wishing to discuss

Physical symptoms
Prognostic awarness
Transplantation preparedness
Advance care planning
Caregiver support
Effects of associated disease and comorbidities
Side effects of PAH-targeted therapies
Emotional spiritual, and existential symptoms
Patient and Caregiver

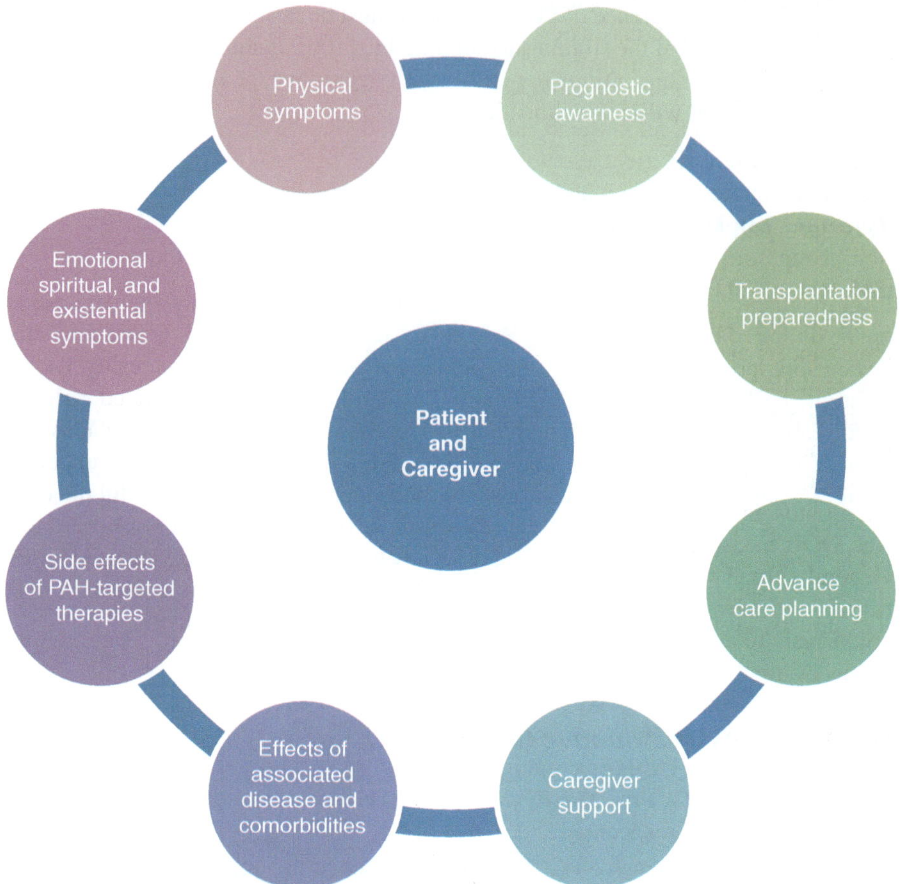

**Fig. 14.3** Illustration depicting the key components of palliative care provision in PAH. (Reproduced with permission of the © ERS 2020: European Respiratory Journal 53 (1) 1801919; DOI: https://doi.org/10.1183/13993003.01919-2018 Published 24 January 2019)

faith, fear of the unknown, and existential distress. Patient support groups and PH associations can provide shared experience, reduce isolation, and improve confidence and outlook on life [113].

Symptoms of anxiety (48%) and depression (33%) are also common in PAH [85]. Undertreatment of depression appears to be frequent with only 24% receiving psychiatric treatment in one study [69]. Management can include pharmacologic therapy and/or referral for psychological or cognitive-behavioral therapy. Psychiatric referral may be required for more severe or refractory disease. Evidence of a direct effect of selective serotonin reuptake inhibitors (SSRIs) on the pulmonary vasculature in PAH is mixed, and appropriate use is encouraged [114, 115]. Altered cerebral oxygenation may impact directly on cognitive and psychological symptoms in PAH [116, 117], but PAH-targeted therapies have not been shown to consistently improve emotional symptoms, as discussed above.

## *Caregiver Support and Bereavement Care*

The majority of caregivers for PAH patients report a very high impact of PAH on their daily life [112]. Time spent caring for an individual and caregiver stress increase with the patient's functional class. Strategies to support caregivers include emotional and informational support, assistance accessing financial help and respite care, and treatment of depressive symptoms, which may occur in up to 14% of PAH caregivers [118].

Bereavement care, both before and after a patient's death, is considered a pillar of PC [39]. Goals should be to assist families in understanding the normal grieving process and seek out resources for support [39]. Meetings between the family and the familiar PAH team can be an opportunity to provide closure, reduce grief or regret, and facilitate acceptance.

## *Prognostic Awareness and Advance Care Planning*

Informing patients of prognosis is critical to advancing care discussions and needs to be done skillfully. Patients appreciate having honest and clear discussion about prognosis. However, PAH patients have reported being given a negative initial outlook but then remaining stable "longer than expected" on medication which can lead to uncertainty and contribute to hopelessness [113]. Thus, frequent reassessment of prognosis and clear communication are required.

In terms of advance care planning (ACP), a survey of patients with PAH identified that only 46% of respondents had discussed ACP with a loved one, 33% had completed living wills, and 24% had a durable power of attorney for health care, while only 13.8% had participated in an ACP discussion with their primary PAH provider [6]. Various models have been applied to ACP, but how to best increase ACP discussions remains uncertain [119]. Earlier integration of PC may result in better preparedness for common end-of-life scenarios [105].

## *Special Considerations*

### Prostanoid Management

Although prostanoids are associated with improved HRQoL due to improvement in PAH symptoms, over time the complexities of prostanoid therapy may pose a burden for patients with PAH and their caregivers [84, 120, 121]. There are scant data to inform PAH patient's preferences regarding prostanoids at end of life. While abrupt discontinuation may lead to sudden death [122], a slow taper may be discussed between patient and provider to lower treatment burden [108]. This may also be required to allow admission to certain long-term care facilities or to hospice. Transition from parenteral to oral or inhaled prostanoid analogues may be helpful but has typically been reserved for those with more favorable prognoses [123].

### Transplant-Eligible Patients

Lung transplantation remains the standard of care for patients with unacceptable QoL or risk of death despite maximal medical therapy. Median wait times for PAH patients range from 87 to 138 days based on 2011–2014 US data [124]. A subset of patients require bridging extracorporeal life support which can last for weeks [125]. Wait-listed individuals may experience substantial anxiety, uncertainty, frustration, and isolation. QoL is lower, and rates of mood and anxiety disorders are higher than in candidates for other kinds of transplantation [126]. Integrated routine involvement of PC may help to manage distressing symptoms, guide advanced care discussions, and improve goal-concordant care in individuals awaiting transplant [127]. Palliative interventions, including the use of opioids in 92% of pretransplant patients in one study, did not appear impact listing eligibility [128].

### Invasive Palliative Therapies

Certain patients may benefit from invasive therapies to improve cardiac output and relieve RV failure. Balloon atrial septostomy is a percutaneous procedure that improves systemic cardiac output and exercise capacity when performed in expert centers [129, 130]. Other invasive treatments include an open Potts shunt (left pulmonary artery to descending aorta conduit), most often in pediatric PAH [131], and, potentially, pulmonary artery denervation [132]. PC may assist in determining whether patient expectations and goals are in keeping with the anticipated outcomes of these of invasive procedures.

### Medical Assistance in Dying

In certain jurisdictions, legislation permits medical assistance in dying (MAiD) for those with advanced disease. In Canada, circulatory/respiratory diseases account for approximately 16% of those receiving MAiD, and specialist PC is likely to be involved in their care at the time of the procedure (74.4%) [133]. The increasing awareness of MAiD coupled with the high symptom burden and poor outlook of advanced PAH suggests physicians should be prepared to discuss this with patients.

## Conclusion and Future Directions

Until such time as prolonged survival with minimal symptoms can be attained for all patients with PAH, there will remain a large role for symptom-based and non-pharmacologic interventions to improve HRQoL. Currently, data would suggest the gap between the HRQoL of PAH patients and a normal or even acceptable HRQoL is large and PC likely has a role to play in narrowing it. Research on PC for PAH is in its infancy. Work is needed to define how, when, and to whom to offer PC, what interventions PC should entail, and, most importantly, how these interventions impact patient and caregivers' symptoms and HRQoL as well as their preparedness for an often unpredictable disease course.

## References

1. Lai YC, Potoka KC, Champion HC, Mora AL, Gladwin MT. Pulmonary arterial hypertension: the clinical syndrome. Circ Res. 2014;115:115–30.
2. Weatherald J, Farina S, Bruno N, Laveneziana P. Cardiopulmonary exercise testing in pulmonary hypertension. Ann Am Thorac Soc. 2017;14:S84–92.
3. Vonk Noordegraaf A, Westerhof BE, Westerhof N. The relationship between the right ventricle and its load in pulmonary hypertension. J Am Coll Cardiol. 2017;69:236–43.
4. Naeije R, Badagliacca R. The overloaded right heart and ventricular interdependence. Cardiovasc Res. 2017;113:1474–85.
5. Hrymak C, Strumpher J, Jacobsohn E. Acute right ventricle failure in the intensive care unit: assessment and management. Can J Cardiol. 2017;33:61–71.
6. Swetz KM, Shanafelt TD, Drozdowicz LB, Sloan JA, Novotny PJ, Durst LA, Frantz RP, MD MG. Symptom burden, quality of life, and attitudes toward palliative care in patients with pulmonary arterial hypertension: results from a cross-sectional patient survey. J Hear Lung Transplant. 2012;31:1102–8.
7. Hoeper MM, Gibbs JSR. The changing landscape of pulmonary arterial hypertension and implications for patient care. Eur Respir Rev. 2014;23:450–7.
8. Dumitrescu D, Sitbon O, Weatherald J, Howard LS. Exertional dyspnoea in pulmonary arterial hypertension. Eur Respir Rev. 2017;26:170039.
9. Sun XG, Hansen JE, Oudiz RJ, Wasserman K. Gas exchange detection of exercise-induced right-to-left shunt in patients with primary pulmonary hypertension. Circulation. 2002;105:54–60.
10. Rich S, Kaufmann E, Levy PS. The effect of high doses of calcium-channel blockers on survival in primary pulmonary hypertension. N Engl J Med. 1992;327:76–81.
11. Rich S, Brundage BH. High-dose calcium channel-blocking therapy for primary pulmonary hypertension: evidence for long-term reduction in pulmonary arterial pressure and regression of right ventricular hypertrophy. Circulation. 1987;76:135–41.
12. Sitbon O, Humbert M, Jaïs X, Ioos V, Hamid AM, Provencher S, Garcia G, Parent F, Hervé P, Simonneau G. Long-term response to calcium channel blockers in idiopathic pulmonary arterial hypertension. Circulation. 2005;111:3105–11.
13. Badesch DB, Tapson VF, McGoon MD, Brundage BH, Rubin LJ, Wigley FM, Rich S, Barst RJ, Barrett PS, Kral KM, Jöbsis MM, Loyd JE. The efficacy of the drug epoprostenol in the treatment of pulmonary hypertension associated with scleroderma. Ann Intern Med. 2000;132:425–34.
14. Barst RJ, Rubin LJ, Long WA, McGoon MD. Conventional therapy for primary pulmonary hypertension. N Engl J Med. 1996;334:296–301.
15. Simonneau G, Barst RJ, Galie N, et al. Continuous subcutaneous infusion of treprostinil, a prostacyclin analogue, in patients with pulmonary arterial hypertension. Am J Respir Crit Care Med. 2002;165:800–4.
16. Olschewski H, Simonneau G, Galie N. Inhaled iloprost for severe pulmonary hypertension. N Engl J Med. 2002;347:322–9.
17. Sitbon O, Channick R, Chin KM, et al. Selexipag for the treatment of pulmonary arterial hypertension. N Engl J Med. 2015;373:2522–33.

18. Channick RN, Simonneau G, Sitbon O, et al. Effects of the dual endothelin-receptor antagonist bosentan in patients with pulmonary hypertension: a randomised placebo-controlled study. Lancet. 2001;358:1119–23.
19. Rubin LJ, Badesch DB, Barst RJ. Bosentan therapy for pulmonary arterial hypertension. N Engl J Med. 2002;3346:896–903.
20. Galiè N, Rubin L, Hoeper M, Jansa P, Al-Hiti H, Meyer G, Chiossi E, Kusic-Pajic A, Simonneau G. Treatment of patients with mildly symptomatic pulmonary arterial hypertension with bosentan (EARLY study): a double-blind, randomised controlled trial. Lancet. 2008;371:2093–100.
21. Mehta S, Channick RN, Delcroix M, et al. Macitentan improves health-related quality of life in pulmonary arterial hypertension: results from the randomized controlled SERAPHIN trial. Chest. 2013;142:47662.
22. Pulido T, Adzerikho I, Channick RN, et al. Macitentan and morbidity and mortality in pulmonary arterial hypertension. N Engl J Med. 2013;369:809–18.
23. Galiè N, Olschewski H, Oudiz RJ, et al. Ambrisentan for the treatment of pulmonary arterial hypertension: results of the ambrisentan in pulmonary arterial hypertension, randomized, double-blind, placebo-controlled, multicenter, efficacy (ARIES) study 1 and 2. Circulation. 2008;117:3010–9.
24. Galiè N, Ghofrani H, Torbicki A. Sildenafil citrate therapy for pulmonary arterial hypertension. N Engl J Med. 2005;353:2148–57.
25. Sastry BKS, Narasimhan C, Reddy NK, Raju BS. Clinical efficacy of sildenafil in primary pulmonary hypertension: a randomized, placebo-controlled, double-blind, crossover study. J Am Coll Cardiol. 2004;43:1149–53.
26. Singh TP, Rohit M, Grover A, Malhotra S, Vijayvergiya R. A randomized, placebo-controlled, double-blind, crossover study to evaluate the efficacy of oral sildenafil therapy in severe pulmonary artery hypertension. Am Heart J. 2006; https://doi.org/10.1016/j.ahj.2005.09.006.
27. Pepke-Zaba J, Gilbert C, Collings L, Brown MCJ. Sildenafil improves health-related quality of life in patients with pulmonary arterial hypertension. Chest. 2008;133:183–9.
28. Galiè N, Brundage BH, Ghofrani HA, et al. Tadalafil therapy for pulmonary arterial hypertension. Circulation. 2009;119:2894–903.
29. Ghofrani H-A, Galiè N, Grimminger F, et al. Riociguat for the treatment of pulmonary arterial hypertension. N Engl J Med. 2013;369:330–40.
30. Christiansen D, Porter S, Hurlburt L, Weiss A, Granton J, Wentlandt K. Pulmonary arterial hypertension: a palliative medicine review of the disease, its therapies, and drug interactions. J Pain Symptom Manag. 2020;59:932–43.
31. Badesch DB, Tapson VF, Mcgoon MD, et al. An uncontrolled trial. German PPH study group. Ann Intern Med. 2000;132:435–43.
32. Kingman M, Archer-Chicko C, Bartlett M, Beckmann J, Hohsfield R, Lombardi S. Management of prostacyclin side effects in adult patients with pulmonary arterial hypertension. Pulm Circ. 2017;7:598–608.
33. Ulrich S, Fischler M, Speich R, Bloch KE. Wrist actigraphy predicts outcome in patients with pulmonary hypertension. Respiration. 2013;86:45–51.
34. Buys R, Avila A, Cornelissen VA. Exercise training improves physical fitness in patients with pulmonary arterial hypertension: a systematic review and meta-analysis of controlled trials. BMC Pulm Med. 2015; https://doi.org/10.1186/s12890-015-0031-1.
35. Mereles D, Ehlken N, Kreuscher S, et al. Exercise and respiratory training improve exercise capacity and quality of life in patients with severe chronic pulmonary hypertension. Circulation. 2006;114:1482–9.
36. Grünig E, Lichtblau M, Ehlken N, et al. Safety and efficacy of exercise training in various forms of pulmonary hypertension. Eur Respir J. 2012;40:84–92.
37. Grünig E, Eichstaedt C, Barberà JA, et al. ERS statement on exercise training and rehabilitation in patients with severe chronic pulmonary hypertension. Eur Respir J. 2019; https://doi.org/10.1183/13993003.00332-2018.

38. Galiè N, Humbert M, Vachiery J-L, et al. 2015 ESC/ERS guidelines for the diagnosis and treatment of pulmonary hypertension. Eur Respir J. 2015;46:903–75.
39. Lanken PN, Terry PB, DeLisser HM, et al. An official American thoracic society clinical policy statement: palliative care for patients with respiratory diseases and critical illnesses. Am J Respir Crit Care Med. 2008;177:912–27.
40. Mahler DA, Selecky PA, Harrod CG, et al. American college of chest physicians consensus statement on the management of dyspnea in patients with advanced lung or heart disease. Chest. 2010;137:674–91.
41. Barnes H, McDonald J, Smallwood N, Manser R. Opioids for the palliation of refractory breathlessness in adults with advanced disease and terminal illness. Cochrane Database Syst Rev. 2014; https://doi.org/10.1002/14651858.CD011008.
42. Ferreira DH, Ekström M, Sajkov D, Vandersman Z, Eckert DJ, Currow DC. Extended-release morphine for chronic breathlessness in pulmonary arterial hypertension—a randomized, double-blind, placebo-controlled, crossover study. J Pain Symptom Manag. 2018;56:483–92.
43. Christiansen D, Wentlandt K, Lew J, Granton J. Late breaking abstract – morphine for dyspnea in advanced pulmonary arterial hypertension. Eur Respir J. 2019;54:Suppl.:PA3948.
44. Matura LA, McDonough A, Carroll DL. Symptom interference severity and health-related quality of life in pulmonary arterial hypertension. J Pain Symptom Manag. 2016;51:25–32.
45. Galiè N, Saia F, Palazzini M, et al. Left main coronary artery compression in patients with pulmonary arterial hypertension and angina. J Am Coll Cardiol. 2017;69:2808–17.
46. Sahay S, Tonelli AR. Pericardial effusion in pulmonary arterial hypertension. Pulm Circ. 2013;3:467–77.
47. Fenstad ER, Le RJ, Sinak LJ, et al. Pericardial effusions in pulmonary arterial hypertension: characteristics, prognosis, and role of drainage. Chest. 2013;144:1530–8.
48. Hemnes AR, Gaine SP, Wiener CM. Poor outcomes associated with drainage of pericardial effusions in patients with pulmonary arterial hypertension. South Med J. 2008;101:490–4.
49. Konstam MA, Kiernan MS, Bernstein D, et al. Evaluation and management of right-sided heart failure: a scientific statement from the American Heart Association. Circulation. 2018; https://doi.org/10.1161/CIR.0000000000000560.
50. Gilotra NA, Princewill O, Marino B, et al. Efficacy of intravenous furosemide versus a novel, pH-neutral furosemide formulation administered subcutaneously in outpatients with worsening heart failure. JACC Hear Fail. 2018;6:65–70.
51. Galiè N, Channick RN, Frantz RP, et al. Risk stratification and medical therapy of pulmonary arterial hypertension. Eur Respir J. 2019; https://doi.org/10.1183/13993003.01889-2018.
52. Liu C, Chen J, Gao Y, Deng B, Liu K. Endothelin receptor antagonists for pulmonary arterial hypertension. Cochrane Database Syst Rev. 2013; https://doi.org/10.1002/14651858.CD004434.pub5.
53. Oudiz RJ, Brundage BH, Gali N, Ghofrani HA, Simonneau G, Botros FT, Chan M, Beardsworth A, Barst RJ. Tadalafil for the treatment of pulmonary arterial hypertension: a double-blind 52-week uncontrolled extension study. J Am Coll Cardiol. 2012;60:768–74.
54. Rubin LJ, Mendoza J, Hood M, McGoon M, Barst R, Williams WB, Diehl JH, Crow J, Long W. Treatment of primary pulmonary hypertension with continuous intravenous prostacyclin (epoprostenol). Results of a randomized trial. Ann Intern Med. 1990;112:485–91.
55. Shapiro SM, Oudiz RJ, Cao T, Romano MA, Beckmann XJ, Georgiou D, Mandayam S, Ginzton LE, Brundage BH. Primary pulmonary hypertension: improved long-term effects and survival with continuous intravenous epoprostenol infusion. J Am Coll Cardiol. 1997;30:343–9.
56. McLaughlin VV, Shillington A, Rich S. Survival in primary pulmonary hypertension: the impact of epoprostenol therapy. Circulation. 2002;106:1477–82.
57. Kitterman N, Poms A, Miller DP, Lombardi S, Farber HW, Barst RJ. Bloodstream infections in patients with pulmonary arterial hypertension treated with intravenous prostanoids: insights from the REVEAL REGISTRY®. Mayo Clin Proc. 2012;87:825–34.

58. Barst RJ, Galie N, Naeije R, Simonneau G, Jeffs R, Arneson C, Rubin LJ. Long-term outcome in pulmonary arterial hypertension patients treated with subcutaneous treprostinil. Eur Respir J. 2006;28:1195–203.
59. Olschewski H, Simonneau G, Galiè N, et al. Inhaled iloprost for severe pulmonary hypertension. N Engl J Med. 2002;347:322–9.
60. White RJ, Jerjes-Sanchez C, Meyer GMB, et al. Combination therapy with oral treprostinil for pulmonary arterial hypertension: a double-blind placebo-controlled clinical trial. Am J Respir Crit Care Med. 2020;201:707–17.
61. Tapson VF, Jing ZC, Xu KF, et al. Oral treprostinil for the treatment of pulmonary arterial hypertension in patients receiving background endothelin receptor antagonist and phosphodiesterase type 5 inhibitor therapy (The FREEDOM-C2 Study): a randomized controlled trial. Chest. 2013;144:952–8.
62. D'Alonzo G, Barst R, Ayres S, et al. Survival in patients with primary pulmonary hypertension. Results from a National Prospective Registry. Ann Intern Med. 1991;115:343–9.
63. Benza RL, Miller DP, Barst RJ, Badesch DB, Frost AE, McGoon MD. An evaluation of long-term survival from time of diagnosis in pulmonary arterial hypertension from the reveal registry. Chest. 2012;142:448–56.
64. Tonelli AR, Arelli V, Minai OA, Newman J, Bair N, Heresi GA, Dweik RA. Causes and circumstances of death in pulmonary arterial hypertension. Am J Respir Crit Care Med. 2013;188:365–9.
65. Grinnan DC, Swetz KM, Pinson J, Fairman P, Lyckholm LJ, Smith T. The end-of-life experience for a cohort of patients with pulmonary arterial hypertension. J Palliat Med. 2012;15:1065–70.
66. Anand V, Vallabhajosyula S, Cheungpasitporn W, Frantz RP, Cajigas HR, Strand JJ, DuBrock HM. Inpatient palliative care use in patients with pulmonary arterial hypertension: temporal trends, predictors, and outcomes. Chest. 2020;158:2568–78.
67. Hoeper MM, Galie N, Murali S, et al. Outcome after cardiopulmonary resuscitation in patients with pulmonary arterial hypertension. Am J Respir Crit Care Med. 2002;165:341–4.
68. Chen H, Taichman DB, Doyle RL. Health-related quality of life and patient-reported outcomes in pulmonary arterial hypertension. Proc Am Thorac Soc. 2008;5:623–30.
69. Löwe B, Gräfe K, Ufer C, Kroenke K, Grünig E, Herzog W, Borst MM. Anxiety and depression in patients with pulmonary hypertension. Psychosom Med. 2004;66:831–6.
70. Banerjee D, Vargas SE, Guthrie KM, Wickham BM, Allahua M, Whittenhall ME, Palmisciano AJ, Ventetuolo CE. Sexual health and health-related quality of life among women with pulmonary arterial hypertension. Pulm Circ. 2018; https://doi.org/10.1177/2045894018788277.
71. Guillevin L, Armstrong I, Aldrighetti R, Howard LS, Ryftenius H, Fischer A, Lombardi S, Studer S, Ferrari P. Understanding the impact of pulmonary arterial hypertension on patients' and carers' lives. Eur Respir Rev. 2013;22:535–42.
72. Armstrong I, Billings C, Kiely DG, Yorke J, Harries C, Clayton S, Gin-Sing W. The patient experience of pulmonary hypertension: a large cross-sectional study of UK patients. BMC Pulm Med. 2019;19:1–9.
73. McGoon MD, Ferrari P, Armstrong I, Denis M, Howard LS, Lowe G, Mehta S, Murakami N, Wong BA. The importance of patient perspectives in pulmonary hypertension. Eur Respir J. 2019; https://doi.org/10.1183/13993003.01919-2018.
74. Taichman DB, Shin J, Hud L, Archer-Chicko C, Kaplan S, Sager JS, Gallop R, Christie J, Hansen-Flaschen J, Palevsky H. Health-related quality of life in patients with pulmonary arterial hypertension. Respir Res. 2005;6:1–10.
75. Delcroix M, Howard L. Pulmonary arterial hypertension: the burden of disease and impact on quality of life. Eur Respir Rev. 2015;24:621–9.
76. McKenna SP, Doughty N, Meads DM, Doward LC, Pepke-Zaba J. The Cambridge Pulmonary Hypertension Outcome Review (CAMPHOR): a measure of health-related quality of life and quality of life for patients with pulmonary hypertension. Qual Life Res. 2006;15:103–15.

77. Twiss J, McKenna S, Ganderton L, Jenkins S, Ben-L'amri M, Gain K, Fowler R, Gabbay E. Psychometric performance of the CAMPHOR and SF-36 in pulmonary hypertension. BMC Pulm Med. 2013; https://doi.org/10.1186/1471-2466-13-45.
78. Gomberg-Maitland M, Thenappan T, Rizvi K, Chandra S, Meads DM, McKenna SP. United States Validation of the Cambridge Pulmonary Hypertension Outcome Review (CAMPHOR). J Hear Lung Transplant. 2008;27:124–30.
79. Coffin D, Duval K, Martel S, Granton J, Lefebvre M-C, Meads DM, Twiss J, McKenna S. Adaptation of the Cambridge Pulmonary Hypertension Outcome Review (CAMPHOR) into French-Canadian and English-Canadian. Can Respir J. 2008;15:77–83.
80. McCollister D, Shaffer S, Badesch DB, Filusch A, Hunsche E, Schüler R, Wiklund I, Peacock A. Development of the Pulmonary Arterial Hypertension-Symptoms and Impact (PAH-SYMPACT®) questionnaire: a new patient-reported outcome instrument for PAH. Respir Res. 2016;17:1–12.
81. Chin KM, Gomberg-Maitland M, Channick RN, et al. Psychometric Validation of the Pulmonary Arterial Hypertension-Symptoms and Impact (PAH-SYMPACT) Questionnaire: results of the SYMPHONY Trial. Chest. 2018;154:848–61.
82. Yorke J, Corris P, Gaine S, Gibbs JSR, Kiely DG, Harries C, Pollock V, Armstrong I. EmPHasis-10: development of a health-related quality of life measure in pulmonary hypertension. Eur Respir J. 2014;43:1106–13.
83. Borgese M, Badesch D, Bull T, et al. EmPHasis-10 as a measure of health-related quality of life in pulmonary arterial hypertension: data from PHAR. Eur Respir J. 2020:2000414.
84. Rival G, Lacasse Y, Martin S, Bonnet S, Provencher S. Effect of pulmonary arterial hypertension-specific therapies on health-related quality of life a systematic review. Chest. 2014;146:686–708.
85. Vanhoof JMM, Delcroix M, Vandevelde E, Denhaerynck K, Wuyts W, Belge C, Dobbels F. Emotional symptoms and quality of life in patients with pulmonary arterial hypertension. J Hear Lung Transplant. 2014;33:800–8.
86. Galiè N, Barberà JA, Frost AE, Ghofrani H-A, Hoeper MM, McLaughlin VV, Peacock AJ, Simonneau G, Vachiery J-L, Grünig RJO E, Vonk-Noordegraaf A, White RJ, Blair C, Gillies H, Miller KL, Harris JHN, Langley J, Rubin LJ. Initial use of ambrisentan plus tadalafil in pulmonary arterial hypertension. N Engl J Med. 2015;373:834–44.
87. Peacock A, Galiè N, Barbera J. Initial combination therapy of ambrisentan and tadalafil and quality of life: SF-36 & CAMPHOR analyses from the AMBITION trial. Am J Respir Crit Care Med. 2017;196:A6905.
88. Barst RJ, Long LJ, WA MG, Rich MD, Badesch S, Groves DB, Tapson BM, Bourge VF, Brundage RC, Others BH. Conventional therapy for primary pulmonary hypertension. N Engl J Med. 1996;334:296–301.
89. Zlupko M, Harhay MO, Gallop R, Shin J, Archer-Chicko C, Patel R, Palevsky HI, Taichman DB. Evaluation of disease-specific health-related quality of life in patients with pulmonary arterial hypertension. Respir Med. 2008;102:1431–8.
90. Matura LA, McDonough A, Carroll DL. Health-related quality of life and psychological states in patients with pulmonary arterial hypertension. J Cardiovasc Nurs. 2014;29:178–84.
91. Ulrich S, Saxer S, Hasler ED, Schwarz EI, Schneider SR, Furian M, Bader PR, Lichtblau M, Bloch KE. Effect of domiciliary oxygen therapy on exercise capacity and quality of life in patients with pulmonary arterial or chronic thromboembolic pulmonary hypertension: a randomised, placebo-controlled trial. Eur Respir J. 2019; https://doi.org/10.1183/13993003.002762019.
92. Fernandes CJCS, Martins BCS, Jardim CVP, Ciconelli RM, Morinaga LK, Breda AP, Hoette S, Souza R. Quality of life as a prognostic marker in pulmonary arterial hypertension. Health Qual Life Outcomes. 2014;12:130.
93. Cenedese E, Speich R, Dorschner L, Ulrich S, Maggiorini M, Jenni R, Fischler M. Measurement of quality of life in pulmonary hypertension and its significance. Eur Respir J. 2006;28:808–15.

94. McCabe C, Bennett M, Doughty N, Ross RM, Sharples L, Pepke-Zaba J. Patient-reported outcomes assessed by the CAMPHOR questionnaire predict clinical deterioration in idiopathic pulmonary arterial hypertension and chronic thromboembolic pulmonary hypertension. Chest. 2013;144:522–30.
95. Favoccia C, Kempny A, Yorke J, Armstrong I, Price LC, McCabe C, Harries C, Wort SJ, Dimopoulos K. EmPHasis-10 score for the assessment of quality of life in various types of pulmonary hypertension and its relation to outcome. Eur J Prev Cardiol. 2019;26:1338–40.
96. Lewis R, Armstrong I, Bergbaum C, et al. EmPHasis-10 health-related quality of life score predicts outcomes in patients with idiopathic and connective tissue disease-associated pulmonary arterial hypertension: results from a UK multi-centre study. Eur Respir J. 2020; https://doi.org/10.1183/13993003.congress-2020.3973.
97. Sahay S, Melendres-Groves L, Pawar L, Cajigas HR. Pulmonary hypertension care center network improving care and outcomes in PH. Chest. 2016; https://doi.org/10.1016/j.chest.2016.10.043.
98. Mitchell S, Tan A, Moine S, Dale J, Murray SA. Primary palliative care needs urgent attention. BMJ. 2019;365:15–6.
99. Quill TE, Abernethy AP. Generalist plus specialist palliative care — creating a more sustainable model. N Engl J Med. 2013;368:1171–3.
100. Meier DE, Beresford L. Outpatient clinics are a new frontier for palliative care. J Palliat Med. 2008;11:823–8.
101. Temel JS, Greer JA, Muzikansky A, et al. Early palliative care for patients with metastatic non-small-cell lung cancer. N Engl J Med. 2010;363:733–42.
102. Ruggiero R, Lynn RF, Reinke LF. Palliative care in advanced lung diseases: a void that needs filling. Ann Am Thorac Soc. 2018;22:1265–8.
103. Kavalieratos D, Corbelli J, Zhang D, et al. Association between palliative care and patient and caregiver outcomes: a systematic review and meta-analysis. JAMA J Am Med Assoc. 2016;316:2104–14.
104. May P, Normand C, Cassel JB, Del Fabbro E, Fine RL, Menz R, Morrison CA, Penrod JD, Robinson C, Morrison RS. Economics of palliative care for hospitalized adults with serious illness: a meta-analysis. JAMA Intern Med. 2018;178:820–9.
105. Qureshi D, Tanuseputro P, Perez R, Pond GR, Seow HY. Early initiation of palliative care is associated with reduced late-life acute-hospital use: a population-based retrospective cohort study. Palliat Med. 2019;33:150–9.
106. Hrustanovic-Kadic M, Ziegler C, El-Kersh K. Palliative care perception in PAH: evaluating the interaction of PPCI, PAH-SYMPACT questionnaire, and REVEAL 2.0 risk score. Ann Am Thorac Soc. 2020; https://doi.org/10.1513/annalsats.202005-552rl.
107. Fenstad ER, Shanafelt TD, Sloan JA, Novotny PJ, Durst LA, Frantz RP, Mcgoon MD, Swetz KM. Physician attitudes toward palliative care for patients with pulmonary arterial hypertension : results of a cross-sectional survey. Pulm Circ. 2015;4:504–10.
108. Sonntag E, Grinnan D. A path forward for palliative care in pulmonary arterial hypertension. Chest. 2020;158:2260–1.
109. Klinger JR, Elliott CG, Levine DJ. Therapy for pulmonary arterial hypertension in adults. Chest. 2019;155:565–86.
110. Galiè N, Humbert M, Vachiéry J-L, et al. 2015 ESC/ERS guidelines for the diagnosis and treatment of pulmonary hypertension. Eur Heart J. 2015;37:67–119.
111. Haddad F, Peterson T, Fuh E, et al. Characteristics and outcome after hospitalization for acute right heart failure in patients with pulmonary arterial hypertension. Circ Hear Fail. 2011;4:692–9.
112. European Pulmonary Hypertension Association. The impact of pulmonary arterial hypertension (PAH) on the lives of patients and carers: results from an international survey; 2012. www.phaeurope.org/wp-content/uploads/International-PAH-patient-and-Carer-Survey-Report-FINAL1.pdf.
113. Kingman M, Hinzmann B, Sweet O, Vachiéry JL. Living with pulmonary hypertension: unique insights from an international ethnographic study. BMJ Open. 2014;4:1–7.

114. Shah SJ, Gomberg-Maitland M, Thenappan T, Rich S. Selective serotonin reuptake inhibitors and the incidence and outcome of pulmonary hypertension. Chest. 2009;136:694–700.
115. Sadoughi A, Roberts KE, Preston IR, Lai GP, McCollister DH, Farber HW, Hill NS. Use of selective serotonin reuptake inhibitors and outcomes in pulmonary arterial hypertension. Chest. 2013;144:531–41.
116. Malenfant S, Brassard P, Paquette M, et al. Compromised cerebrovascular regulation and cerebral oxygenation in pulmonary arterial hypertension. J Am Heart Assoc. 2017; https://doi.org/10.1161/JAHA.117.006126.
117. Somaini G, Stamm A, Müller-Mottet S, Hasler E, Keusch S, Hildenbrand FF, Furian M, Speich R, Bloch KE, Ulrich S. Disease-targeted treatment improves cognitive function in patients with precapillary pulmonary hypertension. Respiration. 2015;90:376–83.
118. Hwang B, Howie-Esquivel J, Fleischmann KE, Stotts NA, Dracup K. Family caregiving in pulmonary arterial hypertension. Heart Lung. 2012;41:26–34.
119. Brinkman-Stoppelenburg A, Rietjens JAC, Van Der Heide A. The effects of advance care planning on end-of-life care: a systematic review. Palliat Med. 2014;28:1000–25.
120. US Food and Drug Administration (FDA). The Voice of the Patient. A series of reports from the U.S. Food and Drug Administration's (FDA's) patient-focused drug development initiative. Pulmonary arterial hypertension; 2014. http://www.fda.gov/downloads/ForIndustry/UserFees/PrescriptionDrugUserFee/UCM4. 1–22.
121. Sitbon O, Morrell NW. Pathways in pulmonary arterial hypertension: the future is here. Eur Respir Rev. 2012;21:321–7.
122. Chebib N, Cottin V, Taharo-Ag-Ralissoum M, Chuzeville M, Mornex JF. Epoprostenol discontinuation in patients with pulmonary arterial hypertension: a complex medical and social problem. Pulm Circ. 2018;8:4–6.
123. Calcaianu G, Calcaianu M, Canuet M, Enache I, Kessler R. Withdrawal of long-term epoprostenol therapy in pulmonary arterial hypertension (PAH). Pulm Circ. 2017;7:439–47.
124. Rosenzweig EB, Gannon WD, Madahar P, Agerstrand C, Abrams D, Liou P, Brodie D, Bacchetta M. Extracorporeal life support bridge for pulmonary hypertension: a high-volume single-center experience. J Hear Lung Transplant. 2019;38:1275–85.
125. Organ Procurement and Transplantation. Organ Procurement and Transplantation Network; 2020. https://optn.transplant.hrsa.gov/data/view-data-reports/national-data/ 1–2.
126. Rosenberger EM, Dew MA, DiMartini AF, DeVito Dabbs AJ, Yusen RD. Psychosocial issues facing lung transplant candidates, recipients and family caregivers. Thorac Surg Clin. 2012;22:517–29.
127. Wentlandt K, Dall'Osto A, Freeman N, Le LW, Kaya E, Ross H, Singer LG, Abbey S, Clarke H, Zimmermann C. The transplant palliative care clinic: an early palliative care model for patients in a transplant program. Clin Transpl. 2016;30:1591–6.
128. Colman R, Singer LG, Barua R, Downar J. Outcomes of lung transplant candidates referred for co-management by palliative care: a retrospective case series. Palliat Med. 2015;29:429–35.
129. Sandoval J, Gaspar J, Pulido T, Bautista E, Martínez-Guerra ML, Zeballos M, Palomar A, Gómez A. Graded balloon dilation atrial septostomy in severe primary pulmonary hypertension: a therapeutic alternative for patients nonresponsive to vasodilator treatment. J Am Coll Cardiol. 1998;32:297–304.
130. Chiu JS, Zuckerman WA, Turner ME, Richmond ME, Kerstein D, Krishnan U, Torres A, Vincent JA, Rosenzweig EB. Balloon atrial septostomy in pulmonary arterial hypertension: effect on survival and associated outcomes. J Hear Lung Transplant. 2015;34:376–80.
131. Aggarwal M, Grady RM, Choudhry S, Anwar S, Eghtesady P, Singh GK. Potts shunt improves right ventricular function and coupling with pulmonary circulation in children with suprasystemic pulmonary arterial hypertension. Circ Cardiovasc Imaging. 2018;11:e007964.
132. Rothman AMK, Vachiery JL, Howard LS, et al. Intravascular ultrasound pulmonary artery denervation to treat pulmonary arterial hypertension (TROPHY1): multicenter, early feasibility study. JACC Cardiovasc Interv. 2020;13:989–99.
133. Downar J, Fowler RA, Halko R, Huyer LD, Hill AD, Gibson JL. Early experience with medical assistance in dying in Ontario, Canada: a cohort study. Can Med Assoc J. 2020;192:E173–81.

# Chapter 15
# Palliative Care for Children with Lung Diseases

**Elisabeth Potts Dellon and Mary G. Prieur**

## Introduction

Children with lung disease are often burdened with distressing physical and emotional symptoms, limitations to achieving typical milestones of growth and development, and complex treatment decisions. Their families face many challenges related to caring for a child with a serious illness: emotional and relationship stressors, financial strain, navigating the health-care system, medical decision-making, and preparing children to manage their own health conditions as they approach adulthood. These children and their families can benefit from palliative care provided directly by their primary clinicians or medical teams, through consultation with palliative care specialists, or a combination [1].

Palliative care is understudied in pediatric lung diseases, with most available literature addressing the palliative care needs of individuals with cystic fibrosis (CF). Within CF, most research is not specific to children, but there are guidelines for models of palliative care delivery, management of advanced CF lung disease, and lung transplant referral which can help guide clinicians in addressing the palliative needs of children with CF [2–4]. Notably, therapeutic advances have brought greater changes in life expectancy and quality of life to children with CF than those with many other childhood lung diseases, but the evolving palliative care in CF remains applicable to many other chronic lung diseases.

E. P. Dellon (✉)
Department of Pediatrics, Division of Pulmonology, University of North Carolina School of Medicine, Chapel Hill, NC, USA
e-mail: elisabeth_dellon@med.unc.edu

M. G. Prieur
Departments of Psychiatry and Pediatrics, University of North Carolina School of Medicine, Chapel Hill, NC, USA
e-mail: mary_grimley@med.unc.edu



K. O. Lindell, S. K. Danoff (eds.), *Palliative Care in Lung Disease*, Respiratory Medicine, https://doi.org/10.1007/978-3-030-81788-6_15

In addition to primary lung diseases, many other conditions have substantial respiratory morbidity. Advances in respiratory support make life extension possible in many conditions that were previously universally fatal in childhood. Further, the availability of lung transplant for some children with advanced lung diseases can affect disease management and care planning. While it is outside the scope of this chapter to describe every condition and associated palliative needs, pediatric pulmonary clinicians are tasked with addressing symptoms, goals, decisions, and prognosis for many children with primary lung diseases as well as a myriad of chronic conditions with significant respiratory morbidity and should be prepared to do this in partnership with other specialists. Table 15.1 outlines characteristics of major childhood respiratory disorders.

In this chapter, we will review key components of palliative care – *symptom management*, *communication*, *emotional support*, and *care coordination* – and describe relevant needs of children with lung disease within each of these [5]. We will also highlight the value added by palliative care specialists and offer examples of opportunities for clinicians from different specialties to partner in addressing the palliative needs of children with lung diseases.

## Symptom Management

As described in other chapters, people with lung diseases experience a variety of physical and emotional symptoms. Approaches to symptom management in children overlaps substantially with that in adults, with special attention to

**Table 15.1** Childhood lung diseases and other conditions marked by significant respiratory morbidity and associated characteristics

| Condition | Characteristics | Indication for lung transplantation[a] |
|---|---|---|
| Cystic fibrosis | Genetic, progressive obstructive lung disease | ✓ |
| Bronchopulmonary dysplasia/chronic lung disease of infancy | Sequela of prematurity, severe forms may be accompanied by pulmonary hypertension | ✓ |
| Childhood interstitial lung disease/diffuse lung disease | Varying onset and severity, may be genetic | ✓ |
| Neuromuscular diseases | Poor cough clearance, respiratory muscle weakness, scoliosis, airway obstruction | |
| Congenital airway malformations | Airway obstruction | |
| Severe neurologic impairment | Poor cough clearance, respiratory muscle weakness, scoliosis, airway obstruction | |
| Pulmonary hypoplasia | May be related to diaphragmatic hernia, congenital kidney disease | ✓ |
| Pulmonary hypertension | Idiopathic or secondary | ✓ |

[a]For patients with severe disease meeting criteria and without contraindications

pharmacological therapies: pediatric-specific dosing, route of administration, side effects, drug interactions, and adherence. Resources for non-pharmacological therapies, particularly complementary and alternative or integrative therapies, may be more limited for children than for adults. It should be noted that many symptoms are managed by primary clinicians or medical teams as a part of routine care, but refractory symptoms and complex symptom clusters should prompt consideration of referral to palliative care specialists, pain specialists, and/or mental health providers.

## *Dyspnea*

Dyspnea in childhood lung diseases may be due to parenchymal disease, airway obstruction, intrathoracic extraparenchymal pathologies, and poor lung mechanics from muscle weakness or scoliosis. While assessment and treatment should target obvious underlying causes, it is important to recognize that symptom clusters – for example, with anxiety, pain, cough, or fatigue – may occur and exacerbate dyspnea. Dyspnea may be mitigated by the use of oxygen or noninvasive respiratory support for children with abnormal gas exchange, airway obstruction, or neuromuscular weakness. A tracheostomy to relieve severe airway obstruction or tracheostomy with ventilator support for children with advanced lung disease or neuromuscular weakness could be a symptom relief strategy, particularly when life extension is a primary goal. Devices to support cough clearance are often beneficial to those with obstructive lung disease and neuromuscular weakness. Adaptation to supportive technologies can be challenging and may be facilitated by pediatric respiratory therapists, physical therapists, child life specialists, and mental health providers. Children who utilize these technologies typically qualify for home health services as well as additional support for their developmental and educational needs; thoughtful counseling about such resources and the impact of these technologies on quality of life and family function should be offered [6, 7].

Though evidence for pharmacological therapies for dyspnea in children is lacking, as with adults, treatment centers on opioids and benzodiazepines. Dosing should be weight-based and adjusted as needed to achieve desired effect, minimize side effects, and with consideration for comorbid conditions. There is often bias – clinician and patient/family – around the use of these classes of medications to treat dyspnea, with less concern about their use as end-of-life approaches. The use of opioids and benzodiazepines may affect lung transplant eligibility in some centers, so communication with transplant centers is advised when prescribing. For those with advanced lung disease due to CF, opioids are recommended for dyspnea in advanced disease and for managing pain and dyspnea at end of life, and benzodiazepines should be considered for dyspnea primarily at end of life [3, 8]. Education for children and families, careful monitoring, and proactive management of side effects should be priorities [9]. For example, in children with CF who are at risk for severe constipation including distal intestinal obstruction syndrome (DIOS), proactive initiation of a bowel regimen is essential. Non-pharmacological therapies for dyspnea may include relaxation-breathing training, distraction, self-hypnosis, use of fans, chest wall vibration, cooler ambient temperatures, and of course addressing other contributors to dyspnea through supportive therapies [10, 11].

## *Cough*

Cough is a common symptom in children with lung diseases and may contribute to pain, dyspnea, fatigue, poor sleep quality, and anxiety, difficulty participating in typical childhood activities, and also being treated differently or even bullied by peers. Treatment for cough should target the underlying condition, particularly when infection, inflammation, or bronchospasm are present. Assessing and treating infection as well as concurrent respiratory conditions like asthma and non-pulmonary causes of cough, including gastroesophageal reflux and postnasal drip, are also important. For children with impaired cough clearance due to disorders of mucociliary clearance or neuromuscular weakness, augmenting clearance with manual or device-based chest physiotherapy can be helpful, sometimes in concert with aerosolized therapies like saline or mucolytics to loosen secretions. For those with muscle weakness, cough facilitation with mechanical insufflation/exsufflation may be beneficial [12, 13].

Pharmacological therapies directed at reducing cough, including honey, over-the-counter antitussives, and antihistamine decongestants, may be helpful for some children but may be contraindicated in very young children and generally have limited benefits [12]. Low-dose opioids can also be considered but should typically be reserved for markedly distressing cough associated with pain and/or dyspnea and for management of cough at end of life.

Hemoptysis, or cough accompanied by bleeding from the respiratory tract, can occur in some children with lung diseases, whether due directly to the underlying condition or associated with infection or comorbid clotting disorders. This tends to be a very distressing symptom, both emotionally and physically. While often self-limited and reversible with rest, treatment for infection if present, and correction of impaired clotting, large volume and even life-threatening hemoptysis may occur. Endoscopic or surgical management may be appropriate depending on a child's stage of illness and prognosis [14].

## *Fatigue*

Many children with lung disease report fatigue. Respiratory insufficiency, cough, impaired gas exchange deconditioning, muscle weakness, and sleep disturbance may be contributing factors depending on a child's underlying condition and stage of illness. Depressed mood and pain are other common associations. Additionally, side effects of treatments may contribute to fatigue. Fatigue may manifest in many ways, from physical tiredness or weakness to mental clouding, poor concentration, or impaired memory to effects on mood including irritability, apathy, and decreased motivation [10]. Sleep may or may not reduce fatigue; sleep quality may be poor such that sleep is not restorative, and unsuccessful attempts to sleep may contribute to poor conditioning and isolation.

Fatigue is highly subjective and thus difficult to measure objectively. Exploring a child's perception of fatigue and its impact on their mood and daily function often yields clues to treatment approaches. Underlying causes should of course be assessed and addressed and additional interventions employed when needed. Goal setting, prioritizing necessary and enjoyable activities that require energy and alertness, and considering ways to conserve energy are important steps. Attending to the emotional impact is critical, and therapy and pharmacological management of mood disorders are recommended. Physical therapists can promote strength and conditioning exercises, and occupational therapists can assist with lifestyle modifications to help conserve energy and optimize function. Sleep hygiene should be assessed and promoted. Finally, pharmacological therapies like stimulants can be considered [10].

## *Sleep Disturbance*

Management of sleep disturbance in children with lung disease centers on improving nocturnal hypoxemia and/or sleep-disordered breathing as well as addressing emotional symptoms and behavioral concerns that might be interfering with sleep. Taking a focused sleep history can inform diagnostic testing and appropriate interventions. While there are no widely accepted tools to measure sleep quality, there are many available tools that could facilitate the evaluation and management of sleep disturbance [15]. As noted throughout this section, poor sleep may be related to dyspnea, cough, anxiety, pain, and other distressing symptoms, with each affecting the other in various ways such that multimodal interventions may be needed.

Children with structural craniofacial or airway abnormalities, neurological conditions, CF, or obesity are particularly at risk for obstructive sleep apnea (OSA), which may be marked by concurrent signs and symptoms like snoring, nasal congestion, pauses in breathing during sleep, nocturnal enuresis, daytime drowsiness, and behavioral issues [16]. Untreated sleep apnea is associated with hypertension, cardiovascular disease, obesity, behavioral issues, and neurodevelopmental concerns. Polysomnography is the gold standard for diagnosis and can be used to guide interventions like lifestyle modifications (positioning during sleep, dietary modification), use of oxygen or noninvasive positive airway pressure, pharmacological management, or surgical intervention such as adenotonsillectomy. Tracheostomy may be indicated for children with severe OSA with craniofacial or airway abnormalities, those who are struggling with growth, who are having life-threatening events, or who have neuromuscular weakness with need for both airway and respiratory support.

While central sleep apnea, caused by dysregulation of central respiratory drive, is more commonly associated with neurological conditions, its presence in children with airway and lung diseases affects recommendations about interventions to support breathing during sleep. Pulmonary clinicians are often involved in shared decision-making with families about the use of noninvasive positive airway pressure or tracheostomy with mechanical ventilation and contribute to the management of these children, sometimes assuming a central role given how common respiratory morbidities are in this population.

Sleep disturbance related to sleep-wake cycle disruption, anxiety, and other symptoms as previously noted typically responds best to behavioral interventions and concurrent management of contributing symptoms. In general, the use of hypnotics is discouraged in favor of non-pharmacological or alternative pharmacological strategies, with melatonin generally felt to be safe and efficacious [17, 18]. Medications like antihistamines, alpha agonists, benzodiazepines, gabapentinoids, and atypical antidepressants are typically best employed to aid sleep when they can be utilized to concomitantly treat other symptoms such that polypharmacy and side effects can be minimized.

## *Pain*

Children with chronic health conditions frequently report pain, which may be acute and related to the underlying condition or to medical procedures, or chronic. Pain is known to negatively impact adherence, quality of life, and survival in CF [19–21], and while data are lacking, it is reasonable to assume a similar impact on children with other progressive lung diseases. The approach to pain assessment requires attention to age and developmental stage, previous experiences with pain, and symptoms with which pain commonly clusters, such as dyspnea, anxiety, and depression [22].

As with any condition, pain management necessitates identifying and targeting underlying causes. A standard approach to pain management, utilizing non-opioid analgesics for milder pain along with adjuncts and non-pharmacological modalities and limiting the use of opioids to more severe pain or episodic pain (acute and procedure-related), is recommended. Children with more advanced lung disease, neuromuscular weakness, or airway obstruction may be at risk for respiratory compromise due to opioids if not dosed with caution and monitored closely, but these conditions should never be considered a contraindication to opioids at the expense of a child's comfort and well-being. Consultation with pain and/or palliative care specialists can be helpful in mitigating discomfort about opioid use on the part of primary clinicians who do not typically prescribe opioids and for children and families who desire additional education and support around opioid use that can be provided by clinicians with more experience prescribing. For children who are awaiting lung transplantation, coordination of care around opioid prescribing with the lung transplant team is encouraged.

## *Emotional Symptoms*

Children with lung disease often experience emotional symptoms in addition to physical ones. Anxiety and symptoms of depression can be quite distressing and can cluster with physical symptoms, negatively affecting function and quality of life for the child and for the family. Please refer to the section entitled “Coping” for discussion of emotional symptom assessment and management in children.

# Communication

Communication is vital to the patient-clinician relationship, and communication needs of a child and family change throughout childhood. Initially centered on parents and caregivers, communication evolves to include the child and, for those who survive into adulthood, to focus on the person living with lung disease who is becoming an independent adult. Hope – for effective treatments, for long-term survival, for a condition to be cured, for realizing all the goals of childhood and emerging independence as a young adult – tends to be central to discussions about diagnosis, prognosis, and treatment decisions. Primary clinicians should be comfortable engaging children in families in these important conversations, calling on palliative care specialists for support when needed [1, 5]. Some general tips for communication offered by Jordan and colleagues [23] is outlined in Table 15.2. In this section, we will review approaches to communicating prognosis, partnering with children and families in decision-making, and advance care planning.

## *Discussing Prognosis*

Childhood mortality has declined with advances in medical care [24], and children with complex medical conditions, including respiratory diseases, are living longer [25]. Prognostication can be challenging, particularly in rare or heterogeneous conditions. An honest, intentional, developmentally appropriate approach to communication about health concerns is recommended for children with serious illnesses [26–30]. Most children develop a gradual awareness and understanding of their illness at rates affected by their social, emotional, and cognitive development [31, 32]. In one study of prognosis communication, adults with CF recalled progressing from understanding that CF is chronic (i.e., affects daily life, makes them different from peers, requires daily treatments and regular medical care) to understanding that it is permanent and finally to understanding that it is progressive [33].

Normal developmental understanding of illness and death occurs on a continuum. Children under age 2 years generally do not have a cognitive understanding of death, often having not yet learned much language, and instead may view it as a

**Table 15.2** Synthesis of recommendations for communication

| | | |
|---|---|---|
| Assessment of quality of life | Ask about child's narrative | "Tell me about Leo"<br>"What has life been like since his diagnosis?" |
| | Ask about child's quality of life | "Describe to us a typical day for Leo when he is well"<br>"What things bring Leo comfort/joy?" |
| Assessment of symptoms | Ask parents/patients about symptoms and response to prior treatments | "What does it look like when he is in pain?"<br>"When he has been in pain before, what has helped?" |
| Goals of care conversations | Ask family how they make decisions for their child | "Who is involved when you have difficult decisions to make in your family?"<br>"How are decisions made in your family?" |
| | Ask family how they want to receive information | "What is most important when you are receiving information from the medical team?" |
| | Involve providers who have long-standing relationship with child/family | "Who are the providers that know Leo best?"<br>"Would you like us to involve them in caring for him at this time?" |
| | Ask parents/patients their hopes and worries | "What are you hoping for Leo?"<br>"What are you most worried about?" |
| | Ask parents/patient their source of strength | "In difficult times what gives you strength?"<br>"How well is that working for you right now?" |
| Talking with child | A child's developmental state and family preference determine communication with the child | Ask the adolescent, "We need to discuss next steps in your care, how would you like to receive this information?"<br>Ask parents, "What does Leo know about his illness?"<br>"How can we partner with you in talking to Leo about his illness?" |

separation from caregivers. From 2 to 6 years of age, though widely variable based on an individual child's emotional and cognitive development, children frequently don't understand the finality of death, may perceive it as a punishment, and engage in magical thinking – believing that wishes may come true. From ages 7 to 12 years, children can understand the difference between contagious and noncontagious illnesses and are solidifying the notions of permanence and irreversibility of death. Children over age 12 typically understand the cause and development of illness and recognize that death is irreversible and universal. This time frame may be shifted earlier for children with chronic conditions [34–36]. There are also numerous individual, familial, and cultural considerations in communicating about prognosis.

The approach to discussing prognosis with children should be tailored to individual children and families, with thoughtful assessment of understanding and attention to emotions. Barriers to these conversations, like clinician reluctance, desire to instill hope, waiting for patients to ask about prognosis, parental hesitation, and difficulty finding time for such conversations, should be proactively addressed [33]. Enlisting help from experts in child development and support, preemptively communicating with parents to allow them time to process information and prepare to share this with their children, and utilizing "conversation-starting" language to help facilitate conversations may relieve anxiety and burden on all parties and enhance the likelihood of effective and supportive communication [30].

Palliative care specialists often prompt communication about prognosis among patients, caregivers, and primary clinicians/teams because of the importance of understanding prognosis when there are treatment decisions to be made. Palliative care specialists can sometimes act as a "third party," creating space and support for these hard conversations and assisting patients and primary team members through shifting goals, conflicts over treatment plans, or new prognostic information that might affect treatment options and/or life expectancy.

## *Decision-Making*

Children with respiratory illnesses and their families may face many decisions about therapies to stabilize, improve, or cure their conditions. Technologies to support respiratory function may be offered as a part of disease and symptom management, and lung transplantation is offered to some children with end-stage lung disease when it has the potential to extend life and improve quality of life and when there are no contraindications.

Complex decisions can come at any time in a child's illness, depending on the condition and its trajectory. For infants and young children, parents are tasked with assessing potential benefits and burdens of their choices for the child within the context of the entire family and often find this to be a tremendous emotional burden. Understanding factual medical information and anticipated outcomes is critical to health-care decision-making, yet the uncertainty about prognosis for an individual child that is so common in childhood diseases complicates decision-making. The values of a child and family are always crucial factors and may bear more weight when there is greater uncertainty about outcomes and when clinicians are reluctant or unable to make specific recommendations. For example, when the goal is life extension and there is more than one treatment option that might achieve this but no one that is superior or guaranteed to produce the desired outcome teams may look more to families to engage in decision-making [37]. More leeway is typically offered for parents to choose less certain interventions when prognosis is particularly difficult to determine.

As a child grows older and become a more engaged stakeholder in his/her own medical care, it is important to gauge how parents wish to incorporate the child into decision-making and encourage them to collaborate with clinicians in educating and supporting the child about his/her diagnosis. Experts in child development can provide helpful assessments of a child's readiness for greater participation in decision-making. Most adolescents wish to be involved in decisions about their health care [38], but the degree of desired involvement may vary depending on age, developmental stage, illness severity, mood, family dynamics, and many other contextual issues [39, 40]. It is also subject to change, not just gradually with time but even fluctuating day to day. Clear communication of medical facts in understandable terms, exploration of goals, dispelling of myths or misperceptions related to illness, and thoughtful involvement of supportive adults are all essential to shared decision-making with children [41]. Many children, even at age 18 years when they become legal adults, rely on parents to support their decision-making and may defer decisions to parents.

Palliative care specialists can support decision-making throughout childhood. They can collaborate with primary medical teams in exploring goals, wishes, and values with parents of infants and young children, assist in assessing a child's readiness to learn more about their condition and work with parents on how to share this information as children get older, and support the needs of older children and adolescents' emerging independence [30]. Palliative care specialists can also be helpful in navigating conflict between children and parents, between parents and other family members, or children/families and primary medical teams [1, 42].

## *Advance Care Planning*

Though advance care planning (ACP) may be less formal in children than adults with serious illness who are encouraged to complete advance directives outlining wishes for their medical care, ACP is recommended for any child with a serious illness [43]. For those with CF, ACP is encouraged across the lifespan to align care with values, preferences, and priorities [4]. Prognostic uncertainty of many lung diseases reinforces the importance of planning ahead for many eventualities so that as children and families gain experience living with a serious illness and learn about emerging therapies, they can thoughtfully consider wishes around interventions, whether the condition is responsive to therapies and improving or whether health is declining.

Involving children in ACP requires an individualized approach with attention to a child's developmental stage, understanding of their condition and treatment options, and support needs. The use of age-appropriate tools to facilitate ACP can be helpful in identifying gaps in information, misperceptions about disease causality, unspoken fears, or complex emotions around communicating concerns with loved ones or clinicians.

Palliative care specialists can be particularly helpful when there is the need for further exploration of goals of care or challenges in patient–/family-clinician communication. By encouraging open communication, revisiting of goals and treatment preferences over time, and documentation of wishes, palliative care specialists can promote continued partnerships among key stakeholders in a child's care through the course of illness. Pediatric palliative care resources to support communication about goals, decisions, and advance care planning are highlighted in Table 15.3.

## Support

While many members of a child's primary medical teams may provide support (e.g., assistance with work, school, insurance), palliative care specialists can offer and advocate for another "layer" of support, helping children and families cope with the

**Table 15.3** Pediatric palliative care resources: communication support and tools

| | Topics addressed | | | | | | | Where to find |
|---|---|---|---|---|---|---|---|---|
| | What is palliative care? | Goals of care | Advance care planning | Decision-making | Symptom management | End of life | Working with palliative specialists | |
| The Conversation Project: Pediatric Starter Kit | | ✓ | ✓ | ✓ | | ✓ | | www.theconversationproject.org |
| My Wishes® Voicing My Choices® | | ✓ | ✓ | ✓ | ✓ | ✓ | | www.agingwithdignity.org |
| The Decision-Making Tool: Information for Families | | ✓ | ✓ | ✓ | | | | www.seattlechildrens.org/pdf/Decision_Making_tool.pdf |
| Palliative Care for Children: Support for the Whole Family When Your Child Is Living with a Serious Illness | ✓ | ✓ | | | ✓ | ✓ | ✓ | https://www.ninr.nih.gov/newsandinformation/conversationsmatter/palliative-care-for-children |
| Courageous Parents Network | ✓ | ✓ | ✓ | ✓ | ✓ | ✓ | ✓ | https://courageousparentsnetwork.org/ |

emotional challenges of lung diseases throughout the course of illness [44]. Emotional support takes many forms throughout a disease course, beginning at diagnosis, a time during which children and their families often feel overwhelmed with medical information [45]. They may be unable to process all that is being shared, instead worrying about "worst-case scenarios." In one retrospective study, parents described feeling high distress, shock, and disbelief regarding the uncertainty of their child's future [46]. Palliative care specialists can help families gather medical information while also attending to and seeking support for their own emotional responses, ranging from anxiety and sadness to grief. Clinicians and staff caring for children with lung diseases also need support around the challenges and emotional toll of this work, and palliative care specialists may provide direct support as well as helpful resources.

## *Grief*

Grief may begin at diagnosis and is not simply related to end of life. Many children and families note numerous losses, from a sense of normalcy to hopes about future goals. Palliative care teams can help explore these losses and their impact on well-being. Anticipatory grief is common and often prevents children and families from enjoying the "rest" of someone's life. Grief is not considered a formal disorder or diagnosis in the DSM-V and no longer precludes a diagnosis of major depressive disorder [47]. Grief is instead conceptualized as an ongoing process, somewhat distinct from mood disorders, allowing a normalization of the experience. The ICD-11 does, however, include persistent complex grief disorder in an attempt to help identify people who may benefit from additional interventions and perhaps be more at-risk, such as those with a previous mental health history [48]. While comorbid MDD and anxiety may be present, grief itself has specialized forms of treatment and may not respond to typical antidepressants. Non-pharmacological treatments specific to grief are less developed for children but may include applications of those for adults (e.g., applying acceptance and commitment therapy skills, narrative therapy, cognitive behavioral therapy [49]).

Although not all families may wish to discuss their grief, preferring to focus on their hopes and/or believing talking about this may be an acknowledgment of their worries for cultural/religious or other reasons, discussing grief related to end of life is another role of palliative care teams. Palliative care specialists can help primary medical teams, children, and family members remember that grief is individualized in how and when it is experienced, although it can be common at certain times such as birthdays and anniversaries [44]. Families may benefit from hearing that grief is both normal and often difficult to acknowledge. Research has demonstrated the positive impact of palliative care teams in aiding with communication and symptom management on parents' long-term grief [50].

## Coping

An illness places many emotional demands on children and families. The rates of anxiety and depression are often higher in this population. For example, an international study found prevalence rates of depression and anxiety to be two to three times those of a community sample for children with CF [51]. Children often report feeling overwhelmed with daily treatments, isolated and different from peers, and prevented from enjoying everyday activities (e.g., sports, social opportunities [52]). Palliative care specialists, along with mental health providers, can help examine the interplay of physical and emotional symptoms. This includes examining symptom clusters (e.g., common for people experiencing shortness of breath to also experience anxiety) and how somatic symptoms are possible characteristics of both physical and mental health (e.g., changes in sleep, eating, and energy are also symptoms of depression [53]). Palliative care specialists emphasize the importance of "whole person care," viewing patients as more than their physical illness and understanding the importance of physical, emotional, and spiritual well-being [54]. They can engage children and families in discussions regarding existential suffering and encourage them to seek additional forms of support if desired. While mental health resources are often limited, new advancements in telehealth have helped improve access to both therapy and psychiatric care [55]. Many palliative care teams have embedded mental health providers, including social workers and psychologists, and may know local providers who have relevant expertise in both individual and group settings [56].

## Family Support

Parental well-being is also important to assess. During infancy, a time when many children are diagnosed, parents are already adjusting to caregiving and may be coping with symptoms such as those related to postpartum depression (PPD). In fact, the rates of postpartum mental health issues in the general population are significant [57, 58]. Parental mental illness can have a substantial impact on children across the lifespan. Research has demonstrated both negative medical effects (e.g., physical health, feeding, sleep, motor functioning [59]) and effects on mental health (e.g., language and social development, bonding, increased rates of neglect and abuse [60, 61]). Rates are also generally higher for parents of children with chronic illnesses [51]. Thus, formal screening of parents' mental health and/or discussion of symptoms is recommended by several organizations [62, 63].

Support from the community has been shown to be particularly helpful for children and families [64]. Despite being aware of or perceiving increased emotional concerns, friends and family may not know how or what to offer as support. This may become increasingly so if a child progresses in their illness course. Thus, children and families may feel isolated and alone. Oftentimes, though, families may feel particularly connected to their faith or school community [65]. Palliative care teams can help and encourage families to connect to these community supports and offer support to these resources as well.

Sibling well-being is often an overlooked part of the family system. Siblings, depending on their developmental stage, may not understand differences in parental attention and concern [44]. They may exhibit changes in behavior (e.g., sleep, eating, school performance) while processing emotions such as anxiety, jealousy, and guilt. Palliative care specialists can offer psychoeducation and support to siblings and to parents regarding sibling adjustment, helping them stay connected to their family and their larger community and support systems [66–68].

### *Support for Clinicians and Staff*

Clinicians themselves identify taking care of chronically and seriously ill children as a significant stressor [69]. This is particularly true when children die, an event many cultures view as traumatic, believing this "isn't supposed to happen" [70]. Various aspects of care may be difficult, from disagreements with families regarding decision-making to witnessing – and not knowing how to support – a child and a family's distress. Palliative care specialists are often able to notice suffering in colleagues, respond empathetically, and work to build a culture of caring and support [71–73]. They can help clinicians and other staff caring for children navigate their own emotions and seek additional resources; within the hospital, these resources may include working with an ethics committee, chaplains, and mental health providers [74–76]. These opportunities allow clinicians and staff to connect, share, and reflect in both individual and group settings. Palliative care specialists can model their own self-care strategies and explore different ways clinicians and staff are coping, in an attempt to help foster well-being and prevent burnout, compassion fatigue, and moral distress [77–79]. They can also help clinicians and staff navigate practical questions as they experience new and challenging emotional scenarios like the first death of a pediatric patient, navigating funeral attendance, and offering bereavement support [80, 81].

## Care Coordination

Children with lung diseases often receive care from many clinicians and teams, including primary care providers, subspecialists, and mental health providers. Effective care coordination requires thoughtful communication among all parties. Palliative care specialists may aid in care coordination through exploration of goals and discussion of preferred approaches to communication and decision-making with children and families, with communication to relevant clinicians in an effort to get everyone "on the same page." Care coordination can reduce confusion caused by conflicting information and changing goals for medical care that can occur with time, disease progression, and greater lived experience with illness. While care coordination is key throughout a child's illness course, times of transition – to adult care, to lung transplant, to end of life – can be especially important for coordination in line with child and family preferences.

## *Transition to Adult Care*

As children are living longer with serious illnesses, there has been increasing attention in the literature and in clinical practice to the process of transition from pediatric to adult care, including the purposeful, planned transfer of care from pediatric to adult-focused clinicians or teams [82]. There is likely to be more support for children with conditions that are managed by multidisciplinary teams with similar structures in pediatric and adult medicine, such as CF, pulmonary hypertension, and neuromuscular diseases [13, 83], children who are dependent on respiratory technology [84], and children who have undergone lung transplantation [85, 86]. Additionally, some centers may offer specialized transition programs or even clinics focused on the disease self-management skills adolescents and young adults should acquire prior to transferring their care to adult clinicians [87]. These include basic disease knowledge, the ability to understand the purpose of and manage one's medications, scheduling and attending medical appointments, knowledge of insurance coverage, managing self-care procedures, understanding nutritional needs, and communicating with health-care providers and personal supports about one's medical condition [88]. Resource assessment is vital, particularly for those who have challenges to accessing care and for those with extensive care needs and technology dependence whose insurance benefits may change as they age into adulthood. While there is limited information in the literature about transition from pediatric to adult palliative care specialists [89], children receiving specialty palliative care should be offered continued care with adult palliative care specialists who can continue working on quality-of-life concerns alongside primary teams and other specialists.

## *Lung Transplantation*

Lung transplantation is an option for select children with some incurable, advanced lung and pulmonary vascular diseases (see Table 15.1). Transplantation is undertaken with the goals of extending life and improving quality of life [90]. The decision to pursue lung transplant is complicated and must include thoughtful evaluation of goals and values in addition to consideration of risks and potential benefits for an individual.

Incorporating specialty palliative care into lung transplant care offers many benefits: support from a third party for decision-making, enhanced physical and emotional symptom management throughout the transplant course, continued exploration of goals as one's illness progresses prior to transplant and as the post-transplant course unfolds, and additional support for family caregivers through what is often an overwhelming process [91]. Views of the role of palliative care in lung transplantation differ among clinicians and centers, with opportunities for holistic, patient- and family-centered care evident to many, but also barriers related to misunderstandings and misperceptions of palliative care. For example, palliative care may be viewed as appropriate only for those who are dying rather than as care that compliments and adds value to disease-directed therapies and transplant-related care [92]. While there is little in the literature to guide palliative care in pediatric lung transplantation, adult data suggest benefits both before and after transplant [93, 94], and specialty palliative care consultation is recommended in CF when unmet palliative care needs are identified [4].

## *End of Life*

End of life is a delicate time when goals and treatment preferences may be changing rapidly along with progression of symptoms, and the family and community around the child often need intensive support. While many clinicians have some experience in caring for dying children, end-of-life care is best delivered with assistance from experts in physical, emotional, and spiritual symptom management, as well as a comfort level with supporting children and families through the dying process [95].

While most children die in the hospital [96], hospice care is the model for quality compassionate care for children who are approaching end of life. Referral should be considered when consistent with a child and family's goals for late-stage illness and end-of-life care [97]. Access to pediatric hospice care may be limited. Palliative care specialists can be helpful in introducing hospice, navigating referral, and assisting with developing a plan of care that can be transferred to the home setting or an inpatient hospice unit. Children in the USA qualify for concurrent care under Section 2302 of the Affordable Care Act [98], such that they can receive hospice care and continued curative or disease-directed therapies as long as they meet criteria for hospice referral, including a terminal diagnosis with a prognosis of 6 months or less. Prognostication can be quite challenging in children, and inconsistencies exist in interpretation of this legislation and application of the hospice benefit to children who are nearing end of life [99], but clinicians are encouraged to explore possibilities given the numerous potential benefits of hospice care – including symptom management and emotional and spiritual support – for dying children and their families [97].

Regardless of location of end-of-life care, general principles of symptom management at end of life should be applied to the childhood lung disease population, with special attention to the interplay between dyspnea, anxiety, and pain (see "Symptom Management" section). Fears of opioid side effects such as respiratory depression, altered mental status, and constipation may limit their use; these fears can be mitigated through careful dose titration and education of family members, fellow clinicians, and staff. Children with complex symptoms typically benefit from consultation with palliative care specialists, pain specialists, mental health providers, and/or others who can address suffering based on an individual patient's values, preferences, beliefs, and culture. Collaborative management with these specialists is likely to enhance symptom control and to reduce stress and anxiety for the child, family, and health-care providers.

Continued connection to primary clinicians and teams can be extremely important to children and families as the end of life draws near. Whether clinicians caring for children with lung diseases "take the lead" in care of the dying child or partner with palliative care specialists or hospice teams, it is recommended that they remain focused on providing active, quality care at end of life [100]. Offering support and identifying resources for grieving and bereaved family members can be helpful, and palliative care specialists can assist with both direct support and appropriate referrals.

## Summary

Children with lung disease and their families face numerous challenges to function and quality of life. Advances in care are leading to better outcomes in many diseases, but many children have extensive palliative care needs that can be addressed by pulmonary clinicians and, when appropriate, palliative care specialists.



## References

1. Quill T, Abernathy A. Generalist plus specialist palliative care--creating a more sustainable model. N Engl J Med. 2013;368(13):1173–5. https://doi.org/10.0056/NEJMp1215620. Epub 2013 Mar 6.
2. Ramos KJ, Smith PJ, McKone EF, Pilewski JM, Lucy A, Hempstead SE, et al. Lung transplant referral for individuals with cystic fibrosis: Cystic Fibrosis Foundation consensus guidelines. J Cyst Fibros. 2019;18(3):321–33.
3. Kapnadak SG, Dimango E, Hadjiliadis D, Hempstead SE, Tallarico E, Pilewski JM, et al. Cystic Fibrosis Foundation consensus guidelines for the care of individuals with advanced cystic fibrosis lung disease. J Cyst Fibros. 2020;
4. Kavalieratos D, Georgiopoulos AM, Dhingra L, Basile MJ, Rabinowitz E, Hempstead SE, et al. Models of palliative care delivery for individuals with cystic fibrosis: Cystic Fibrosis Foundation evidence-informed consensus guidelines. J Palliat Med. 2020;
5. Kavalieratos D, Gelfman LP, Tycon LE, Riegel B, Bekelman DB, Ikejiani DZ, et al. Palliative Care in Heart Failure: rationale, evidence, and future priorities. J Am Coll Cardiol. 2017;70(15):1919–30.
6. Sherman JM, Davis S, Albamonte-Petrick S, Chatburn RL, Fitton C, Green C, et al. Care of the child with a chronic tracheostomy. This official statement of the American Thoracic

Society was adopted by the ATS Board of Directors, July 1999. Am J Respir Crit Care Med. 2000;161(1):297–308.

7. Sterni LM, Collaco JM, Baker CD, Carroll JL, Sharma GD, Brozek JL, et al. An Official American Thoracic Society Clinical Practice Guideline: pediatric chronic home invasive ventilation. Am J Respir Crit Care Med. 2016;193(8):e16–35.
8. Lanken PN, Terry PB, Delisser HM, Fahy BF, Hansen-Flaschen J, Heffner JE, et al. An official American Thoracic Society clinical policy statement: palliative care for patients with respiratory diseases and critical illnesses. Am J Respir Crit Care Med. 2008;177(8):912–27.
9. Dowell D, Haegerich TM, Chou R. CDC Guideline for Prescribing Opioids for Chronic Pain - United States, 2016. Contract No.: (No. RR-1).
10. Ullrich CK, Mayer OH. Assessment and management of fatigue and dyspnea in pediatric palliative care. Pediatr Clin N Am. 2007;54(5):735–56, xi.
11. Wolfe J, Sourkes B, Hinds P. Textboook of interdisciplinary pediatric palliative care. 1st ed. Saunders; 2011.
12. Craig F, Henderson EM, Bluebond-Langner M. Management of respiratory symptoms in paediatric palliative care. Curr Opin Support Palliat Care. 2015;9(3):217–26.
13. Bushby K, Finkel R, Birnkrant DJ, Case LE, Clemens PR, Cripe L, et al. Diagnosis and management of Duchenne muscular dystrophy, part 1: diagnosis, and pharmacological and psychosocial management. Lancet Neurol. 2010;9(1):77–93.
14. King CS, Brown AW, Aryal S, Ahmad K, Donaldson S. Critical care of the adult patient with cystic fibrosis. Chest. 2019;155(1):202–14.
15. Erwin AM, Bashore L. Subjective sleep measures in children: self-report. Front Pediatr. 2017;5:22.
16. Gipson K, Lu M, Kinane TB. Sleep-disordered breathing in children. Pediatr Rev. 2019;40(1):3–13.
17. de Castro-Silva C, de Bruin VM, Cunha GM, Nunes DM, Medeiros CA, de Bruin PF. Melatonin improves sleep and reduces nitrite in the exhaled breath condensate in cystic fibrosis--a randomized, double-blind placebo-controlled study. J Pineal Res. 2010;48(1):65–71.
18. Ivanenko A, Crabtree VM, Tauman R, Gozal D. Melatonin in children and adolescents with insomnia: a retrospective study. Clin Pediatr. 2003;42(1):51–8.
19. Lee AL, Rawlings S, Bennett KA, Armstrong D. Pain and its clinical associations in individuals with cystic fibrosis: a systematic review. Chron Respir Dis. 2016;13(2):102–17.
20. Lechtzin N, Allgood S, Hong G, Riekert K, Haythornthwaite JA, Mogayzel P, et al. The association between pain and clinical outcomes in adolescents with cystic fibrosis. J Pain Symptom Manag. 2016;52(5):681–7.
21. Blackwell LS, Quittner AL. Daily pain in adolescents with CF: effects on adherence, psychological symptoms, and health-related quality of life. Pediatr Pulmonol. 2015;50(3):244–51.
22. McGrath PA. Pain in the pediatric patient: practical aspects of assessment. Pediatr Ann. 1995;24(3):126–33, 37–8.
23. Jordan M, Keefer PM, Lee YA, Meade K, Snaman JM, Wolfe J, et al. Top ten tips palliative care clinicians should know about caring for children. J Palliat Med. 2018;21(12):1783–9.
24. Feudtner C, Christakis DA, Connell FA. Pediatric deaths attributable to complex chronic conditions: a population-based study of Washington State, 1980–1997. Pediatrics. 2000;106(1 Pt 2):205–9.
25. Tennant PW, Pearce MS, Bythell M, Rankin J. 20-year survival of children born with congenital anomalies: a population-based study. Lancet. 2010;375(9715):649–56.
26. Faulkner KW. Talking about death with a dying child. Am J Nurs. 1997;97(6):64. 6, 8-9
27. Nyborn JA, Olcese M, Nickerson T, Mack JW. "Don't try to cover the sky with your hands": parents' experiences with prognosis communication about their children with advanced cancer. J Palliat Med. 2016;19(6):626–31.
28. van der Geest IM, van den Heuvel-Eibrink MM, van Vliet LM, Pluijm SM, Streng IC, Michiels EM, et al. Talking about death with children with incurable cancer: perspectives from parents. J Pediatr. 2015;167(6):1320–6.

29. Levetown M. Communicating with children and families: from everyday interactions to skill in conveying distressing information. Pediatrics. 2008;121(5):e1441–60.
30. Rosenberg AR, Wolfe J, Wiener L, Lyon M, Feudtner C. Ethics, emotions, and the skills of talking about progressing disease with terminally ill adolescents: a review. JAMA Pediatr. 2016;170(12):1216–23.
31. Bibace R, Walsh ME. Development of children's concepts of illness. Pediatrics. 1980;66(6):912–7.
32. Piaget J. Cognitive development in children: piaget development and learning. J Res Sci Teach. 1964;2:176–80.
33. Farber JG, Prieur MG, Roach C, Shay R, Walter M, Borowitz D, et al. Difficult conversations: discussing prognosis with children with cystic fibrosis. Pediatr Pulmonol. 2018;53(5):592–8.
34. The pediatrician and childhood bereavement. American Academy of Pediatrics. Committee on psychosocial aspects of child and family health. Pediatrics. 2000;105(2):445–7.
35. Freyer DR. Care of the dying adolescent: special considerations. Pediatrics. 2004;113(2):381–8.
36. Bluebond-Langner M. The private worlds of dying children. Princeton, NJ: Princeton University Press; 1978.
37. Krick JA, Hogue JS, Reese TR, Studer MA. Uncertainty: an uncomfortable companion to decision-making for infants. Pediatrics. 2020;146(Suppl 1):S13–s7.
38. Hinds PS, Drew D, Oakes LL, Fouladi M, Spunt SL, Church C, et al. End-of-life care preferences of pediatric patients with cancer. J Clin Oncol. 2005;23(36):9146–54.
39. Wiener L, Zadeh S, Wexler LH, Pao M. When silence is not golden: engaging adolescents and young adults in discussions around end-of-life care choices. Pediatr Blood Cancer. 2013;60(5):715–8.
40. Wiener L, Zadeh S, Battles H, Baird K, Ballard E, Osherow J, et al. Allowing adolescents and young adults to plan their end-of-life care. Pediatrics. 2012;130(5):897–905.
41. Lyon ME, Jacobs S, Briggs L, Cheng YI, Wang J. Family-centered advance care planning for teens with cancer. JAMA Pediatr. 2013:1–8.
42. Rosenberg AR, Starks H, Unguru Y, Feudtner C, Diekema D. Truth telling in the setting of cultural differences and incurable pediatric illness: a review. JAMA Pediatr. 2017;171(11):1113–9.
43. American Academy of Pediatrics. Committee on Bioethics and Committee on Hospital Care. Palliative care for children. Pediatrics. 2000;106(2 Pt 1):351–7.
44. Hutton N, Levetown M, Frager G. The hospice and palliative medicine approach to caring for pediatric patients. Glenview, IL; 2008.
45. Mack JW, Wolfe J. Early integration of pediatric palliative care: for some children, palliative care starts at diagnosis. Curr Opin Pediatr. 2006;18(1):10–4.
46. Brown AR, Prieur MB, Sangvai AC, Penta E. Family needs during child's first year of life for parents of children with cystic fibrosis. Pediatr Pulmonol. 2020;55(S2):281.
47. Pies RW. The bereavement exclusion and DSM-5: an update and commentary. Innov Clin Neurosci. 2014;11(7–8):19–22.
48. Killikelly C, Maercker A. Prolonged grief disorder for ICD-11: the primacy of clinical utility and international applicability. Eur J Psychotraumatol. 2017;8(Suppl 6):1476441.
49. Shear MK, Reynolds CF 3rd, Simon NM, Zisook S, Wang Y, Mauro C, et al. Optimizing treatment of complicated grief: a randomized clinical trial. JAMA Psychiat. 2016;73(7):685–94.
50. van der Geest IM, Darlington AS, Streng IC, Michiels EM, Pieters R, van den Heuvel-Eibrink MM. Parents' experiences of pediatric palliative care and the impact on long-term parental grief. J Pain Symptom Manag. 2014;47(6):1043–53.
51. Quittner AL, Goldbeck L, Abbott J, Duff A, Lambrecht P, Sole A, et al. Prevalence of depression and anxiety in patients with cystic fibrosis and parent caregivers: results of The International Depression Epidemiological Study across nine countries. Thorax. 2014;69(12):1090–7.
52. Ernst MM, Johnson MC, Stark LJ. Developmental and psychosocial issues in cystic fibrosis. Child Adolesc Psychiatr Clin N Am. 2010;19(2):263–83. viii
53. APA. Diagnostic and statistical manual of mental disorders. 5th ed. Washington, DC: American Psychiatric Association; 2013.

54. Puchalski C, Ferrell BR, Viriani R, Otis-Green S, Baird P, Bull J, et al. Improving the quality of spiritual care as a dimension of palliative care: the report of the consensus conference. Palliat Med. 2009;12(10)
55. Winegard B, Miller EG, Slamon NB. Use of telehealth in pediatric palliative care. Telemed J e-Health. 2017;23(11):938–40.
56. Get Palliative Care: Center to Advance Palliative Care; 2020. Available from: https://getpalliativecare.org/whatis/pediatric/the-pediatric-palliative-care-team/.
57. O'Hara MW, McCabe JE. Postpartum depression: current status and future directions. Annu Rev Clin Psychol. 2013;9:379–407.
58. Paulson JF, Bazemore SD. Prenatal and postpartum depression in fathers and its association with maternal depression: a meta-analysis. JAMA. 2010;303(19):1961–9.
59. Fallon V, Groves R, Halford JC, Bennett KM, Harrold JA. Postpartum anxiety and infant-feeding outcomes. J Human Lactat. 2016;32(4):740–58.
60. Babenko O, Kovalchuk I, Metz GA. Stress-induced perinatal and transgenerational epigenetic programming of brain development and mental health. Neurosci Biobehav Rev. 2015;48:70–91.
61. Slomian J, Honvo G, Emonts P, Reginster JY, Bruyère O. Consequences of maternal postpartum depression: a systematic review of maternal and infant outcomes. Women's Health (London, England). 2019;15:1745506519844044.
62. Quittner AL, Abbott J, Georgiopoulos AM, Goldbeck L, Smith BA, Hempstead SE, et al. International Committee on Mental Health in Cystic Fibrosis: Cystic Fibrosis Foundation and European Cystic Fibrosis Society consensus statements for screening and treating depression and anxiety. Thorax. 2016;71(1):26–34. https://doi.org/10.1136/thoraxjnl-2015-207488. Epub 2015 Oct 9.
63. Earls MF, Yogman MW, Mattson G, Rafferty J. Incorporating recognition and management of perinatal depression into pediatric practice. Pediatrics. 2019;143(1)
64. Greeff AP, Vansteenwegen A, Herbiest T. Indicators of family resilience after the death of a child. Omega. 2011;63(4):343–58.
65. Hexem KR, Mollen CJ, Carroll K, Lanctot DA, Feudtner C. How parents of children receiving pediatric palliative care use religion, spirituality, or life philosophy in tough times. J Palliat Med. 2011;14(1):39–44.
66. Chin WL, Jaaniste T, Trethewie S. The role of resilience in the sibling experience of pediatric palliative care: what is the theory and evidence? Children (Basel, Switzerland). 2018;5(7)
67. Gaab EM, Owens GR, MacLeod RD. Siblings caring for and about pediatric palliative care patients. J Palliat Med. 2014;17(1):62–7.
68. Chudleigh J, Browne R, Radbourne C. Impact of cystic fibrosis on unaffected siblings: a systematic review. J Pediatr. 2019;210:112–7.e9.
69. Garcia TT, Garcia PC, Molon ME, Piva JP, Tasker RC, Branco RG, et al. Prevalence of burnout in pediatric intensivists: an observational comparison with general pediatricians. Pediatr Crit Care Med. 2014;15(8):e347–53.
70. Institute of Medicine Committee on P, End-of-Life Care for C, Their F. In: Field MJ, Behrman RE, editors. When Children Die: Improving Palliative and End-of-Life Care for Children and Their Families. Washington (DC): National Academies Press (US). Copyright 2003 by the National Academy of Sciences. All rights reserved.; 2003.
71. Granek L, Buchman S. Improving physician well-being: lessons from palliative care. CMAJ. 2019;191(14):E380–e1.
72. Rushton CH, Reder E, Hall B, Comello K, Sellers DE, Hutton N. Interdisciplinary interventions to improve pediatric palliative care and reduce health care professional suffering. J Palliat Med. 2006;9(4):922–33.
73. Jonas DF, Bogetz JF. Identifying the deliberate prevention and intervention strategies of pediatric palliative care teams supporting providers during times of staff distress. J Palliat Med. 2016;19(6):679–83.
74. Feudtner C, Nathanson PG. Pediatric palliative care and pediatric medical ethics: opportunities and challenges. Pediatrics. 2014;133(Suppl 1):S1–7.

75. Santoro JD, Bennett M. Ethics of end of life decisions in pediatrics: a narrative review of the roles of caregivers, shared decision-making, and patient centered values. Behavioral sciences (Basel, Switzerland). 2018;8(5)
76. Radwany SM, Mann P, Myerscough R, Jencius A. Resilience, compassion, and communication: how the Schwartz Center Rounds promotes primary palliative care. J Pain Symptom Manag. 2017;53(2):395.
77. Sanchez-Reilly S, Morrison LJ, Carey E, Bernacki R, O'Neill L, Kapo J, et al. Caring for oneself to care for others: physicians and their self-care. J Support Oncol. 2013;11(2):75–81.
78. Sansó N, Galiana L, Oliver A, Pascual A, Sinclair S, Benito E. Palliative care professionals' inner life: exploring the relationships among awareness, self-care, and compassion satisfaction and fatigue, burnout, and coping with death. J Pain Symptom Manag. 2015;50(2):200–7.
79. Kase SM, Waldman ED, Weintraub AS. A cross-sectional pilot study of compassion fatigue, burnout, and compassion satisfaction in pediatric palliative care providers in the United States. Palliat Support Care. 2019;17(3):269–75.
80. Beaune L, Muskat B, Anthony SJ. The emergence of personal growth amongst healthcare professionals who care for dying children. Palliat Support Care. 2018;16(3):298–307.
81. Baer TE, Feraco AM, Tuysuzoglu Sagalowsky S, Williams D, Litman HJ, Vinci RJ. Pediatric resident burnout and attitudes roward patients. Pediatrics. 2017;139(3)
82. Council NR, Medicine Io. Challenges in adolescent health care: workshop report. Washington, DC: The National Academies Press; 2007. 90 p.
83. Onofri A, Tan HL, Cherchi C, Pavone M, Verrillo E, Ullmann N, et al. Transition to adult care in young people with neuromuscular disease on non-invasive ventilation. Ital J Pediatr. 2019;45(1):90.
84. Agarwal A, Willis D, Tang X, Bauer M, Berlinski A, Com G, et al. Transition of respiratory technology dependent patients from pediatric to adult pulmonology care. Pediatr Pulmonol. 2015;50(12):1294–300.
85. LaRosa C, Glah C, Baluarte HJ, Meyers KE. Solid-organ transplantation in childhood: transitioning to adult health care. Pediatrics. 2011;127(4):742–53.
86. Benden C. Pediatric lung transplantation. J Thorac Dis. 2017;9(8):2675–83.
87. Crowley R, Wolfe I, Lock K, McKee M. Improving the transition between paediatric and adult healthcare: a systematic review. Arch Dis Child. 2011;96(6):548–53.
88. Reed-Knight B, Blount RL, Gilleland J. The transition of health care responsibility from parents to youth diagnosed with chronic illness: a developmental systems perspective. Fam Syst Health. 2014;32(2):219–34.
89. Doug M, Adi Y, Williams J, Paul M, Kelly D, Petchey R, et al. Transition to adult services for children and young people with palliative care needs: a systematic review. Arch Dis Child. 2011;96(1):78–84.
90. Kirkby S, Hayes D Jr. Pediatric lung transplantation: indications and outcomes. J Thorac Dis. 2014;6(8):1024–31.
91. Wentlandt K, Weiss A, O'Connor E, Kaya E. Palliative and end of life care in solid organ transplantation. Am J Transplant. 2017;17(12):3008–19.
92. Nolley E, Fleck J, Kavalieratos D, Dew MA, Dilling D, Colman R, et al. Lung transplant pulmonologists' views of specialty palliative care for lung transplant recipients. J Palliat Med. 2020;23(5):619–26.
93. Colman R, Singer LG, Barua R, Downar J. Characteristics, interventions, and outcomes of lung transplant recipients co-managed with palliative care. J Palliat Med. 2015;18(3):266–9.
94. Colman R, Singer LG, Barua R, Downar J. Outcomes of lung transplant candidates referred for co-management by palliative care: a retrospective case series. Palliat Med. 2015;29(5):429–35.
95. Johnson LM, Snaman JM, Cupit MC, Baker JN. End-of-life care for hospitalized children. Pediatr Clin N Am. 2014;61(4):835–54.
96. Basu RK. End-of-life care in pediatrics: ethics, controversies, and optimizing the quality of death. Pediatr Clin N Am. 2013;60(3):725–39.

97. Friebert S, Williams C. NPHCO facts and figures: pediatric palliative and hospice care in America. Alexandria, VA; 2015.
98. Social Security Act. Available from: https://www.ssa.gov/OP_Home/ssact/ssact-toc.htm.
99. Lotstein DS. Concurrent care is not enough: more hospice reforms are needed for children with serious illness. J Pediatr. 2020;225:11–2.
100. Back AL, Young JP, McCown E, Engelberg RA, Vig EK, Reinke LF, et al. Abandonment at the end of life from patient, caregiver, nurse, and physician perspectives: loss of continuity and lack of closure. Arch Intern Med. 2009;169(5):474–9.

# Chapter 16
# Specialty Palliative Care Program ILD

**Meena Kalluri**

> "I believe palliative care should be with you from when you're diagnosed, saying, "You know what, you're terminal but we're going to help you live until you die." I figure you should enjoy every minute of your life. We don't know, you could live two years, three years, (or) you could live 6 months or a month. But if you could access somebody and say, "This is the disease I have. What steps can I (take) to stay in my home, be happy in my home and as my disease progresses, who can I have, whether it be nursing staff, any access to anything that's going to make my life at home easier for myself and my caregivers." (A bereaved caregiver on the need for early palliative care in ILD) [1]

*Interstitial lung disease* (ILD) is a diverse group of entities that affect the interstitium, alveoli, and distal airways of the lung. The classification of such diseases is complex, and variable based on etiology, histopathology as well as clinical behavior, and continues to evolve with advancing knowledge. The pathology in ILD is characterized by inflammation and fibrosis. This process of injury and scarring frequently results in unrelenting progression that leads to a poor quality of life, high levels of patient distress, and subsequent morbidity and mortality. This phenotype is recognized as progressive fibrosing ILD (PF-ILD) [2].

## IPF: An Incurable, Progressive, and Terminal Reality

Idiopathic pulmonary fibrosis (IPF) is a prototypical ILD of PF-ILD phenotype. On average, patients die 3–5 years post-diagnosis from respiratory failure [3]. The unpredictable course means lung deterioration can be slow, rapid, or marked by

M. Kalluri (✉)
Division of Pulmonary Medicine, Department of Medicine, University of Alberta, Edmonton, AB, Canada

Alberta Health Services, Edmonton, AB, Canada
e-mail: Kalluri@ualberta.ca



K. O. Lindell, S. K. Danoff (eds.), *Palliative Care in Lung Disease*, Respiratory Medicine, https://doi.org/10.1007/978-3-030-81788-6_16

precipitous declines, while patients experience a poor quality of life characterized by its heavy symptom burden (i.e., dyspnea, cough, fatigue, anxiety, depression) [4, 5]. Timely and accurate diagnosis and access to disease-specific therapies are necessary first steps but not sufficient. This is because neither do the indicated antifibrotic therapies that slow down disease progression address symptoms, nor do they positively affect patient quality of life [6]. It is becoming increasingly clear that patient-centered or comprehensive IPF/ILD care cannot be delivered without addressing symptoms, informational needs, and improving care coordination and support throughout the disease trajectory. In the absence of such a comprehensive approach, IPF care is resource-intensive because patients are more likely to rely on costly, non-beneficial acute care services for symptom crises and end-of-life care [7, 8]. Therefore, guidelines have recommended early adoption of palliative care (PC) [9]. Palliative care is a multidisciplinary approach prioritizing prevention and relief of suffering experienced by patients afflicted by a terminal disease and their families [10]. It focuses on symptom relief, improving communication, care coordination, and ensuring care delivery is congruent with patient goals and preferences. Unfortunately, PC remains widely misunderstood in medical and public domains as singularly end-of-life (EOL) care. Therefore, PC is often treated as a last resort option, if at all, instead of early adoption in the disease trajectory [8].

## Traditional ILD Care: What Is Missing?

Sampson and colleagues documented patient perceptions of what can be termed traditional clinic-based ILD care [11]. Patients, recruited from specialist ILD clinics, described the clinic consultation as being disconnected from their lived experience of disease. This perceived disconnect stems from the clinical emphasis on physiological lung function measures and CT scans that do not directly correlate with patient experience dominated by dyspnea. Thus, dyspnea itself remains invisible, subsumed by objective measurements that are disconnected from patient's subjective experience. The clinical focus is on diagnosis and disease-specific treatments, appropriately so, but often ignoring patient narratives (experience of symptoms and impact). This is likely due to the lack of time in clinics and/or culture of practice. Thus, many patient and family concerns remain unaddressed during clinic visits [12]. Symptom management is not routinely integrated in care; self-management is not emphasized, and patient and caregiver information needs are not fully addressed during routine encounters [13]. The clinical focus on objective measurements of IPF progression, and prescribed treatments that do not directly improve patient condition or meet needs, result in profound consequences for health-related quality of life (HRQol) even at presentation [6], as many IPF patients have a poor HRQoL early in the disease trajectory [14]. Even though they leave clinics with diagnosis and guidelines-based treatments, patients and their families continue to suffer the heavy burden of untreated symptoms; new knowledge of a fatal prognosis coupled with anxiety, depression, and social isolation; and lack education and comprehensive support for living and coping with their disease.

Having a progressive disease, IPF patients are likely to decline and suffer a worsening HRQoL between clinic visits. Remote monitoring and symptom management as part of clinic outreach could expeditiously address needs and alleviate distress but are not available to most patients. The lack of such a case management approach is identified by patients as an unmet need [11]. In addition, communication gaps between patients and care providers and among care providers themselves, and poor care coordination have also been noted within current care models [15].

The limits of a disease-centric approach became increasingly clear with disease progression, when symptom-based therapies and advance care planning (ACP) are obviously required but not undertaken [12, 16, 17]. Patients and their families experience overwhelming distress from unmet physical and psychosocial and emotional needs, resulting in decline in health and HRQol [18]. Care providers appear unwilling to engage in conversations about prognosis, practical realities of disease progression, dying, and death even though many patients desire explicit EOL discussions [12, 19]. Many do not receive palliative support even at EOL; as a result, patients receive inappropriate care and die in hospitals with untreated symptoms leading to a poor quality of dying and death [8, 20]. Families frequently express fear, hopelessness, and helplessness and are unprepared to deal with what is coming their way [21].

Traditional clinic models cannot fully address the diverse spectrum of rapidly changing IPF/ILD care needs and, therefore, cannot facilitate comprehensive patient-centered care. IPF may be a lung-limited disease, but it affects all domains of health, the whole person. Therefore, a holistic approach to address distress from the physical, psychosocial, emotional, and spiritual domains is required in addition to usual care. Consequently, many clinical guidelines endorsed by professional societies, patient advocacy bodies, and lung associations have advocated for early integration of PC in IPF/PF-ILD [22, 23]. Despite the recognition of patient distress and loud calls to action, PC remains conspicuously absent in most outpatient ILD care settings. For a disease like IPF, marked by a poor quality of life at clinic presentations and a median survival of 3.8 years, unmet patient and family needs and symptom relief must be prioritized at the earliest opportunity [3].

## Why Is Palliative Care Not Integrated in ILD Clinical Practice?

There are several barriers to integration of palliative care, both as an approach and as a service in ILD. Many providers and patients mistakenly believe that palliative care is giving up of all care, a passive process, untenable with curative therapy or transplantation. Many also view PC as a last resort when "nothing more can be done"; many frequently associate it with futile feelings of failure, loss, and surrender. Given the negative perceptions and emotions the name evokes, some have suggested changing it to supportive care [24]. There is also a lingering misperception that patients need to be at the end of life, or that accurate prognostication and timeline predictions are needed to identify suitable patients, and that the physician inability to do so impedes timely provision of palliative care [22]. Fortunately, PC is not limited by a physician's estimate of life expectancy or a patient's preference for curative medication. The 2008 American Thoracic Society's clinical policy statement on PC clearly states that PC is for supporting patients and families during any stage of illness whether acute, chronic, or terminal and that "all patients receiving curative or restorative health care should receive palliative care concurrently, the elements and intensity of which are individualized to meet the patient's and family's needs and preferences" [25]. Therefore, PC is appropriate at any stage in a serious illness with unmet patient needs and suffering, and can be provided together with a life-extending treatment like lung transplantation [26]. In a terminal illness like IPF and other PF-ILD, it is essential to introduce PC early and gradually increase delivery as needs progress over time. There is overwhelming evidence that delivery of PC improves outcomes in people with other serious illnesses including cancer, and specifically early PC access is better than late [26, 27]. A randomized controlled trial showed that early integration of PC for patients with advanced lung diseases including ILD improved breathlessness mastery and survival (94% vs 75%; overall survival $p = 0.048$) [28]. Unfortunately, despite such evidence, most clinicians today are not well prepared by education or experience to recognize patients' palliative care needs, the obvious care gaps, or how palliative care strategies can address their patients' suffering [29].

Many providers, including ILD specialists, have not experienced the real-world transformative power of palliative care. This can only be appreciated through first-hand observation of PC and its impact on patients, families, and providers themselves. Very few encounters in clinical medicine rival the deep and profound impact of palliative care on the shared human experience between those who provide it and those who receive it. Education and real-world experience of this palliative approach may hold the key to changing perception in both public and professional domains.

In a large Belgian physician survey, the most common reasons for not referring to specialty PC were the perception that PC needs were being met (56%) and that PC was not meaningful (26%) [30]. In another survey of Japanese pulmonologists and a UK-based qualitative study, both pulmonologists and ILD experts acknowledged the lack of competency in basic palliative approach: lack of education and training in symptom management (83%) as well as ACP communication skills (75%) [12, 31]. They perceived many barriers to PC delivery and felt less confident in PC for IPF when compared to cancer. In contrast, in a recent survey of providers in the UK that included ILD and respiratory nurses, ILD specialists, and respirologists, many indicated a high degree of provider confidence in discussing PC (97%), providing generalized PC (88%), addressing PC needs (82%), and understanding the roles of specialists PC teams in ILD management (91%) [11]. This suggests a mismatch between self-reported confidence and competence as literature shows that majority of ILD patients do not receive PC despite expressed provider confidence.

This signals the need for mandatory primary PC approach education and training to avoid inadvertent neglect stemming from misplaced confidence. This is also recommended by professional society guidelines. Other described barriers including clinicians' personalities, discomfort in discussing palliative needs, fear of depriving patients of hope, and their own beliefs and fears about mortality may lead to avoidance of PC [32]. Patient factors such as unrealistic expectations, misunderstanding of the role and scope of PC, fear of dying, giving up hope and physician abandonment, unwillingness to engage, and barriers to PC access are also reported [22, 33]. Most of these factors are a result of lack of patient understanding of PC role and related benefits. Providers, including specialists, may also lack the needed infrastructure, trained support staff, dedicated time in clinics, or appropriate remuneration. Absence of strong leadership support and community resources may further add to this complex problem. Most IPF patients, therefore, have to not only contend with a dreadful prognosis but also accept care that does not fully address what matters to them the most, relief from distressing symptoms and declining function, and need for information and support.

## Palliative Care Delivery Models for Community Dwelling ILD Patients

### *Who Is Responsible for PC Delivery?*

While there is agreement on the need for a palliative care in ILD, the ideal way to deliver PC is still unclear [22]. There are two described levels of PC: (1) primary- or generalist-level PC, provided by professionals who are not palliative care specialists, but are equipped with core palliative care competencies allowing them to activate a PC approach themselves, and (2) specialist-level palliative care, provided by clinicians and services with in-depth training and experience in PC, for whom palliative care makes up all or the majority of their work. The former model, referred to as "PC approach," is widely endorsed given the shortage of PC experts and growing volumes of non-oncology patients needing PC [34]. Many professional societies have also endorsed this approach and long regarded competency development in basic PC skills as part of training in pulmonary medicine [25].

A recent Delphi survey of US-based ILD expert centers and patient focus group analysis clearly outlined that provision of comprehensive, patient-centered care must include comprehensive support for living and coping with ILD [35]. This is a clarion call for adopting a primary PC approach by all providers including the expert centers. PC approach is fundamentally an approach to patient-centered care in ILD where all the unmet domains of care can be adequately addressed [36]. Unfortunately, there are few real-world descriptions of any PC models in ILD [37]. Some ILD centers employ a consultative model where patients are referred to specialist PC services for all PC needs without initiating a PC approach themselves. This approach, however, is untenable given the limited number of PC specialist and difficulty in identifying the appropriate time to refer in IPF/PF-ILD. Even where such supportive care clinics exist, the referral rates are low (11 patients over 2 years) and mostly delayed (MRC 4–5 at referral) [38]. This study team found that most patients struggled to attend yet another appointment due to dyspnea and frailty. There are limited descriptions of ILD centers providing integrated or primary-level PC approach [37, 39]. Unfortunately, this type of care is hampered by several factors including the lack of basic PC skills among clinicians; many physicians do not see PC delivery as their responsibility and fear using opioids in lung diseases [40]. The importance of updating or upskilling clinicians and the whole team, including physicians, nurses, allied health staff, social workers, and pharmacists, on the PC approach cannot be overstated. In Canada, for example, Pallium Canada is a nonprofit organization that provides such training for all health-care professionals. Sometimes a simple 1 or 2-day course or short online course is all that is required to make a difference. Major professional bodies have also called for basic PC training for all care providers including respirologists to address this need [25, 41].

In addition to the shortage of PC specialists, there is also a growing concern that PC experts may not have adequate expertise in non-oncology disciplines. In 2015 Canadian survey, 57% of palliative medicine physicians reported that fewer than 20% of their palliative patients had a noncancer diagnosis [42]. In 2020 UK-based survey of ILD care providers, 58% felt that specialist PC team was unlikely to add additional benefits to ILD patient management [43]. It is possible that PC specialists have limited experience with conditions like IPF/PF-ILD [30]. Even among those who have some experience, it may be limited to EOL care in hospitals and hospice with minimal to no experience in meeting care needs earlier in the trajectory [8]. Many PC subspecialty-training programs now include dedicated training in nonmalignant diseases as part of the curricula to address this gap. Expanding collaborations between ILD and PC teams may also help in mutual learning and building competence [43]. The gaps in PC expertise with IPF/ILD further highlight the need to adopt a primary-level PC approach in ILD. Disease experts, with core palliative skills, are well poised to provide a PC approach, only calling on their PC colleagues for assistance with complex cases. Some examples where specialist PC input may be especially useful in ILD include patients with refractory symptoms despite targeted therapies, existential distress, challenging family dynamics or situations that preclude effective ACP conversations, and facilitation of hospice or complex home deaths. All respirologists and primary care teams, however, must develop basic PC competency and be comfortable in initiating and titrating symptom management, and facilitating ACP in their respective practices. A recent international consensus definition of PC also highlights the need for all providers to have basic competency to provide PC and only refer complex patients to specialist PC services [44]. It is particularly important that ILD centers develop pilot programs based on local resources and model this approach as best practice. ILD centers have an educational mandate for raising awareness and improving knowledge of other care providers and can play an important role in moving the related PC field forward [22].

## ILD Clinic: Transition to Multidisciplinary Collaborative

### *How Do We Move from Disease-Centered to Patient-Centered Care?*

In 2012, our ILD clinic was reorganized with a goal to deliver patient-centered ILD care through the adoption of an early-integrated palliative approach from diagnosis to end of life with outreach extending to patient homes. The shift from disease-centered to patient-centered care requires not only a structural change but also a deliberate psychological and philosophical shift in thinking necessary to support behavior change. This transition was powered by firsthand observation of palliative approach in action and the impact on patients' HRQoL. The transformative effect of relieving symptom distress; improving communication through open and honest conversations around issues of uncertainty, dying, and death; and, most of all, adding an extra layer of practical support at home was truly striking. The approach allayed patient anxiety, sensitively addressed concerns, and helped sustain hope, meaning, and dignity in living.

An IPF qualitative literature review and local practice audit also supported this self-reflection. These led to the understanding that PF-ILD are multifaceted conditions that require attention to the patient's total being and journey in addition to addressing their medical needs. Moreover, the responsibility for delivery of such comprehensive care must fall upon all providers involved and not just on palliative care. Arriving at this practice agreement is the first step to changing practice culture. Clinicians need to prioritize PC tasks when faced with many competing activities of ILD care. A cognitive shift is required to achieve the needed practice change to integrate a PC approach. While the needed structural changes require time and health system resources, all clinicians have the freedom to individually adopt patient-centered thinking and make necessary changes at any time.

Our care redesign process is described in the New England Journal Catalyst online publication [45]. We developed an integrated PC approach for ILD with focus on symptom assessment and personalized management and proactive care through self-management education. Shared decision-making through advance care planning conversations was emphasized in clinic. Delivery of such care, guided by patient and family needs, necessitated creation of specialized multidisciplinary allied health teams in the ILD clinic and the community. Team composition and member roles are described in the following section. The teams worked collaboratively to identify and address patient needs from diagnosis to transplantation or death across care settings [46]. Multidisciplinary collaborative practice is necessary in our opinion to meet patients' escalating needs that demand appropriate and timely care, education, and support from different disciplines [15, 47]. Hence, our model design is multidisciplinary and collaborative (Fig. 16.1). The integration of palliative approach over referral to specialist PC was purposefully chosen to avoid adding another layer of specialized care for ILD/IPF patients. This approach is more patient-centric in our opinion as it preserves continuity of care, helps maintain

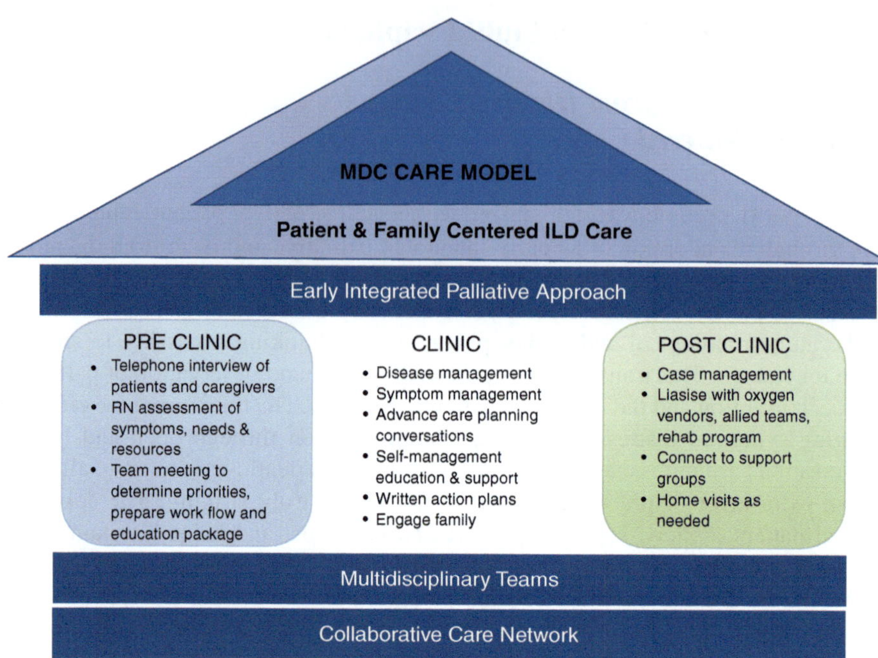


**Fig. 16.1** Multidisciplinary collaborative care model. Legend: *MDC* multidisciplinary collaborative care, *ILD* interstitial lung disease, *RN* nurse

existing therapeutic relationships, and retains expertise of the ILD clinicians. We do engage PC specialists when transferring patients to hospice.

In order to execute our goal, we received an operational grant to hire a dedicated ILD nurse (RN), engaged part-time allied clinic staff, and identified the community team from within existing provincial home care teams in the patients' vicinity. Composition of community teams was based on patient needs (Fig. 16.2). We dedicated time in clinic to implement PC protocols as part of a quality improvement approach. Training was provided to the team members through workshops and applied training experiences in clinic and during joint home visits. The teams were trained in symptom management protocols created by us. We also created patient and caregiver education material that was shared with the extended teams. An ACP conversation guide was developed and shared. Ongoing post implementation audits inform changes to practice. There was no formal memorandum of understanding between clinic and community teams, and the network continues to develop organically, shaped by patient needs and care provider desire to deliver patient-centered care.

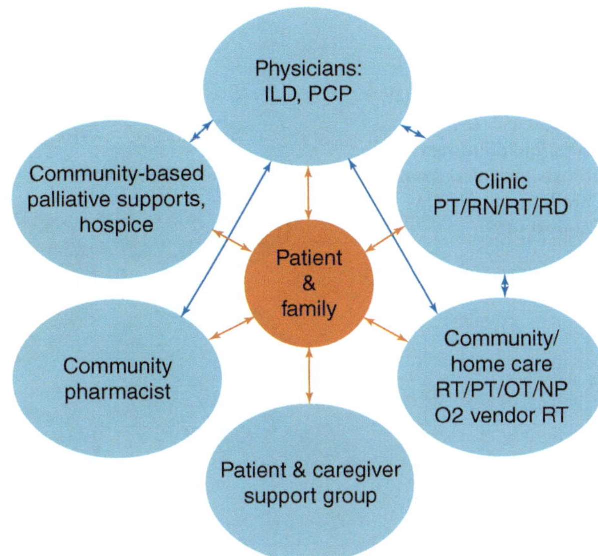


**Fig. 16.2** ILD clinic and community-based teams. Legend: *ILD* interstitial Lung disease, *PCP* primary care physician, *PT* physiotherapist, *RN* nurse, *RT* respiratory therapist, *RD* registered dietitian, *OT* occupational therapist, *O2* oxygen. Reproduced from IPF Care Redesign NEJM Catalyst [45]

## What Are the Components of a Palliative Care Approach in ILD?

A PC approach starts by (1) identifying patients with unmet needs who could benefit from this approach, (2) followed by systematic needs identification and assessment, (3) personalized care plan development, (4) self-management education delivery, and (5) ACP and providing access to various supports (Fig. 16.3). We provide anticipatory guidance to patients, their families, and involved allied care teams to prepare everyone for future events/crises. These PC components are based on identified patient needs [13, 22, 48].

### *Identifying Patients Who Will Benefit from a Palliative Approach*

There are few ILD-specific screening questionnaires such as NAT-ILD to help identify palliative needs and trigger specialist PC referrals [49]. We use a locally developed needs-based tool to trigger integrated palliative approach that is implemented at first visit. The tool screens for needs related to symptoms, function, psychosocial needs, and support. The use of a decision aid in another ILD clinic also led to greater integration of PC approach, triggered timely referral to PC, and related support services [50]. Implementation of decision aids in clinics can change practice by improving recognition of patient needs, documentation of decisions and discussions

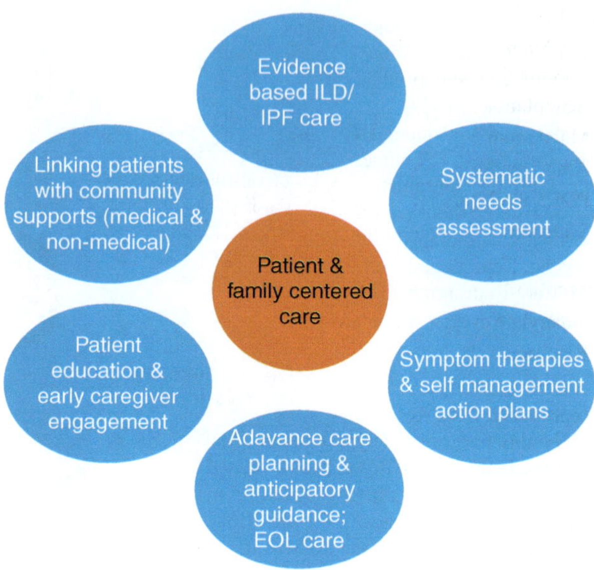


**Fig. 16.3** Integrated palliative approach to ILD – care components. Legend: *ILD* interstitial lung disease, *IPF* idiopathic pulmonary fibrosis. Adapted from IPF Care Redesign NEJM Catalyst [45]

related to PC and EOL management, and patients' preferences. This is a necessary step to implement a PC approach in ILD.

## *Systematic Needs Identification and Assessment*

Patients with identified needs undergo systematic assessment of symptoms and resources. We use the locally developed needs-based assessment tool discussed previously; this also includes the multidimensional dyspnea scale (MDDS, adapted pilot tool, not validated) and a numeric rating scale for cough and fatigue [51, 52]. The dyspnea scale serves to differentiate resting, incident/anticipated/exertional, and crisis dyspnea and understand the triggers. Understanding dyspnea intensity, context, and triggers forms the basis of a personalized treatment plan. Many validated dyspnea scales exist, but none has led to improvement in clinical practice and management. MDDS embedded within our palliative approach led to early recognition and treatment of dyspnea in a preliminary analysis [53, 54]. We also use it for patient self-management education. Our tool also elicits patient and caregiver concerns and goals. This information can help guide ACP conversations. The ILD RN collects the data during preclinic telephone assessment and documents in the electronic medical record. All team members review this data to develop respective care plans and determine workflow in preclinic meetings. This helps improve efficiency in clinics.

Edmonton symptom assessment scale, a widely used symptom assessment battery, can also be considered for use in ILD [55]. There is a need for standardized, validated needs assessment instruments and patient-reported outcome measures for

PC in ILD. Pilot instruments can be developed and implemented within a quality improvement methodology based on local needs.

## *Personalized Symptom Management*

Dyspnea, cough, fatigue, and pain are common physical symptoms in ILD [56]. IPF and fibrotic ILD patients also describe psychosocial concerns such as depression, anxiety, social isolation, anger, frustrations, and hopelessness [21, 57]. Practical guidelines for symptom management in IPF/ILD are not available. Thus, we developed strategies that are personalized for and by patients.

### Dyspnea

Dyspnea is the most pervasive and distressing symptom that leads to a poor HRQoL in IPF and is also an independent predictor of mortality [3]. IPF patients afflicted by dyspnea often describe the shrinking world syndrome and frustrations of being "tethered" to oxygen that limits activities and their life [58]. Despite its pervasiveness, dyspnea remains invisible and is frequently underdiagnosed and undertreated from diagnosis to death as most care providers lack necessary competency in basic PC [17, 59]. Our approach to dyspnea management is similar to other described breathlessness services [45, 52, 60]. It includes the following elements: (1) a structured interview approach that includes input from family and the use of MDDS to assess dyspnea in the context of patients' daily life, needs, and goals; (2) an interdisciplinary team for dyspnea assessment, care, and monitoring; (3) stepwise approach to development of personalized care and action plans to achieve patient goals; (4) collaboration among formal and informal caregivers, in clinic and the community for continuity of care and meeting needs in real time throughout the disease trajectory; and (5) ongoing patient education and support both in clinic and outside.

We use data from ILD RN preclinic interview that includes patient's MDDS intensity scores to guide initiation of non-pharmacologic interventions, oxygen, and medications in an iterative fashion (Fig. 16.4). The use of individual dyspnea scores and the knowledge of triggers allows the team to develop personalized plans. Therapies are titrated to decrease dyspnea intensity as measured by the scale and/or improve function while decreasing associated unpleasantness or distress. We review non-pharmacologic interventions like pacing and energy conservation with all patients with dyspnea. Dyspnea profoundly affects daily life leading to frustrations; hence, IPF patients seek personalized practical advice on how to improve function and how to perform daily activities like showering, dressing, walking, using stairs with less distress, and engaging safely in exercise and outdoor recreational activities while on oxygen. As disease advances and oxygen needs increase, patients need advice on walking aids with necessary modifications to carry extra tanks that

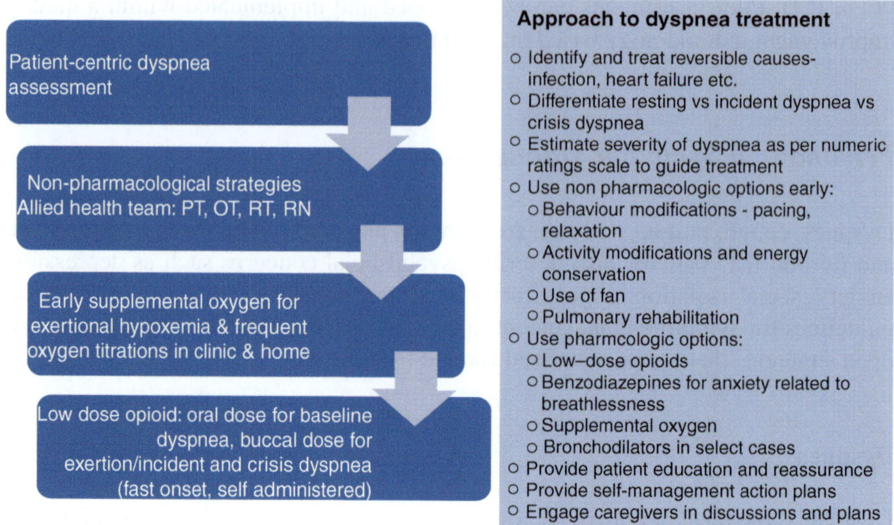


**Fig. 16.4** Multidisciplinary collaborative approach to dyspnea management. Legend: *MDC* multidisiplinary collaborative, *PT* physiotherapist, *OT* occupational therapist, *RT* respiratory therapist, *RN* nurse

facilitate ambulation. Home environment modifications are needed as part of dyspnea management. This requires the services of home occupational therapists (OT) and physiotherapists (PT) and cannot be provided in clinics alone. The ILD RN provides information and education at the outset, and home care allied staff further supplement this during home visits to reinforce strategies. Hence, engaging homecare teams is necessary for effective and ongoing dyspnea management. We also refer patients to pulmonary rehabilitation programs for symptom education and support.

Supplemental oxygen for exertional hypoxemia is another important and underutilized strategy in ILD. There are no guidelines on the use of oxygen for isolated exertional hypoxemia in ILD [61]. A short-term randomized, open-label crossover study of supplemental oxygen in fibrotic ILD suggested benefit including improvement in HRQoL and reduction of symptoms (dyspnea) with the use of oxygen [62]. Our practice is to routinely assess for exertional hypoxemia (nadir Spo2 < 90% on walk tests) at clinic visits. We aim to start supplemental oxygen early, but local payment criteria based on COPD does not support early use despite patient willingness to use oxygen in many cases. Once initiated, we ensure timely flow titrations to meet needs, at rest and exertion, and provide ongoing education and self-management support. In addition to clinic support, we engage respiratory therapists (RT) in the community to assess oxygen needs and flow titrations at home, reinforce education, address equipment problems, and advocate for patients as needed. Frequent titrations are necessary to meet needs, as with any other medication, if the right dose is not used, the therapy is unlikely to have the intended effect. This can lead to the perception of ineffectiveness among both patients and providers.

Collaborative care with community teams including oxygen vendor companies is essential to support patient adherence and sustained benefit. We developed oxygen education material and provide self-management education, which involves teaching patients how to use a pulse oximeter, monitor oxygen flow needs, and call for advice if frequent desaturations and worsening symptoms are noted. Similar to published trials, we have noted reductions of symptoms, increased endurance, and other effects not previously described such as improvements in cough, fatigue, sleep, pain, mood, and general well-being. We have jointly developed processes with the oxygen vendor companies to enable patients on high flow oxygen (up to 25 to 30 liters per minute) to live at home and remain independent until death [63, 64]. Besides limited evidence, there are several challenges to be overcome with oxygen therapy including restrictive oxygen payment policies, patient perceived embarrassment and reluctance to use cumbersome therapy, equipment problems (including lack of portability), and personal belief that oxygen is addictive and not useful [61, 65].

We optimize non-pharmacologic strategies and oxygen titrations iteratively, but as dyspnea intensity worsens over time despite these measures, we add low-dose opioids. Opioids are the mainstay pharmacologic therapies for refractory dyspnea in addition to strategies as described above. They can safely decrease dyspnea without respiratory depression [66]. The key to oral opioid use is to start with low doses and slowly titrate up while managing side effects like constipation. Oral morphine is widely used and has good evidence for dyspnea relief (10–30 mg daily sustained release) [66]. The clinical evidence base for other non-oral routes, particularly for episodic dyspnea management, is growing [66]. Non-oral routes like buccal or nasal have a rapid onset of action and, therefore, can be useful in management of episodic and crisis dyspnea. We use liquid hydromorphone in a combination of oral and buccal routes to treat different "types" of dyspnea (resting, exertional, or crisis), as the buccal route is conducive to rapid self-management in the community settings. We use off label hydromorphone formulations; even though effectiveness data is limited, our experience suggests benefit. We assess each patient's dyspnea profile as baseline (rest, continuous), anticipated dyspnea (exertional, episodic), and crisis dyspnea at every visit. We prescribe oral opioid to treat baseline dyspnea that requires a steady-state opioid level. Buccal route is used to achieve a rapid onset of action for anticipated dyspnea (exertional dyspnea), as well as for crisis dyspnea episodes. We have described this approach to opioid initiation, titration to treat dyspnea, and cough through disease progression to end of life [52, 63, 64]. We do not use oral long-acting opioids although there is good evidence for this approach [66]. It is important to address underlying mood issues as they may blunt response to opioids. Written action plans for crisis dyspnea provide directions for opioid use, oxygen and relaxation, and instructions for patients and caregivers as well.

**Other Symptoms**

*Cough* is another common and distressing symptom in fibrotic ILD without effective therapies [56]. We assess for other cough etiologies (GERD, upper airway cough syndrome, etc.) and treat as needed. Additional therapies initiated include early oxygen to treat exertional hypoxemia when possible, opioids, and gabapentin to decrease cough sensitivity. Patients also report benefit from the use of over-the-counter cough suppressants and cough drops [67]. For productive cough, we sometimes employ airway clearance techniques like huff coughing and breathing techniques and use the oscillating positive expiratory pressure device like Aerobika® (off label) although controlled studies are lacking. We do not use corticosteroids for IPF-related cough.

*Fatigue* and deconditioning are commonly reported symptoms in IPF, and evidence-based therapies are needed [56]. We screen for and treat comorbidities like sleep apnea and contributing factors like dyspnea, cough, and exertional hypoxemia. Patient education for setting realistic expectations, pacing and energy conservation, and referral to pulmonary rehabilitation programs are beneficial strategies for many patients.

*Depression and anxiety* are common comorbidities in IPF that can have a reciprocal relationship with dyspnea, cough, and social isolation [56]. The key to management is early recognition and intervention. We screen for depression using the previously described assessment tool. We treat associated conditions (sleep apnea, hypothyroidism) and address informational and educational needs. The latter helps to relieve confusion, fear, and uncertainty that can worsen mental health. We also address poor symptom control and social isolation to the extent possible as these can also affect mental health. We refer patients to support groups and rehabilitation programs and consult psychiatrists for complex cases. Pharmacologic therapies are prescribed in partnership with primary care.

## *Self-Management Education*

Self-management education is an important strategy in any chronic disease and is also necessary for patient empowerment in PF-ILD [6, 68]. IPF patients and caregivers lack symptom self-management efficacy. They often express confusion, hopelessness, helplessness, and fear stemming from uncertainty and not knowing what to do and who to call for help [12, 21]. Therefore, self-management education is integral to an effective palliative approach in IPF and other PF-ILD. It can facilitate patient self-efficacy in managing their disease and treatments. Self-management action plans can help patients cope with antifibrotic adverse effects and promote adherence, exercise plans can educate them on effective oxygen use and safely increase physical activity which is an independent predictor of mortality, and nutrition education can help with reflux management and maintaining ideal body weight. Anticipatory guidance can also be provided through such education to help prepare patients and families for managing crisis at home. Symptom crises drive hospitalizations and cost in IPF and overwhelm patients and their families [69]. Other examples of action plan are provided (Box 16.1). An example of crisis dyspnea action plan is also provided (Box 16.1.1). A proactive approach to care is required to anticipate such events, develop contingency plans, connect patients to needed supports, and thereby mitigate risks, adverse events, and costs.

**Box 16.1 ILD action plans**

Action plans for

- Symptoms
  - Dyspnea: baseline, incident (anticipated), crisis (unanticipated)
  - Cough
  - Anxiety/panic
  - Sinus congestion
  - Constipation
- Worsening lung disease
- Chest infection
- Heart failure

**Box 16.1.1 MDC ILD clinic crisis dyspnea action plan**

1. Stop what you're doing and call for help.
2. Find your recovery position (sit and lean forward or rest standing with back against the wall).
3. Use your breathing technique to calm yourself down. (Breathe in for a few counts, breathe out for a few counts, or breathe around the rectangle: focus on a door/window in the room and breathe as you trace the edges.)
4. Use a fan for relief. (Use either a hand-held, free standing, or desk top fan or open windows/doors.)
5. Increase your oxygen flow if levels are low.
6. If breathlessness persists (>5 min), take (insert) ml of hydromorphone syrup in the cheek.
7. Wait for 10 min.
8. If breathlessness persists, take (insert) mg of hydromorphone syrup in your cheek.
9. Wait for 10 min.
10. If breathlessness persists, take (insert) mg of hydromorphone syrup in your cheek, and take (insert) mg lorazepam under your tongue.
11. Other advice (personalize).
12. Call your clinic or home care contact if breathlessness has not resolved (insert contact #).
13. When crisis has resolved, reflect on what triggered the episode and how to avoid it. Discuss incident with your providers at the next opportunity.

Development of self-management action plan starts with understanding patients' daily life, limitations, crises, and their triggers as well as patient and clinician goals. We use patient responses to questionnaires and patient narratives to inform this process. We anticipate escalation of symptoms, dyspnea crisis, oxygen flow needs, and death. Significantly, we openly discuss these potential events with patients and their families. We develop action plans for such contingencies and provide education to patients and families, so they know what to expect and what to do in such situations. These action plans provide systematic instructions including what to do and who to call for help in a crisis. These personalized action plans are developed collaboratively in clinic. Caregivers also need self-management education, as patients may not be able to enact the action plan in crisis and increasingly depend on family support. The ILD RN provides this type of education and training during the clinic visit. Face to face, sensitive, honest, and empathic communication is an important strategy to support patients with dyspnea [70]. In a recent audit, we noted that 83% of our patients received some form of self-management education at first visit in our model [53]. A recently published qualitative study supports this approach to self-management; our patients were able to adopt these practical strategies, internalize and personalize them, and change behaviors. They reported 80% confidence in symptom self-management [71]. Self-management education is also provided through a variety of other formats (virtual, and both written and verbal) and in different venues, including group sessions through the clinic, ILD pulmonary rehabilitation, and at home [1, 64]. The other area of need is EOL self-management and related caregiver education [16]. We anticipate EOL symptom needs and prescribe needed crises medications in advance (hydromorphone, lorazepam, methotrimeprazine, olanzapine) and written instructions on their use and what to do when home death occurs [63]. Action plans are also shared with community allied teams and primary care, so they are prepared to help patients at home as and when needed.

## *Advance Care Planning: More than Do Not Resuscitate (DNR) Orders*

IPF patients perceive large communications gaps at all stages of disease starting from diagnosis, throughout follow-up and at end of life. Patients often do not receive needed education and information to understand their disease and care options; they desire information on prognosis, how to live well and prepare for decline, EOL planning, management of psychosocial needs, and access to other supports [13]. Caregivers also express dissatisfaction with the lack of information and are unprepared for what is coming their way. IPF patients and families need personalized, timely, and appropriate information at all stages including open and honest discussions on difficult topics like EOL. All these gaps can be addressed by adopting good communication practices that include ACP conversations. ACP is a patient-centered process designed to facilitate patient understanding, reflection, sharing, and documentation of their wishes and preferences for care including at EOL [72]. It provides direction to the health-care teams to ensure delivery of care aligned to patient values. While desired by many, ACP is often not implemented in ambulatory clinics [17, 59]. In the absence of ACP, EOL care remains poor with uncontrolled symptoms, with high rates of hospitalizations and hospital deaths despite patient preference for home deaths [8]. Lack of structured communication not only results in poor patient care but also increases caregiver distress and burden. If EOL planning is not undertaken, patients' goals of care (GoC) and their preferences for care and death are not known. Substitute decision-makers, who know patient values and wishes and can make decision on their behalf, often cannot be identified in a timely manner [16].

We, therefore, prioritize early and ongoing ACP in our care model (Fig. 16.5). We engage both patients and family members in these conversations. Iterative discussions are preferable and necessary as disease progresses. ACP is not just EOL planning but also a comprehensive discussion about patient values, wishes, and their preferences for care in general. We identify patient goals, discuss facilitating strategies to achieve these goals, and improve HRQoL in addition to talking about the future EOL needs. This addresses unmet informational needs and also sustains hope [73]. It is important to address patient fears and concerns particularly around the dying process. Many have stated that they do not fear death but suffocation. Hence, we specifically discuss how effective self-management action plans can address suffocation; this allays their fears. This is further complemented by GoC discussions to identify specific treatment choices informed by patient values. GoC may change as the disease progresses. In particular, the decision to continue antifibrotics at EOL should be addressed as it may further worsen HRQoL due to known

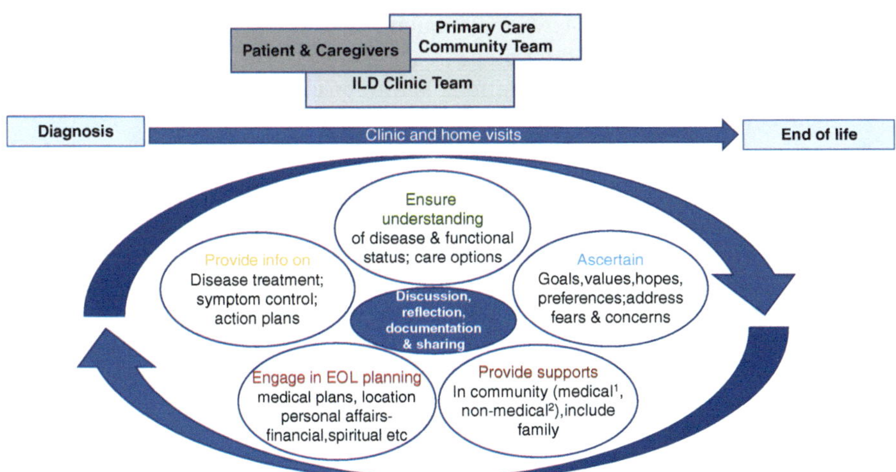


**Fig. 16.5** Advance care planning – MDC approach. Legend: *EOL* end of life;[1] *medical* remote monitoring, allied health support, psychologists, home care services, physician home visits;[2] nonmedical – patient support groups, caregiver respite services, spiritual support

adverse effects in some cases. This risk-benefit analysis must be done on an individual basis. We proactively plan for EOL medical care and provide anticipatory guidance to patients and their families as discussed above [63, 64]. Anticipating symptom worsening and functional decline, and openly discussing these issues facilitates care planning, avoids "unexpected deaths," and meets psychological and emotional EOL needs. We document patient preferences for location for death, specific choices like ICU care and life support, and withdrawal of care as informed by ACP discussions. We include primary care teams in the circle of care from the beginning and encourage them to assist with ACP conversations throughout the course.

Clinicians often avoid ACP in IPF due to its unpredictable course and difficulty in identifying EOL. Inability to predict timelines does not preclude these necessary conversations; using an ACP framework (Fig. 16.5) has allowed us to increase documentation rates in our clinic. The absence of a proactive approach and ACP leads to "unexpected deaths" in IPF/ILD. This is very distressing to the patients' families. Good EOL care must start early. Some practical ACP tips are provided in Box 16.2. A checklist developed by our clinic is provided (Box 16.2.1).

**Box 16.2 Advance care planning tips**

1. Prioritize time for conversations during clinics.
2. Develop competency in ACP communication skills for physicians and nurses through dedicated training.
3. Create an ACP documentation template to ensure consistent quality and delivery if institutional template is not available.
4. Assess patient readiness: Initial reluctance can be overcome through thoughtful conversations to explore reasons for reluctance, addressing fears and explaining the pros and cons of ACP.
5. Allow silence and explore and acknowledge emotions including fear and anxiety and uncertainty.
6. Engage family members, and address their fears and questions.
7. Provide written information or direct patients to online resources [84].
8. Recognize that ACP is an ongoing, dynamic conversation that happens

**Box 16.2.1 Serious illness conversation and ACP checklist for care providers**

1. *Provider documentation (to be completed in EMR)*

   I. Goals of care medical orders
   II. Preferred place of care and death
   III. Medical proxy or power of attorney

2. *Provider ACP discussion contents (personalize to patient and family needs)*

I. *Provide* information and discuss and review the following:

- Current medical status
- Goals of care designations and medical orders
- What decline looks like
- What death looks like

II. *Discuss* symptom management with advanced stage lung disease

- Develop and share action plans with patients/family/community teams
  - For example, symptoms action plan: dyspnea, baseline, incident (anticipated), crisis (unanticipated), cough, and anxiety/panic provide education and training

III. *Discuss Options* for care at the end of life

- Locations: Home, hospice, ER/acute care; others: patient medical home/Treat in Place EMS program
- Engage Informal Caregivers and discuss their role in care
- Review implications of location on symptom management
- Review home care supports and respite services for caregivers
- Care options at EOL: symptom management/discontinuation of meds/withdrawal of therapies/forgoing antibiotics, bloodwork and investigations and implications

IV. *Address fears* about dying process

V. *Encourage reflection* on unfinished business/unspoken words

VI. *Discuss End of life planning*

- Will; state of affairs (including finances)
- Funeral type/place; Funeral home; Ceremony/memorial
- List of family/friends to notify
- List of things to be done after (eg. Banking, Life insurance etc)
- For planned home deaths review what to do once death occurs

VII. *Review and discuss spiritual care support needs*

VIII. *Review family supports for coping with loss*

Creation of ILD Collaborative Teams: Defining Responsibility, Workflow, and Communication to Enhance Teamwork

Patient-centered care delivery in ILD/IPF requires interprofessional teams, because diverse patient and family needs cannot be addressed by a physician-nurse dyad alone. Our adaptive network consists of clinic and community teams and nonmedical supports (Fig. 16.2). The ILD clinic team includes physicians with expertise in ILD and palliative approach, RN, and a registered dietitian (RD). Individualized community teams emerge from patient needs and available resources. Nurse practitioners (NP), RN, PT, OT, RT, and social workers are recruited as applicable. Private partners, like the oxygen vendor company RTs, are essential members of the community network. Member roles and responsibilities are outlined in Fig. 16.6. We have described how an interprofessional team with the right mix of experts can help meet patient needs and provide personalized strategies and education [63, 64, 74, 75].

The ILD nurse, a key player in this network, facilitates care coordination and communication between patients, families, and teams. The ILD RN also helps determine clinic workflow for members of the team to facilitate efficiency. A specialist nurse can assist with medications, side effect management, and facilitation of referrals to services and provide education and navigation advice. Patients overwhelmingly support this type of service [76]. The ILD nurse provides self-management education including advice on titration of oxygen and opioids under physician supervision. The ILD RN uses a case management approach to problem solve, update action plans, and communicate with patients and the community teams between clinic visits. As care needs escalate and EOL approaches, rapid and seamless communication between patients and all care teams is ensured by ILD RN. This is done through in-person or virtual clinic meetings and telephone communication with community partners. This is a key aspect of our palliative approach and necessary to achieve patient-centered goals.

Allied expertise is essential for effective symptom management; the roles of RT, PT, OT, and RD are listed in Fig. 16.6 and previously discussed [75]. Their presence in clinic and within home care teams is essential to meet needs in this population.

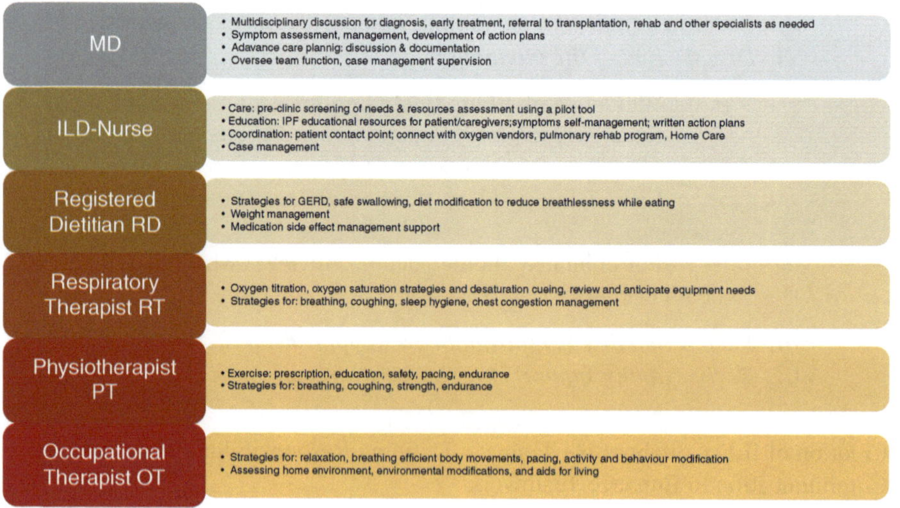


**Fig. 16.6** Team member roles and responsibility. Legend: *ILD* interstitial lung disease

We also work closely with the primary care doctors and community pharmacists. We communicate via phone calls to avoid delays and discuss anticipated decline so that primary care can arrange home visits where possible and assist in ACP; pharmacists help ensure home delivery of crisis meds and provide education, as necessary. Community-based pulmonary rehabilitation program are important partners, and we rely on them to provide additional tailored education in many cases. Home palliative care is engaged to support patients and families when preferred. Nonmedical supports such as respite services, support groups, and spiritual guidance also play an important role.

## Collaborative Practice Among Clinic and Community Teams

The increasingly complex nature of ILD care and escalating patient needs between clinic appointments necessitate a case management approach that relies on community resources. Patients themselves desire more supports in their local communities [77]. We refer patients to home care services and leverage the expertise of the allied community health professionals to extend the reach of the clinic's palliative approach. As previously described, we provided training to these team members at the outset of our program. We also work with family physicians who do home visits to support patients at home. This collaborative practice allows us to meet patient needs in real time, outside clinic and across the disease continuum as much as possible [63, 64]. We have described this approach in case studies [64]. Frequently, patients will call our clinic with worsening symptoms, and after appropriate triaging, the ILD RN can trigger the community team to assess and co-manage patients at home with ILD physician guidance. Figure 16.7 demonstrates how our collaborative approach with community teams results in safe de-escalation of crisis and avoids emergency use. Crisis dyspnea episodes often trigger acute care use in IPF, and a collaborative approach using community teams is recommended to manage such episodes [69, 78]. A proactive approach in clinic is needed to create action plans and provide self-management education, this helps in preparing patients and family, and ongoing communication between clinic and community allied teams (via phone calls) prepares the community teams to act whenever needed. Thus, when a crisis occurs, all stakeholders are prepared to respond rapidly and collaboratively with physician oversight, in many cases avoiding unnecessary hospitalizations and clinic visits. This is particularly important at EOL, where timely support is critical. Rapid symptom management, ensuring equipment support (oxygen and other aids), coordination of services, and hospice referrals are critical needs for ILD home palliation addressed through this collaborative approach. The ILD nurse, with physician oversight, directs, coordinates, supports, and sustains this collaboration.

We have shown that collaborative home care with family caregiver engagement are important aspects of palliative approach in ILD and are deterministic for patient location of death [74]. Our model of interprofessional collaboration has helped develop PC competency with respect to IPF/PF-ILD within home care teams

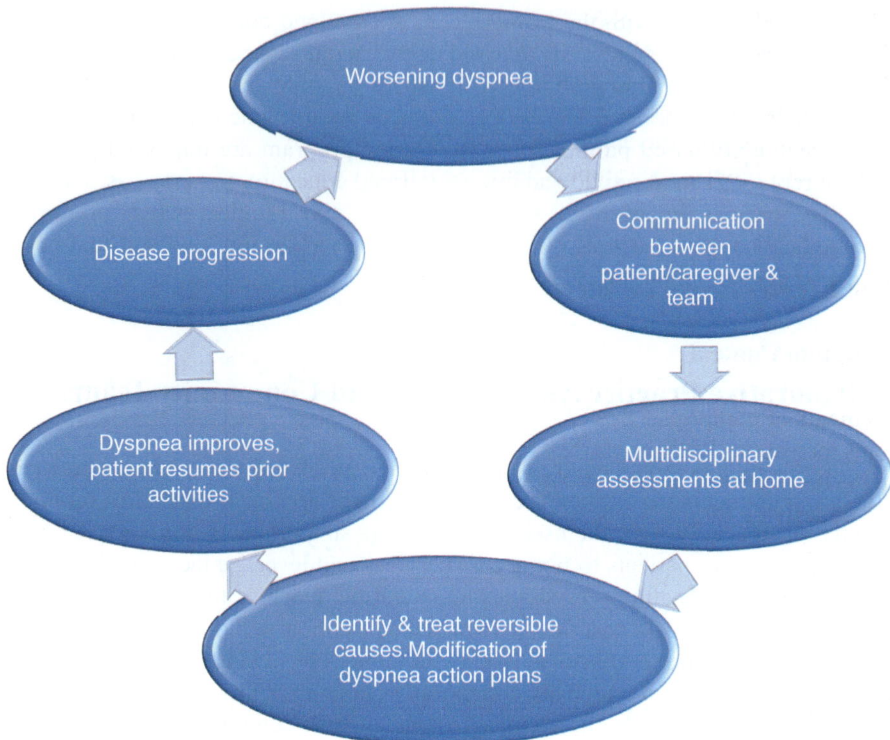


**Fig. 16.7** Collaboration with community teams – addressing symptom crisis outside clinic visits. Legend: Collaborative care – this approach facilitates home assessments and management, helps maintain HRQol, avoids needless acute care use, and increases days spent at home – a patient-centered goal

(including remote communities) as demonstrated by homecare NPs who now manage complex EOL patients at home [63, 64]. This has allowed us to task shift this aspect of care to the community safely and effectively. Training and developing competency are an ongoing process as we extend our reach into new communities.

## Palliative Care and Lung Transplantation

Integrated palliative approach can be applied with life-extending therapies including transplantation in IPF/PF-ILD patients [79]. In our cohort, 28 (7%) patients have undergone transplantation to date, 27 (96%) of them received integrated PC, and 7 (25%) were on opioids at the time of transplantation for dyspnea management. Effective symptom self-management support including using oral buccal opioids and high flow supplemental oxygen allowed these patients to remain at home until transplantation (unpublished data). Similar outcomes have been reported in an ILD transplant cohort at the University of Toronto [80].

## What Is the Impact of Our Integrated Palliative Approach in ILD?

Preliminary model audits show improvements in care, increased rates of symptom therapies, increase in ACP documentation, and better EOL care that is concordant with patient preferences [74, 81]. Ninety percent of patients' preferences for location of death were met with 62% hospice/home deaths in our model. Our symptom management approach utilizing MDDS results in early identification and appropriate dyspnea treatments when compared to other published studies [53]. Our novel dyspnea self-management action plans using buccal opioids are acceptable to patients, increase symptom control, facilitate self-management, and decrease acute care use [54, 81]. In contrast to published studies describing poor symptom control at EOL in ILD, our caregivers report effective patient symptom self-management [1]. Another recent qualitative study suggests positive impact of our self-management education and improved symptom self-efficacy that supports engaged coping [71]. The ILD RN-led case management and collaborative home care as part of a palliative approach led to improved care outcomes like reduction of hospitalization rates and hospital deaths with an economic analysis confirming cost savings when compared to traditional care models [54]. Qualitative studies show that patients and caregivers perceive improved quality of life and death, better communication and experience care satisfaction [1]. Bereaved caregivers reported good quality of death and dying, less anxiety and distress with EOL preparation, and enhanced support through homecare services and collaborative care as facilitators [1]. These preliminary analyses make a compelling clinical, economic, and humanitarian argument for supporting integrated PC models for ILD and the need for further work in this direction. The Canadian Foundation for Healthcare Improvement recognized our approach as an emerging innovation in palliative and end-of-life care delivery. The model also received a clinical innovation award from the Department of Medicine, University of Alberta, in 2019.

## Challenges and Future Direction for Our Program

Our care model continues to face challenges despite early data suggesting benefit to patients and caregivers, and improvement in care, and cost savings at end of life. ILD is less known than other chronic diseases or cancers and requires administrative and leadership support, which in turn influences access to resources, wider systemic organizational support, and policy. Awareness and commitment to this population hold implications for operational funding for program survival, ongoing quality improvement, and research. Our collaborative faces the constant threat of staff turnover through loss of financial support. This is a huge challenge as training staff and building experience takes time and is crucial to excellent care delivery and sustaining a good team culture.

While numerous challenges and barriers to consistent implementation of PC exist at micro-, meso-, and macro-levels, the one desire that unites us at all such levels is the need to improve patient well-being, relieve their distress, and provide excellent quality care that is equitable and accessible to all. The 2020 World Hospice Day slogan of "My care, My right" is a powerful endorsement of this shared vision. PC can no longer be ignored and considered optional. Care teams looking after patients with terminal diseases must develop competency and resources to provide basic PC to all patients who need it. Some recommendations are provided in Box 16.3 for teams desiring to adopt an integrated approach to PC in ILD clinics. There is early evidence to suggest that PC in ILD can improve care, patient and caregiver satisfaction, perceived quality of life, and death and reduce costs. Studies in oncology and ILD further suggest survival benefit from integrating PC [28, 82]. In addition, interprofessional patient-centered collaborative practice can also improve job satisfaction, relieve burden and burn out in the health professionals [83]. In a stressful health-care environment, palliative approach, by enabling deeper, more meaningful relationships with patients across the care continuum, can nourish not only the patients but also the care providers. Correct understanding of PC and its deeply human impact are needed to rectify misperceptions and address the prevailing culture of neglect. A cognitive shift that enables health-care providers to treat the whole person and not just the disease will propel us in the right direction.

**Box 16.3 Recommendations for implementing PC in outpatient ILD care**

1. Prioritize palliative approach in care. Palliative care is everybody's business so care teams must dedicate time and resources for implementation, education and training.
2. Providers who want to implement PC may wish to identify and partner with teams that have a proven track record in palliative care delivery specific to ILD.
3. Identify and partner with local palliative specialists to build expertise and capacity
4. Create interdisciplinary teams: a dedicated ILD nurse (case management, outreach and support) and allied staff with palliative care competency.
5. Establish protocols for treatments, documentation, patient education, and collaborative care.
6. Invite caregivers to attend appointments with patients and engage them in shared decision-making.
7. Explicitly identify patient goals and concerns at clinics visits.
8. Actively assess symptoms & needs in clinic- create personalized action plans & provide self-management education.
9. Invite and engage in advance care planning conversations: use open-ended questions to ask about goals/fears/concerns. Discuss care preferences including end of life preferences. Discuss concerns around death and dying openly, honestly, and sensitively.
10. Connect patients to community resources: Allied health, home care, palliative care services and hospice, patient support groups, rehab programs, and respite services
11. Garner institutional and administrative leadership support.

**Acknowledgment** I thank Dr. Janice Richman-Eisenstat for sharing protocols and her unwavering support, wisdom, and inspiration; the ILD clinic staff and Alberta Health Services Continuing care services (community teams – home care, rehab, and palliative care) for their exceptional service, and all ILD patients and their families, who, through their feedback, generosity, and efforts, allow us to learn and improve the program to better serve their needs.

## References

1. Pooler C, Richman-Eisenstat J, Kalluri M. Early integrated palliative approach for idiopathic pulmonary fibrosis: a narrative study of bereaved caregivers' experiences. Palliat Med. 2018;32:1455–64.
2. Cottin V, Hirani NA, Hotchkin DL, et al. Presentation, diagnosis and clinical course of the spectrum of progressive-fibrosing interstitial lung diseases. Eur Respir Rev. 2018; https://doi.org/10.1183/16000617.0076-2018.
3. Lederer DJ, Martinez FJ. Idiopathic pulmonary fibrosis. N Engl J Med. 2018;378:1811–23.
4. Martinez FJ, Collard HR, Pardo A, Raghu G, Richeldi L, Selman M, Swigris JJ, Taniguchi H, Wells AU. Idiopathic pulmonary fibrosis. Nat Rev Dis Prim. 2017;3:1–19.
5. Swigris JJ, Gould MK, Wilson SR. Health-related quality of life among patients with idiopathic pulmonary fibrosis. Chest. 2005;127:284–94.
6. Van Manen MJG, Geelhoed JJM, Tak NC, Wijsenbeek MS. Optimizing quality of life in patients with idiopathic pulmonary fibrosis. Ther Adv Respir Dis. 2017;11:157–69.
7. Collard HR, Chen SY, Yeh WS, Li Q, Lee YC, Wang A, Raghu G. Health care utilization and costs of idiopathic pulmonary fibrosis in U.S. Medicare beneficiaries aged 65 years and older. Ann Am Thorac Soc. 2015;12:981–7.
8. Lindell KO, Liang Z, Hoffman LA, Rosenzweig MQ, Saul MI, Pilewski JM, Gibson KF, Kaminski N. Palliative care and location of death in decedents with idiopathic pulmonary fibrosis. Chest. 2015;147:423–9.
9. Raghu G, Collard HR, Egan JJ, Martinez FJ, Behr J, Brown KK. An official ATS/ERS/JRS/ALAT statement: idiopathic pulmonary fibrosis: evidence-based guidelines for diagnosis and management. Am J Respir Crit Care Med. 2011;183:788–824.
10. WHO. WHO definition of palliative Care. https://www.who.int/cancer/palliative/definition/en/. Accessed 28 Oct 2020.
11. Sampson C, Gill BH, Harrison NK, Nelson A, Byrne A. The care needs of patients with idiopathic pulmonary fibrosis and their carers (CaNoPy): results of a qualitative study. BMC Pulm Med. 2015;15:155.
12. Bajwah S, Higginson IJ, Ross JR, Wells AU, Birring SS, Riley J, Koffman J. The palliative care needs for fibrotic interstitial lung disease: a qualitative study of patients, informal caregivers and health professionals. Palliat Med. 2013;27:869–76.
13. Lee JYT, Tikellis G, Corte TJ, et al. The supportive care needs of people living with pulmonary fibrosis and their caregivers: a systematic review. Eur Respir Rev. 2020; https://doi.org/10.1183/16000617.0125-2019.
14. Kreuter M, Swigris J, Pittrow D, et al. The clinical course of idiopathic pulmonary fibrosis and its association to quality of life over time: longitudinal data from the INSIGHTS-IPF registry. Respir Res. 2019; https://doi.org/10.1186/s12931-019-1020-3.
15. Masefield S, Cassidy N, Ross D, Powell P, Wells A. Communication difficulties reported by patients diagnosed with idiopathic pulmonary fibrosis and their carers: a European focus group study. ERJ Open Res. 2019;5:00055–2019.
16. Bajwah S, Koffman J, Higginson IJ, Ross JR, Wells AU, Birring SS, Riley J. "I wish I knew more..." the end-of-life planning and information needs for end-stage fibrotic interstitial lung disease: views of patients, carers and health professionals. BMJ Support Palliat Care. 2013;3:84–90.

17. Bajwah S, Higginson IJ, Ross JR, Wells AU, Birring SS, Patel A, Riley J. Specialist palliative care is more than drugs: a retrospective study of ILD Patients. Lung. 2012;190:215–20.
18. Rajala K, Lehto JT, Sutinen E, Kautiainen H, Myllärniemi M, Saarto T. Marked deterioration in the quality of life of patients with idiopathic pulmonary fibrosis during the last two years of life. BMC Pulm Med. 2018; https://doi.org/10.1186/s12890-018-0738-x.
19. Bajwah S, Ross JR, Peacock JL, Higginson IJ, Wells AU, Suresh Patel A, Koffman J, Riley J. Interventions to improve symptoms and quality of life of patients with fibrotic interstitial lung disease: a systematic review of the literature. Thorax. 2013;68:867–79.
20. Ahmadi Z, Wysham NG, Lundstrom S, Janson C, Currow DC, Ekstrom M. End-of-life care in oxygen-dependent ILD compared with lung cancer: a national population-based study. Thorax. 2016. thoraxjnl-2015-207439 [pii].
21. Belkin A, Albright K, Swigris JJ. A qualitative study of informal caregivers' perspectives on the effects of idiopathic pulmonary fibrosis. BMJ Open Respir Res. 2014;1:e000007.
22. Kreuter M, Bendstrup E, Russell AM, et al. Palliative care in interstitial lung disease: living well. Lancet Respir Med. 2017; https://doi.org/10.1016/S2213-2600(17)30383-1.
23. Canadian Pulmonary Fibrosis Foundation. Toward exceptional care: a Canadian IPF patient charter; 2016.
24. Fadul N, Elsayem A, Palmer JL, Del Fabbro E, Swint K, Li Z, Poulter V, Bruera E. Supportive versus palliative care: what's in a name? Cancer. 2009;115:2013–21.
25. Lanken PN, Terry PB, DeLisser HM, et al. An official American thoracic society clinical policy statement: palliative care for patients with respiratory diseases and critical illnesses. Am J Respir Crit Care Med. 2008;177:912–27.
26. Parikh RB, Kirch RA, Smith TJ, Temel JS. Early specialty palliative care — translating data in oncology into practice. N Engl J Med. 2013;369:2347–51.
27. Hearn J, Higginson IJ. Do specialist palliative care teams improve outcomes for cancer patients? A systematic literature review. Palliat Med. 1998;12:317–32.
28. Higginson IJ, Bausewein C, Reilly CC, Gao W, Gysels M, Dzingina M, McCrone P, Booth S, Jolley CJ, Moxham J. An integrated palliative and respiratory care service for patients with advanced disease and refractory breathlessness: a randomised controlled trial. Lancet Respir Med. 2014;2:979–87.
29. Professional Education in Palliative and End-of-Life Care for Physicians, Nurses, and Social Workers – Improving Palliative Care for Cancer – NCBI Bookshelf. https://www.ncbi.nlm.nih.gov/books/NBK223527/. Accessed 30 Sept 2020.
30. Beernaert K, Deliens L, Pardon K, Van den Block L, Devroey D, Chambaere K, Cohen J. What are physicians' reasons for not referring people with life-limiting illnesses to specialist palliative care services? A nationwide survey. PLoS One. 2015;10:e0137251.
31. Akiyama N, Fujisawa T, Morita T, et al. Palliative care for idiopathic pulmonary fibrosis patients: pulmonary physicians' view. J Pain Symptom Manag. 2020; https://doi.org/10.1016/j.jpainsymman.2020.06.012.
32. Mcateer R, Wellbery C. Palliative care: benefits, barriers, and best practices; 2013.
33. Kim JW, Atkins C, Wilson AM. Barriers to specialist palliative care in interstitial lung disease: a systematic review. BMJ Support Palliat Care. 2018; https://doi.org/10.1136/bmjspcare-2018-001575.
34. Quill TE, Abernethy AP. Generalist plus specialist palliative care — creating a more sustainable model. N Engl J Med. 2013;368:1173–5.
35. Graney BA, He C, Marll M, et al. Essential components of an interstitial lung disease clinic. Chest. 2020:1–14.
36. Rocker GM, Simpson AC, Horton R. Palliative care in advanced lung disease: the challenge of integrating palliation into everyday care. Chest. 2015;148:801–9.
37. Kalluri M, Younus S, Adamali H, Barratt S, Morales MG, Rippon N. Description of palliative care models in ILD clinics and their impact on IPF care. In: American Thoracic Society International Conference Abstracts. American Thoracic Society; 2019. p. A4776.

38. Reipas KM, Grossman DL, Lock K, Caraiscos VB. Examining the characteristics of patients with non-malignant lung disease at the time of referral to an inter-professional supportive care clinic. Am J Hosp Palliat Med. 2021;104990912110056
39. Barratt SL, Morales M, Spiers T, et al. Specialist palliative care, psychology, interstitial lung disease (ILD) multidisciplinary team meeting: a novel model to address palliative care needs. BMJ Open Respir Res. 2018; https://doi.org/10.1136/bmjresp-2018-000360.
40. Brown CE, Jecker NS, Curtis JR. Inadequate palliative care in chronic lung disease. An issue of health care inequality. Ann Am Thorac Soc. 2016;13:311–6.
41. Selecky PA, Eliasson AH, Hall RI, Schneider RF, Varkey B, McCaffree DR. Palliative and end-of-life care for patients with cardiopulmonary diseases: American College of Chest Physicians position statement. Chest. 2005;128:3599–610.
42. Chauhan, Tara NATIONAL PALLIATIVE MEDICINE SURVEY DATA REPORT Canadian Society of Palliative Care Physicians Human Resources Committee Partners Canadian Medical Association College of Family Physicians of Canada Royal College of Physicians and Surgeons of Canada Technology Evaluation in the Elderly Network.
43. National Palliative Medicine Survey Data Report Human Resources Committee Survey Date November 2014 Report Date: May 2015 website: https://cspcp.ca/wp-content/uploads/2015/04/PM-Survey-Data-Report-EN.pdf.
44. Kim JW, Olive S, Jones S, et al. Interstitial lung disease and specialist palliative care access: a healthcare professionals survey. BMJ Supportive & Palliative Care Published online first: 19 June 2020. https://doi.org/10.1136/bmjspcare-2019-002148.
45. Kalluri M. From consulting to caring: care redesign in idiopathic pulmonary fibrosis. https://catalyst.nejm.org/doi/full/10.1056/CAT.19.0682. Accessed 30 Sep 2020.
46. Kalluri M, Luppi F, Ferrara G. What patients with idiopathic pulmonary fibrosis and caregivers want: filling the gaps with patient reported outcomes and experience measures. Am J Med. 2020;133:281–9.
47. Sepúlveda C, Marlin A, Yoshida T, Ullrich A. Palliative care: the World Health Organization's global perspective. J Pain Symptom Manage. 2002;24(2):91–6.
48. Wijsenbeek MS, Holland AE, Swigris JJ, Renzoni EA. Comprehensive supportive care for patients with fibrosing interstitial lung disease. Am J Respir Crit Care Med. 2019;200:152–9.
49. Boland JW, Reigada C, Yorke J, et al. The adaptation, face, and content validation of a needs assessment tool: progressive disease for people with interstitial lung disease. J Palliat Med. 2016;19:549–55.
50. Sharp C, Lamb H, Jordan N, Edwards A, Gunary R, Meek P, Millar AB, Kendall C, Adamali H. Development of tools to facilitate palliative and supportive care referral for patients with idiopathic pulmonary fibrosis. BMJ Support Palliat Care. 2017:1–7.
51. Kalluri M, Bakal J, Ting W, Younus S. Comparison of MRC breathlessness scale to a novel multidimensional dyspnea scale (MDDS) for clinical use. In: American Thoracic Society International Conference Abstracts. American Thoracic Society; 2019. p. A3371.
52. Fong S, Richman-Eisenstat J, Kalluri M. Buccal hydromorphone syrup for managing dyspnea in idiopathic pulmonary fibrosis. Am J Hosp Palliat Med. 2020;104990912096912
53. van den Bosch L, Kalluri M. Dyspnea management in interstitial lung disease: an early integrated palliative care approach in a multidisciplinary setting. In: American Thoracic Society International Conference Abstracts. American Thoracic Society; 2019. p. A4757.
54. Kalluri M, Lu-Song J, Younus S, Nabipoor M, Richman-Eisenstat J, Ohinmaa A, Bakal JA. Health care costs at the end of life for patients with idiopathic pulmonary fibrosis. Evaluation of a pilot multidisciplinary collaborative interstitial lung disease clinic. Ann Am Thorac Soc. 2020;17:706–13.
55. Hui D, Bruera E. The Edmonton symptom assessment system 25 years later: past, present, and future developments. J Pain Symptom Manag. 2017;53:630–43.
56. Garibaldi BT, Danoff SK. Symptom-based management of the idiopathic interstitial pneumonia. Respirology. 2016;21:1357–65.

57. Carvajalino S, Reigada C, Johnson MJ, Dzingina M, Bajwah S. Symptom prevalence of patients with fibrotic interstitial lung disease: a systematic literature review. BMC Pulm Med. 2018;18:78.
58. Ramadurai D, Corder S, Churney T, Graney B, Harshman A, Meadows S, Swigris JJ. Understanding the informational needs of patients with IPF and their caregivers: 'You get diagnosed, and you ask this question right away, what does this mean?'. BMJ Open Qual. 2018;7:e000207.
59. Rajala K, Lehto JT, Saarinen M, Sutinen E, Saarto T, Myllärniemi M. End-of-life care of patients with idiopathic pulmonary fibrosis. BMC Palliat Care. 2016;15:85.
60. Bausewein C, Schunk M, Schumacher P, Dittmer J, Bolzani A, Booth S. Breathlessness services as a new model of support for patients with respiratory disease. Chron Respir Dis. 2018;15:48–59.
61. Khor YH, Smith DJF, Johannson KA, Renzoni E. Oxygen for interstitial lung diseases. Curr Opin Pulm Med. 2020;26:464–9.
62. Visca D, Mori L, Tsipouri V, et al. Effect of ambulatory oxygen on quality of life for patients with fibrotic lung disease (AmbOx): a prospective, open-label, mixed-method, crossover randomised controlled trial. Lancet Respir Med. 2018;6:759–70.
63. Kalluri M, Richman-Eisenstat J. Early and integrated palliative care to achieve a home death in idiopathic pulmonary fibrosis. J Pain Symptom Manag. 2017;53:1111–5.
64. Kalluri M, Richman-Eisenstat J. Breathing is not an option; dyspnea is. J Palliat Care. 2014;30:188–91.
65. Lindell KO, Collins EG, Catanzarite L, Garvey CM, Hernandez C, Mclaughlin S, Schneidman AM, Meek PM, Jacobs SS. Care of adults with pulmonary disorders equipment, access and worry about running short of oxygen: key concerns in the ATS patient supplemental oxygen survey. Heart Lung. 2019;48(3):245–9. https://doi.org/10.1016/j.hrtlng.2018.12.006.
66. Johnson MJ, Currow DC. Opioids for breathlessness: a narrative review. BMJ Support Palliat Care. 2020;10:287–95.
67. Ryan NM, Birring SS, Gibson PG. Gabapentin for refractory chronic cough: a randomised, double-blind, placebo-controlled trial. Lancet. 2012;380:1583–9.
68. van Manen MJG, van't Spijker A, Tak NC, Baars CT, Jongenotter SM, van Roon LR, Kraan J, Hoogsteden HC, Wijsenbeek MS. Patient and partner empowerment programme for idiopathic pulmonary fibrosis. Eur Respir J. 2017; https://doi.org/10.1183/13993003.01596-2016.
69. Vaidya S, Hibbert CL, Kinter E, Boes S. Identification of key cost generating events for idiopathic pulmonary fibrosis: a systematic review. Lung. 2017;195:1–8. https://doi.org/10.1007/s00408-016-9960-6.
70. van Vliet LM, Harding R, Bausewein C, Payne S, Higginson IJ. How should we manage information needs, family anxiety, depression, and breathlessness for those affected by advanced disease: development of a clinical decision support tool using a Delphi design. BMC Med. 2015; https://doi.org/10.1186/s12916-015-0449-6.
71. Kalluri M, Younus S, Archibald N, Richman-Eisenstat J, Pooler C. Action plans in idiopathic pulmonary fibrosis: a qualitative study—'I do what I can do'. BMJ Support Palliat Care. 2021. bmjspcare-2020-002831.
72. Sudore RL, Lum HD, You JJ, et al. Defining advance care planning for adults: a consensus definition from a multidisciplinary Delphi panel. J Pain Symptom Manage. 2017;53:821–832.e1.
73. Wright AA, Zhang B, Ray A, et al. Associations between end-of-life discussions, patient mental health, medical care near death, and caregiver bereavement adjustment. JAMA J Am Med Assoc. 2008;300:1665–73.
74. Archibald N, Bakal JA, Richman-Eisenstat J, Kalluri M. Early integrated palliative care bundle impacts location of death in interstitial lung disease: a pilot retrospective study. Am J Hosp Palliat Med. 2020; https://doi.org/10.1177/1049909120924995.
75. Mcdermott L, Kalluri M, Fox K, Richman-eisenstat J. Redesigning interstitial lung disease clinic care through interprofessional collaboration. J Interprof Care. 2021:1–11.

76. Burge G, Moore V. The value of a specialist nurse-lead interstitial lung disease clinic, patients' views. In: European Respiratory Journal. European Respiratory Society (ERS); 2015. p. PA332.
77. Breathless for Change Report 2020 – Canadian Pulmonary Fibrosis Foundation. https://cpff.ca/get-involved/advocate/breathless-for-change-report-2020/. Accessed 7 Oct 2020.
78. Mularski RA, Reinke LF, Carrieri-Kohlman V, et al. An official American Thoracic Society workshop report: assessment and palliative management of dyspnea crisis. Ann Am Thorac Soc. 2013;10:S98–106.
79. Pawlow PC, Doherty CL, Blumenthal NP, Matura LA, Christie JD, Ersek M. An integrative review of the role of palliative care in lung transplantation. Prog Transplant. 2020;30:147–54.
80. Colman R, Singer LG, Barua R, Downar J. Outcomes of lung transplant candidates referred for co-management by palliative care: a retrospective case series. Palliat Med. 2015;29:429–35.
81. Kalluri M, Claveria F, Ainsley E, Haggag M, Armijo-Olivo S, Richman-Eisenstat J. Beyond idiopathic pulmonary fibrosis diagnosis: multidisciplinary care with an early integrated palliative approach is associated with a decrease in acute care utilization and hospital deaths. J Pain Symptom Manag. 2018;55:420–6.
82. Temel JS, Greer JA, Muzikansky A, et al. Early palliative care for patients with metastatic non-small-cell lung cancer. N Engl J Med. 2010;363:733–42.
83. Carney PA, Thayer EK, Palmer R, Galper AB, Zierler B, Eiff MP. The benefits of interprofessional learning and teamwork in primary care ambulatory training settings. J Interprofessional Educ Pract. 2019;15:119–26.
84. Home - Speak Up. Parlons en. https://www.advancecareplanning.ca/. Accessed 25 Aug 2020.

# Chapter 17
# Withdrawal of Mechanical Ventilation: Considerations to Guide Patient and Family Centered Care and the Development of Health Care Policy

**Lynn F. Reinke and Alice M. Boylan**

## Introduction

Discussions regarding withdrawal of mechanical ventilation can be the most challenging and distressing conversations held between health care providers, patients, and families. Using a case-based approach, barriers to communication and achievement of consensus regarding withdrawal of life support are discussed including religious, cultural, and lack of provider training in end of life communication. We also discuss the additional challenges generated by the ambiguity and lack of consistency of laws regarding withdrawing and withholding life support between states and differences in interpretation of those laws within states. A better understanding of barriers and strategies shown to successfully overcome those barriers may help inform development of health care policies that advance these discussions and improve satisfaction of all involved.

L. F. Reinke (✉)
Department of Veterans Affairs, Puget Sound Health Care System, Health Services R&D, Seattle, WA, USA

University of Washington, School of Nursing, Department of Biobehavioral Nursing and Health Informatics, Seattle, WA, USA
e-mail: reinkl@uw.edu

A. M. Boylan
Medical University of South Carolina, Division of Pulmonary and Critical Care, Mt Pleasant, SC, USA
e-mail: boylana@musc.edu


K. O. Lindell, S. K. Danoff (eds.), *Palliative Care in Lung Disease*, Respiratory Medicine, https://doi.org/10.1007/978-3-030-81788-6_17

## Case

A 65-year-old female with history of metastatic adenocarcinoma of unknown primary origin who had completed whole brain radiation therapy 6 months previously for leptomeningeal metastasis was admitted with septic shock, aspiration pneumonia, and encephalopathy. Based on previously expressed wishes she was intubated and received aggressive care. Over the next few days vasopressors were weaned and she was liberated from the ventilator. She was still encephalopathic but appeared able to protect her airway. The patient's next of kin, a son and daughter, were both attorneys. They requested continued aggressive care including resuscitation if she suffered a cardiac arrest and re-intubation if she developed respiratory failure. She was transferred out of the ICU, but two days later was found with pulseless electrical activity. She was intubated and resuscitated with return of spontaneous circulation after approximately 10 minutes. That afternoon and evening she was comatose but had brainstem reflexes. In the morning, these reflexes were absent. CT scan of the brain confirmed edema and herniation. An apnea test was performed and confirmed brain death. Her family was informed of these findings and withdrawal of life support was recommended. However, they refused and, when challenged about this decision, threatened litigation. They requested to confer with their own rabbi, who initially advised that they should not allow withdrawal of mechanical ventilation. This was based on the religious belief that human intervention such as cessation of mechanical ventilation to end the life of a patient is unethical. Subsequently, a senior rabbi was consulted who recommended that a timer be installed on the ventilator and set to shut power off at a randomly selected time. The family agreed with the rabbi's recommendation, however before this was implemented, the patient experienced cardiac death and was not resuscitated.

This case illustrates some of the potential barriers to end of life discussions and withdrawal of mechanical ventilation which include both patient/family barriers as well as physician barriers. The attending in this case was unaware of the religious beliefs of the family and their distrust of medical professionals, which the team eventually learned had developed during their father's illness and death. In addition, the threat of litigation made the physician fearful of repercussions should support be withdrawn without the family's consent.

### *Patient and Family Barriers*

One barrier to consent to withdrawal of mechanical ventilation that has been reported by multiple investigators is religiousness or positive religious coping. Religiousness has been found to be significantly associated with wanting all measures to extend life in advanced cancer patients [1]. Specifically, this type of coping is associated with receipt of mechanical ventilation and intensive life-prolonging care in the last week of life [2]. In addition, racial differences in religiousness and associated preference for aggressive care have been found with African Americans and Hispanics with these groups rating religion as important in end of life treatment preferences more frequently than whites [1].

As in this case, the religious beliefs of the patient or family may impact decisions regarding withdrawal of care and these beliefs may not be uniform across a specific religion. For example, the United Kingdom Muslim Law Council in 1996 officially supported organ donation and recognized brain death as true irreversible death [3]. This perspective has since been embraced by the Islamic Fiqh Academies of the Organization of the Islamic Conference and the Muslim World League, the Islamic Medical Association of North America, and legal rulings by multiple Islamic nations. Despite this, there is not uniform consensus, and many Muslims only accept cardiopulmonary death as true death [4]. Similarly, many types of Buddhism do not accept brain death as true death as well as most groups of Haredi Judaism (ultra-orthodox) [5]. The diversity within and among religions on termination of care were confirmed in a meta-analysis examining the major religions. The authors concluded views within a religion can shift among those who set the guidelines, those who provide the care, the patients, and their families [6]. Thus, understanding the specific religious beliefs of a patient is critical in approaching discussions of withdrawal of mechanical ventilation in cases of very poor prognosis.

In addition to family, the individual patient's clergy may participate in these discussions. Terminally ill patients with high levels of support from their religious community are generally more likely to receive aggressive care in an ICU rather than hospice [9]. In a survey regarding the values promoted by US clergy regarding end of life decisions for patients with terminal cancer, most agreed that god performs miracles despite a terminal diagnosis. In addition, more than half would encourage treatment due to the sanctity of life, some would postpone medical decisions due to god being in control, and some would encourage painful treatment due to the redemptive nature of suffering. Furthermore, clergy with less medical knowledge were more likely to embrace life-prolonging values [10].

Racial differences in end of life choices may extend beyond religious differences. African Americans have consistently been found to have a preference for life support compared to whites [7]. More specifically, a study found significantly more African Americans and Hispanics would choose mechanical ventilation to extend life for 1 week than would whites. Some of this was attributed to a more optimistic belief in the benefit of mechanical ventilation and intensive care [8].

Medical mistrust may be seen in all racial and socio-economic groups, but has consistently been found in African Americans. This is understandable given the history of mistreatment of African Americans at the hands of the US medical establishment as epitomized by the Tuskegee Syphilis Study where therapy was withheld from patients. Adjusted for sex, education, age, income and insurance status, African American race was associated with mistrust [11] and the belief that hypervigilance is required to receive high-quality care [12].

Finally, the patient and family members may have difficulty accepting a poor prognosis. In a survey of clinicians regarding barriers to end of life discussions, this was cited as the most frequent barrier [13]. Other factors included difficulty understanding the limits of life-sustaining treatment, disagreement among family members regarding goals of care, and the patient's inability to participate in goals of care discussions. All of these factors underscore the need for effective and regular communication between patients/family and knowledgeable members of the health care team.

## *Physician Barriers*

Multiple barriers to these discussions exist on the provider side, as well. Often goals of care discussions are not pursued or occur late in the course of care. In a Canadian multicenter study of seriously ill hospitalized patients and family members only 22% of patients and 24% of family members reported any discussion about preferences for end of life care during their stay [13]. Some of this may be attributed to lack of provider skills and training in communication related to end of life. Many feel unprepared for these discussions [14]. In a review of 36 studies, an important factor was providers' lack of communication training and skills, specifically their communication of the futility of further treatment [15]. In addition, the survey found that current medical education leaves physicians feeling unprepared for these discussions. In fact, in one large survey, less than 18% of medical students and residents had received education regarding end of life discussions [14].

Fear of litigation usually is less of a factor in general goals of care discussions, but rises in importance when discussions involve withdrawal of life support. In a survey of neurologists asked about their reasons to continue supportive care in the event of brain death if a family objected for religious reasons, 48% stated they would continue due to fear of litigation [16]. Although the likelihood of criminal or civil litigation is low if internal standards and guidelines are followed, there is theoretical risk of withdrawing a ventilator from a nonconsenting patient including a risk of criminal homicide charges [17]. In addition, although federal and state statutes provide limited immunity to physicians in some circumstances such as emergency situations, they do not specifically address withholding or withdrawing mechanical ventilation, and usually do not provide immunity to criminal charges [17].

Adding to physician insecurity regarding vulnerability to litigation is the fact that laws regarding withholding and withdrawing life support vary from state to state [18] and few states provide immunity to criminal charges [17]. In addition, practice generally varies across states because it is left up to the individual hospital to interpret the state's statutes regarding withholding or withdrawing life support [19]. Finally, most states do not directly address objection to withdrawal of life support even in patients deemed brain dead based on religious beliefs. In Illinois, the directive is to take religious beliefs into account, but no specifics are given. Taking a slightly different stance, a New Jersey statute states that death should be solely declared based on cardiac death if determination of death by brain death criteria violates a patient's religious beliefs [19].

## *Facilitators: Clinician Training in End-of Life Discussions*

Training positively impacts provider willingness to initiate goals of care conversations. Those who have received training were more likely to report having advance care planning discussions with patients (19% vs 12%), although still notably a minority. They were also more likely to find those conversations rewarding (46% [20] vs 30% [21]). Effective communication in the ICU specifically focused on family members is important since often patients are too ill to accurately communicate their goals of care or may be on ventilators or sedated, thus unable to communicate.

As critically ill patients often lack decision-making capacity, providers ask family members to act as surrogates for the patient in discussions about the goals of care. Therefore, clinician-family communication is a central component of medical decision making in the ICU, and the quality of this communication has direct bearing on decisions made regarding care for critically ill patients. In addition, studies suggest that clinician-family communication can have profound effects on the experiences and long-term mental health of family members [22]. Azoulay and colleagues [22] found that family members of critically ill patients who felt information was incomplete, who shared in decision making and whose relative died after end of life decisions experienced higher rates of post traumatic stress disorder.

The specific language and semantics that clinicians use to explain a patient's prognosis may influence family members' decisions to either prolong life sustaining treatments or transition to comfort care. A qualitative study conducted focus groups with community members to gain perspectives about the meaning of futile treatment including the term "medically inappropriate" care [23]. Laypersons did not clearly understand the meaning of "medically inappropriate", equating this to a wrong treatment that may result in malpractice. The lack of clarity about medical terms reinforces the importance of clinicians' mastering communication skills. Some laypersons suggest employing ICU facilitators to foster medical translation from providers to family members [24]. An ICU facilitator is usually a nurse or social worker trained in how to conduct family conferences and mediation amongst the health care team. Studies have demonstrated that ICU facilitators may improve patient and family satisfaction of care and decrease length of ICU days. Focus group members believed it was important for providers to be honest and give guidance on the utility of treatments. However, in situations of conflict between providers and families, the families should ultimately decide on treatments, reinforcing the principle of autonomy. The practice of shared decision-making is usually preferred among patients. Some patients and families, however, prefer to have physicians make treatment decisions, while others prefer to make independent decisions. Thus, asking patients and families how they prefer to make decisions is an important aspect of treating patients with respect [25].

There are essential evidence-based components of family-centered communication that can facilitate positive outcomes. These include: (1) applying a shared decision-making model; (2) discussing prognosis and treatments in clear, lay terms;

**Table 17.1** Risk factors for potentially challenging goals of care discussions

| |
|---|
| No documented advance directives or advance directives are "old or outdated" at the time when a patient's medical condition rapidly declines |
| Disagreement among treating professionals re: patient's prognosis |
| Disagreement among family members/surrogates re: aggressive care vs withdrawal of life support or allowing a natural death |
| Family members/surrogates that "want everything" done despite poor prognosis |
| No legal surrogate available |
| Family/surrogate voices concern that medical decisions are being based on financial "savings" for the hospital or unequitable allocation of resources |
| Patients or providers from different ethnic or cultural backgrounds and/or language barriers |
| Patient and families whose religious beliefs oppose withdrawal of life support |

(3) including all members of the interdisciplinary team; (4) addressing spiritual and/or religious beliefs; (5) ensuring cross-cultural communication by inviting a medical interpreter if the patient or family members does not speak English; and (6) using empathic language [26]. Risk factors or "red flags" for goals of care conversations that may be challenging for clinicians are identified in Table 17.1.

In the case we describe, a family meeting including all members of the interdisciplinary team (physicians, nurses, social service, an ethics team member and a palliative care team member), family members and their rabbi may have helped clarify the family's decision making preference. It would have allowed the clinicians and other team members to "get to know" who the patient was as a "person" and discover the basis of mistrust that stemmed from the father's illness. This approach may have increased the family's trust in the medical team. Acknowledging the family's strict religious beliefs, while at the same time helping them to understand her poor prognosis, may have helped align the patient and family preferences with her treatment and mitigated the family's litigation threat.

## *Effective Communication Tools for the Clinical Team*

The intentional use of empathic and supportive statements such as the mnemonic "NURSES", N = naming, U = understanding, R = respect, S = support, E = explore and S = silence, are simple yet effective statements that clinicians can use during patient and family conversations [5]. Table 17.2 offers examples of NURSE statements.

The use of NURSE statements was studied in a large ICU trial with over 1400 patients. Critical care nurses regularly met with family members and applied NURSE statements [26]. The study resulted in improvement in family members satisfaction of care ratings, decreased use of aggressive treatments, and decreased ICU length of stay. The researchers posit that addressing emotional aspects of a critically ill patient with family members facilitates trust with the medical team and helps align patient and family care preferences with treatments [26].

**Table 17.2** NURSE statements. (Copyright © 2021 Vital Talk. All rights reserved. (vitaltalk.org))

| NURSE(S) responding to emotion with empathy | | |
|---|---|---|
| | What you say or do | Comments |
| *N*-Name | "You sound frustrated" | Acknowledges the emotion. Be careful to suggest only, most people don't want to be told how they feel. In general, mm down the intensity (e.g., scared→concerned). Can use third person neutral to take emphasis off person. |
| | "This situation is overwhelming" | |
| *U*-Understand | "I can't imagine what you are going through" | Acknowledges or normalizes the emotion or situation |
| | "I could imagine many people in your situation might feel…" | Avoid suggesting you understand their experience, because we often can't |
| *R*-Respect | "I can see you really care about your daughter" | Expression of praise or gratitude about the things they are doing. This can be especially helpful when there is conflict |
| *S*-Support | "We will do everything we can to support you through this process" | Expression of what you can do for them and a good way to express nonabandonment. Making this kind of commitment can be a powerful statement |
| *E*-Explore | "Can you tell me more about…" | Emotion cues can be expressions of underlying concerns or meaning. Combining this with another NURSE statement can be very effective and help you understand their reasoning or actions. Make sure to avoid judgment and come from a place of curiosity |

Furthermore, VALUE statements can be essential components of effective communication among the clinical staff and family members. These statements can be used in one on one conversations and in family meetings [24]. "VALUE": *V*alue family statements; *A*cknowledge emotions; *L*isten to the family; *U*nderstand the patient as a person; *E*licit family questions. Some examples of VALUE statements are: *V* Thank you for sharing this information about your loved one with us…it is very helpful; *A* - This news must be very hard; *L* - listen more than talk, give information in small amounts then be quiet and pause; *U* – Tell me about your mother, what kinds of activities or hobbies did she enjoy; *E* – We went over a lot…what questions do you have for us?

Addressing emotion and learning about the patients' personhood by using NURSE and VALUE statements will help ensure that complex decisions about medical treatments are based on a person's values and goals. Thus, it is important clinicians incorporate these communication skills into their practice. Using exploratory questions when initiating goals of care discussions may ease introducing this topic to patients and families. See Table 17.3 for examples.

Finally, researchers have identified essential components of a family meeting that may improve the chances of reaching consensus among the interdisciplinary team members and the family members (Table 17.4) [24].

**Table 17.3** Helpful exploratory questions that can be used in palliative care for the advanced care planning process

| |
|---|
| Have you had someone close to you/had your own experience with serious illness or death? If you were in that situation (again), what would you hope for? |
| Can you think of circumstances in which living longer might be more burdensome than dying? |
| When you think of becoming critically ill, what worries you the most? |
| If you were to become critically ill and unable to speak on your own behalf, is there anyone you trust to make medical decisions for you? Are your preferences documented/in writing? |
| Have you given any thought to whether you'd like cardiopulmonary resuscitation if you were to die suddenly? May I explain what CPR entails in your circumstances and what are your estimated chances of benefiting from it? |
| What kind of treatments would you want, and which ones might you decline if you were to become critically ill and unable to speak for yourself? |

**Table 17.4** Communication components shown to be associated with increased quality of care, decreased family psychological symptoms, or improved family ratings of communication

| |
|---|
| Conduct family conference within 72 h of ICU admission |
| Identify a private place for communication with family members |
| Provide consistent communication from different team members |
| Increase proportion of time spent listening to family rather than talking |
| Empathic statements |
| Statements about the difficulty of having a critically ill loved one |
| Statements about the difficulty of surrogate decision-making |
| Statements about the impending loss of a loved one |
| Identify commonly missed opportunities |
| Listen and respond to family members |
| Acknowledge and address family emotions |
| Explore and focus on patient values and treatment preferences |
| Explain the principle of surrogate decision-making to the family |
| Affirm nonabandonment of patient and family |
| Assure family that the patient will not suffer |
| Provide explicit support for decisions made by the family |

Reprinted with permission from Elsevier [24]

## *Key Ethical Concepts Related to Withdrawal of Life Sustaining Treatment*

Three main ethical principles help to shape the current U.S. consensus around the withdrawal of life-sustaining treatment. While not all clinicians personally agree with each of them, these principles have broad-based support within the U.S. legal system and accepted clinical practice and thereby form the basis for the specific recommendations. The three principles are: (1) withholding and withdrawing life support are equivalent; (2) there is an important distinction between killing and allowing to die; and (3) the doctrine of "double effect" provides an ethical rationale for providing relief of pain and other symptoms with sedatives even when this may have the foreseen (but not intended) consequence of hastening death [25].

## Decision Making Capacity

Legal guidelines regarding end-of-life decision making are less clear when patients without capacity lack an appropriate surrogate. One option is to ask the court to appoint a guardian for the patient. Another option is for institutions to develop a clear procedural guideline, including safeguards to protect the patient's interests, such as mandatory ethics committee review. The lack of consensus among institutions, states and professional societies on how to make treatment decisions on behalf of unrepresented patients led the ATS to convene an interdisciplinary, multi-society taskforce to address this issue. These recommendations (Table 17.5) are designed to help clinicians and hospital administrators make fair and practical decisions for patients in the ICU setting [27].

## Definition of Death

Controversy on the definition of death adds to the complexity of decision making about withdrawal of life sustaining treatments. Examples of some of these controversies include whether there is a right to refuse apnea testing, which set of criteria

**Table 17.5** Policy recommendations for medical decision-making for unrepresented patients in intensive care medicine

| | |
|---|---|
| 1. | Institutions should promote advance care planning to prevent patients at high risk for becoming unrepresented from meeting this definition, both (1) by helping adult patients with decision-making capacity to identify a preferred surrogate decision-maker and to record their preferences and values in an advance directive and (2) by ensuring that such documents are widely available to clinicians at the point of care |
| 2. | Institutions should implement strategies to determine whether seemingly unrepresented patients are, in fact, unrepresented, including (1) carefully assessing capacity, (2) diligently searching for potential surrogates among the patient's family and friends, and (3) involving any nonhospital individuals who have shown care and concern for the patient's welfare and are familiar with the patient's preferences and values |
| 3. | Institutions should manage decision-making for unrepresented patients using collaboration between the clinical team and a diverse interprofessional, multidisciplinary committee rather than ad hoc by treating clinicians |
| 4. | Institutions should use all available information on the patient's preferences and values to guide treatment decisions. If such information is not available, the committee should collaborate with the treatment team to make decisions in the patient's best interest |
| 5. | Institutions should manage decision-making for unrepresented patients using a fair process that comports with procedural due process, such as transparency, legitimacy, and consistency |
| 6. | Institutions should employ this fair process even when state law authorizes procedures with less oversight |

Reprinted with permission of the American Thoracic Society

Cite: Pope et al. [27]

should be chosen to measure the death of the brain, and how the problem of erroneous testing should be handled [28]. These controversies leave little hope of consensus on how to define death for social and public policy purposes. Compounding these controversies are patients and family members' belief systems including cultural and religious aspects. Given the multifactorial complexities of end of life decisions, public policy should allow individuals and their valid surrogates to choose the definition of death, thus medical treatments. Health care professionals can promote goal alignment and trust with the patient and family by being aware of our own implicit and explicit biases, conducting values based goals of care conversations upon admission to the ICU, or earlier if possible, and include ethics and palliative care teams to participate as members of the care team.

In summary, there are multiple factors that play a role in the decision to withdraw life support for critically ill patients. These factors may include patient and family's religious and cultural beliefs, differences in decision making approaches and lack of clear communication from the medical team about the patients' condition and likely prognosis. We highlight the importance of clinician's being trained how to conduct goal of care and end of life discussions with patients and family members and offer practical guides to improve skills and mitigate conflict.

## References

1. Balboni TA, Vanderwerker LC, Block SD, Paulk ME, Lathan CS, Peteet JR, et al. Religiousness and spiritual support among advanced cancer patients and associations with end-of-life treatment preferences and quality of life. J Clin Oncol. 2007;25(5):555–60.
2. Phelps AC, Maciejewski PK, Nilsson M, Balboni TA, Wright AA, Paulk ME, et al. Religious coping and use of intensive life-prolonging care near death in patients with advanced cancer. JAMA. 2009;301(11):1140–7.
3. Choo V. UK Shariah Council approves organ transplants. Lancet. 1995;346(8970):303.
4. Miller AC, Ziad-Miller A, Elamin EM. Brain death and Islam: the interface of religion, culture, history, law, and modern medicine. Chest. 2014;146(4):1092–101.
5. www.vitaltalk.org/. 2020. Available from: https://www.vitaltalk.org/.
6. Muishout G, van Laarhoven HWM, Wiegers G, Popp-Baier U. Muslim physicians and palliative care: attitudes towards the use of palliative sedation. Support Care Cancer. 2018;26(11):3701–10.
7. Phipps E, True G, Harris D, Chong U, Tester W, Chavin SI, et al. Approaching the end of life: attitudes, preferences, and behaviors of African-American and white patients and their family caregivers. J Clin Oncol. 2003;21(3):549–54.
8. Barnato AE, Anthony DL, Skinner J, Gallagher PM, Fisher ES. Racial and ethnic differences in preferences for end-of-life treatment. J Gen Intern Med. 2009;24(6):695–701.
9. Balboni TA, Balboni M, Enzinger AC, Gallivan K, Paulk ME, Wright A, et al. Provision of spiritual support to patients with advanced cancer by religious communities and associations with medical care at the end of life. JAMA Intern Med. 2013;173(12):1109–17.
10. Balboni MJ, Sullivan A, Enzinger AC, Smith PT, Mitchell C, Peteet JR, et al. U.S. Clergy religious values and relationships to end-of-life discussions and care. J Pain Symptom Manage. 2017;53(6):999–1009.

11. Brandon DT, Isaac LA, LaVeist TA. The legacy of Tuskegee and trust in medical care: is Tuskegee responsible for race differences in mistrust of medical care? J Natl Med Assoc. 2005;97(7):951–6.
12. McCleskey SG, Cain CL. Improving end-of-life care for diverse populations: communication, competency, and system supports. Am J Hosp Palliat Care. 2019;36(6):453–9.
13. You JJ, Downar J, Fowler RA, Lamontagne F, Ma IW, Jayaraman D, et al. Barriers to goals of care discussions with seriously ill hospitalized patients and their families: a multicenter survey of clinicians. JAMA Intern Med. 2015;175(4):549–56.
14. Sullivan AM, Lakoma MD, Block SD. The status of medical education in end-of-life care: a national report. J Gen Intern Med. 2003;18(9):685–95.
15. Visser M, Deliens L, Houttekier D. Physician-related barriers to communication and patient- and family-centred decision-making towards the end of life in intensive care: a systematic review. Crit Care. 2014;18(6):604.
16. Aad G, Abbott B, Abdallah J, Abdinov O, Aben R, Abolins M, et al. Determination of the ratio of b-quark fragmentation fractions f(s)/f(d) in pp collisions at radicals=7 TeV with the ATLAS detector. Phys Rev Lett. 2015;115(26):262001.
17. Cohen IG, Crespo AM, White DB. Potential legal liability for withdrawing or withholding ventilators during COVID-19: assessing the risks and identifying needed reforms. JAMA. 2020;323(19):1901–2.
18. Aad G, Abbott B, Abdallah J, Abdel Khalek S, Abdinov O, Aben R, et al. Two-particle Bose-Einstein correlations in pp collisions at [Formula: see text] 0.9 and 7 TeV measured with the ATLAS detector. Eur Phys J C Part Fields. 2015;75(10):466.
19. Lewis A, Greer D. Current controversies in brain death determination. Nat Rev Neurol. 2017;13(8):505–9.
20. John A. Hartford Foundation CHF, California HealthCare Foundation Physicians' views toward advance care planning and end-of-life care conversations. 2016:1–28. Available from: https://www.johnahartford.org/images/uploads/resources/ConversationStopper_Poll_Memo.pdf.
21. Keating NL, Landrum MB, Rogers SO Jr, Baum SK, Virnig BA, Huskamp HA, et al. Physician factors associated with discussions about end-of-life care. Cancer. 2010;116(4):998–1006.
22. Azoulay E, Pochard F, Kentish-Barnes N, Chevret S, Aboab J, Adrie C, et al. Risk of post-traumatic stress symptoms in family members of intensive care unit patients. Am J Respir Crit Care Med. 2005;171(9):987–94.
23. Neville TH, Tarn DM, Pavlish CL, Wenger NS. The community perspective on potentially inappropriate treatment. Ann Am Thorac Soc. 2020;17(7):854–9.
24. Curtis JR, White DB. Practical guidance for evidence-based ICU family conferences. Chest. 2008;134(4):835–43.
25. Truog RD, Campbell ML, Curtis JR, Haas CE, Luce JM, Rubenfeld GD, et al. Recommendations for end-of-life care in the intensive care unit: a consensus statement by the American College [corrected] of Critical Care Medicine. Crit Care Med. 2008;36(3):953–63.
26. White DB, Angus DC, Shields AM, Buddadhumaruk P, Pidro C, Paner C, et al. A randomized trial of a family-support intervention in intensive care units. N Engl J Med. 2018;378(25):2365–75.
27. Pope TM, Bennett J, Carson SS, Cederquist L, Cohen AB, DeMartino ES, et al. Making medical treatment decisions for unrepresented patients in the ICU. An official American Thoracic Society/American Geriatrics Society policy statement. Am J Respir Crit Care Med. 2020;201(10):1182–92.
28. Veatch RM. Controversies in defining death: a case for choice. Theor Med Bioeth. 2019;40(5):381–401.

# Chapter 18
# Palliative Care During a Pandemic

Shelli Feder, Dena Schulman-Green, and Kathleen M. Akgün

## Introduction

Palliative care plays a central role in the care of patients during public health crises including epidemics and pandemics. We discuss the role of palliative care during pandemics caused primarily by droplet or airborne pathogens. We begin with a historical description of the use of palliative care during the 1918–1919 flu pandemic and the 2002–2003 Severe Acute Respiratory Syndrome (SARS) outbreak in the early 2000s. We next focus on palliative care use in patients during the pandemic caused by the novel severe acute respiratory syndrome-coronavirus-2 (SARS-CoV-2), the coronavirus strain that causes COVID-19. We discuss how palliative care delivery models have been challenged during the COVID-19 pandemic, how the field responded and adapted to the challenges, and identify ongoing questions to be answered. We conclude with critical considerations for the delivery of

S. Feder
Yale School of Nursing, New Haven, CT, USA; Palliative Care Service, VA Connecticut Healthcare System, West Haven, CT, USA
e-mail: shelli.feder@yale.edu

D. Schulman-Green
New York University Rory Meyers College of Nursing, New York, NY, USA
e-mail: dena.schulman-green@nyu.edu

K. M. Akgün (✉)
Department of Medicine, Section of Pulmonary, Critical Care and Sleep Medicine (PCCSM), VA Connecticut Healthcare System, West Haven, CT, USA

Department of Internal Medicine, Section of PCCSM, Yale University School of Medicine, New Haven, CT, USA
e-mail: kathleen.akgun@yale.edu



K. O. Lindell, S. K. Danoff (eds.), *Palliative Care in Lung Disease*, Respiratory Medicine, https://doi.org/10.1007/978-3-030-81788-6_18

palliative care during pandemics including barriers and opportunities to preserve patient-centeredness, symptomatic management considerations, ethical considerations, the role of the family caregiver, palliative communication, and shared decision-making.

## Defining Public Health Crises

The terms *outbreak, epidemic,* and *pandemic* refer to the degree of spread of a disease across populations (Table 18.1). An outbreak refers to a greater-than-expected increase in cases of a disease within a specific population or setting. An epidemic is when a disease affects a larger than expected number of people and is actively spreading within a specific community, population, or region. When epidemics spread over multiple countries or continents, they become pandemics. For the purposes of this chapter, we focus on palliative care for patients during pandemics, but many principles can likely be applied to any significant spread of disease.

## The Role of Palliative Care in Past Pandemics

Palliative care has long played an essential role in the care of patients during public health crises such as infectious outbreaks, epidemics, and pandemics. Historical texts going back to the fourteenth century reference treatments to palliate symptoms such as pain for patients dying from the Bubonic Plague, the disease caused by the bacteria *Yersinia pestis* [4]. Regional and global communicable diseases have continued to contribute to widespread suffering and death from diseases that may be alleviated by palliative care. Since 1900, at least seven airborne and/or droplet-based epidemies or pandemics have spread across the globe (Table 18.2).

**Table 18.1** Common terms and definitions

| Term | Definition | Example |
|---|---|---|
| Outbreak | Greater than expected number of cases of the disease within a specific population or setting. | Measles Outbreak, Clark County, Washington, 2018–1019 [1] |
| Epidemic | An epidemic is a disease that affects a larger than expected number of people at the same time and is actively spreading within a specific community, population, or region | Middle East Respiratory Syndrome [2], 2012–2015 |
| Pandemic | An epidemic that spreads across multiple countries or continents. | COVID-19 (SARS-CoV-2) [3], 2019-present |

**Table 18.2** Examples of Droplet and Airborne Pathogen Health Crises since 1900

| Public Health Crisis | Years | Pathogen | Level | Number of Deaths |
|---|---|---|---|---|
| 1918 Influenza [5–8] | 1918–1920 | Influenza A | Pandemic | 50 Million+ |
| 1957 H2N2 Influenza [9, 10] | 1957–1958 | Influenza A | Pandemic | 1–4 Million |
| 1968 H3N2 Influenza | 1968–1970 | Influenza A | Pandemic | 1–4 Million |
| Severe Acute Respiratory Syndrome Coronavirus (SARS-CoV) [11] | 2002–2003 | Coronavirus | Epidemic | 774 |
| Novel H1N1 Influenza [12, 13] | 2009–2010 | Influenza A | Pandemic | 151,700 – 575,400 |
| Middle East Respiratory Syndrome (MERS) [2] | 2012 – present 2015 (largest outbreak) | Coronavirus | Epidemic | 835 |
| COVID-19 (SARS-CoV-2) [3] | 2019 - present | Coronavirus | Pandemic | 1.23 Million[a] |

[a]Mortality as of November 5, 2020 [3]

## *1918–1919 Influenza Pandemic ("The 1918 Flu")*

The 1918 influenza pandemic was one of the deadliest pandemics in recorded history, quickly spreading worldwide over 12 months. By the end of the pandemic in 1919, an estimated 500 million people had been infected and more than 50 million people had died [8]. The 1918 influenza pandemic spread quickly in part because of the mass mobilization of military personnel and civilians as a result of the First World War. Young adults ages 20–40 years had the highest mortality rate from the 1918 influenza pandemic relative to other age groups and represented nearly 50% of all deaths [14]. The case fatality rate, defined as the proportion of deaths from a specific disease relative to the total number of people diagnosed with the disease for a specified time period, was so high in young adult populations that average life expectancy in the United States (U.S.) dropped by approximately 12 years [15].

The widespread rapid onset and high lethality of the 1918 influenza pandemic, coupled with limited supportive or curative treatment options at the time, led to a high demand for palliative services. Patients frequently died within 24 hours of symptom onset. As hospitals were quickly overrun, medical care frequently occurred in patients' homes, increasing demands for nurses who could provide home-based palliative care [8, 14]. Training of family caregivers by nurses to deliver palliative and supportive care became a priority. Palliative interventions included reducing fever, alleviating pain, keeping the patient warm and hydrated, and providing psychological support to patients and caregivers [8, 14]. The 1918 flu pandemic demonstrates the importance of having trained and available clinicians who are competent and skilled in providing palliative care interventions to patients in a variety of clinical and non-clinical settings during public health emergencies.

## *Severe Acute Respiratory Syndrome (SARS) 2002–2003*

First identified in 2002 in China, SARS was the first deadly epidemic caused by a coronavirus, the RNA-virus family that also causes COVID-19. SARS is a viral respiratory disease with symptoms including fever, cough, and difficulty breathing. SARS carries a case fatality rate of 9.7% [16]. Once identified, SARS quickly spread from China to other regions, including Singapore, Viet Nam, Hong Kong, and eventually Toronto, Canada. By the end of the epidemic, SARS had resulted in 8098 reported cases and 774 deaths [16].

Palliative care teams identified several challenges to providing care to SARS patients. For example, Leong and colleagues [17] interviewed palliative care clinicians working in Tan Tock Seng Hospital, the hospital designated to manage all SARS cases in Singapore. Researchers found that disruptions in therapeutic communication between patients, clinicians, and families due to visitation restrictions and isolation precautions were common, often increasing distress for the patient and family. Difficulties with prognostication and uncertainties over the clinical course of SARS also made discussions about patient preferences and goals of care difficult. Ultimately, the authors concluded that these challenges only underscored the importance of integrating palliative care teams into the care of all patients suffering with SARS [17].

The 1918–1919 Flu pandemic and the SARS epidemic illustrates the importance of palliative care during epidemics and pandemics and highlight several historical challenges. Personnel challenges, assuring adequate staffing of clinicians with palliative expertise who are able to provide palliative interventions to patients, can seem insurmountable in a crisis. Palliative medicine leaders in local, regional, national and international professional settings must learn to respond quickly to rapidly changing patient loads and to develop strategies to manage disruptions to bedside care due to isolation precautions. Discussions about prognosis and mapping out patients' goals of care in the setting of uncertainty and shifts in available resources is also essential in the face of a poorly understood pathogen. Notably, these challenges have also been observed and experienced during the COVID-19 pandemic. We next describe these challenges as they relate to care for patients during the COVID-19 pandemic and report on innovations and potential solutions to these challenges identified by palliative care teams across the U.S.

## The Surge Framework of Palliative Care Delivery and General Considerations during Pandemics

This section describes the Downar and colleagues' palliative care Surge Framework, a framework based on critical care surge planning during crises [18] developed to inform palliative care delivery during pandemics [19]. The framework was modified by Etkind in a systematic review in response to COVID-19 (Fig. 18.1) [18–20]. The

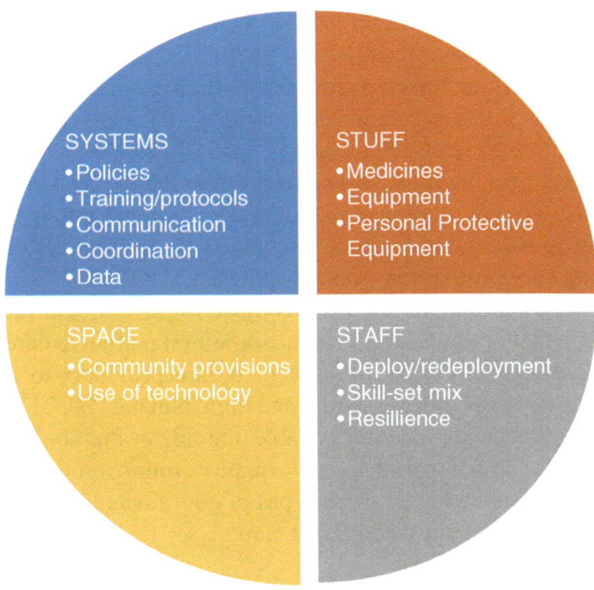


**Fig. 18.1** The Surge Framework adapted from Downar and Etkind [18–20] for palliative care delivery during pandemics includes four components: systems, stuff, staff and space. (With Permission from Elsevier [18–20])

Surge framework includes four components of the delivery of palliative care that require adjustments to facilitate patient care during pandemics: systems; stuff; staff; and space. We describe each component below.

## *Systems: Flexibility, Transparency, and Accountability*

Systems provide overarching structure and context to the delivery of palliative care and direct how the team functions during the pandemic. Effective system responses to pandemics must address communication strategies, coordination, and data collection procedures to track changing health care needs. Systems also must consider training to meet the demands for palliative care as a result of the pandemic [20], from up-training of non-specialist palliative staff in the delivery of palliative interventions (i.e., primary palliative care) to infection prevention practices for specialty palliative care teams. Increased demands for palliative care services, high patient acuity, and patient and provider turnover and subsequent staffing pressures may inevitably lead to non-specialist staff delivering primary palliative care interventions including symptom management, therapeutic communication, discussions of goals of care, and bereavement counseling. Additional requirements involve training of palliative care team members in infection prevention practices and procedures. Systems also include hospital and palliative care team policies and protocols. Policies may include visitation restrictions (such as who is allowed at the bedside of a hospitalized patient, under what circumstances and for what length of time), availability of remote access telehealth technologies (i.e., video-enabled tablets) for expanded home monitoring, and changes to hospital admission criteria.

High functioning systems of palliative care delivery during pandemics embrace and facilitate communication within and across organizations [20]. For example, institutions and organizations may share protocols and procedures specifically developed and/or tested to respond to the pandemic. These systems may establish institutional relationships that allow palliative care teams to share patient care practices and lessons learned, disseminating experiences that may blunt the steep learning curves of systems not yet exposed to pandemic strains. The creation of standard operating procedures, such as those for safe opioid prescribing to relieve dyspnea, and that organize and structure common palliative care tasks, can streamline workload and allow for non-palliative care providers to perform palliative care tasks during times of low staffing and high demand [20, 21]. Finally, uniform data collection tools and procedures enable ongoing evaluation and iterative care quality monitoring, benchmarking, and quality improvement. However, it has not been determined whether these types of coordinated efforts to reduce unknowns is associated with improved patient care.

## *Stuff: Supplies, Medications and Equipment*

As with all aspects of the healthcare response to a pandemic, palliative care providers require essential supplies: the "stuff" to assure evidence-based, patient-centered delivery of palliative care. Acquiring appropriate amounts of supplies also requires planning and contingency planning for projected or anticipated increases in the demand for supplies and addressing supply shortages while proposing alternate regimens. Healthcare providers, whether palliative medicine specialists or general/frontline clinicians, require adequate supplies of palliative medications like opioids for pain or dyspnea and scopolamine for the management of secretions. Supplies to administer medications, such as intravenous line insertion kits, tubing and flushes for intravenous access, are also essential for palliative support of patients during a pandemic. Finally, adequate personal protective equipment (PPE) supplies must be available as well to ensure the safety and effectiveness of palliative support during a pandemic.

## *Staff: Personnel, Skill Sets, Alternative Deployment and Resilience*

Ensuring adequate staffing of the palliative care team during a pandemic is essential. Planning for staffing needs includes considerations of community needs, staff skill mix, and staff resilience [20]. While immediate staffing needs during a pandemic take priority, staffing considerations must also include the ability to scale staffing up or down, or the ability to have trainees function independently when warranted, to meet fluctuating demands for services, risk for staff absences due to illness, and to prepare for potential initial and secondary surges in infection rates. Hiring clinicians to join the palliative care team who have the skills necessary to meet patient needs is also an important consideration. Staffing may also involve training non-specialist clinicians to provide primary palliative care during times of high staffing demands. Addressing the palliative care needs of patients during a pandemic requires a mix of skills and clinicians, including services provided by psychologists and chaplains. For example, these team members may be able to help address increased patient and caregiver psychological distress related to isolation precautions, rapid and unexpected decompensation of infected patients, as well as increased spiritual and/or existential distress [22].

Heightened anxiety and risks of depression during pandemics not only affect patients and families, but also clinicians [22–26]. Clinicians may feel stressed, overworked, or fearful of infecting themselves or others [27]. Support for palliative care providers is critical to facilitating ongoing patient care and to avoid burnout [28]. Supporting clinician resilience requires helping them to find meaning in their work personally, clinically, and structurally, with opportunities for engagement with healthcare systems to enact needed changes in real time (Table 18.3). Responsive staffing models that incorporate "down time" for clinicians even in times of highest demand and provide staff with opportunities for self-care are two strategies to build resilience among clinicians [29].

## *Space: Meeting the Demands of Patients in the Community and the Role of Technology*

Space encompasses both the in-person and virtual, or telehealth, space needed for palliative clinicians to deliver their care. Telehealth is the use of telecommunication to provide healthcare using telephone and/or videoconference technologies [30–32]. Due to infection control practices required during pandemic responses, space

**Table 18.3** Strategies to build resilience among palliative care clinicians during a pandemic

| |
|---|
| Responsive staffing models that allow for "down time" |
| Provide opportunities for self-care |
| Offer mental health and/or employee health services |
| Think "outside the box" for the delivery of self-care services<br>Virtual chaplain and/or mental health services<br>Virtual social gatherings (e.g., book clubs, happy hours) |
| Offer opportunities to express themselves, channel creativity (e.g., poetry writing) |
| Give clinicians agency in how care is delivered and how it can be improved<br>Daily "huddles" focused on care improvement<br>Opportunities for advocacy at the local, state, and federal level |

to practice palliative care may be limited to telephone or virtual telehealth visits as necessary. For example, during the COVID-19 pandemic, many palliative care teams moved to using telehealth as infection rates surged across the U.S., only to return to gradually phased increases in-person visits as infection rates declined [33]. Palliative care teams used several techniques to make telehealth visits more patient-centered, including discussing pitfalls of remote technology upfront, scheduling "test calls" with patients and families to familiarize them with the technology [34], and prioritizing videoconference over telephone visits when feasible so that the body language and emotions of the patient and family could be seen and empathy more effectively shared by the clinician [35]. These examples highlight that during a pandemic, palliative care teams need space to work, but also flexibility to provide services in several settings as the pandemic enters different phases.

## Surge Framework Case Example: Palliative Care Workforce and Delivery During the COVID-19 Pandemic

The COVID-19 pandemic has exposed ongoing workforce and delivery challenges in palliative care. Care of patients with COVID-19 illuminated the importance of palliative care for acutely and critically ill patients suffering from the disease. Using the essential elements of palliative care described in the prior section, we highlight several challenges to palliative care delivery using the Surge Framework [18–20]. In each section, we describe challenges experienced by palliative care teams, and in many cases the solutions developed by these teams, in response to the COVID-19 pandemic.

### *Systems*

Fundamental to palliative care teams' ability to respond to and care for patients during a pandemic are the systems, policies, and procedures that determine care delivery. While pandemics are unquestionably times of great duress, novel models of palliative care delivery have emerged as a result of the COVID-19 pandemic. For example, in New York City, Mount Sinai's Palliative Care Team created the PAlliaTive Care Help (PATCH-24) [21] telephone line to support clinicians on the frontlines caring for COVID-19 patients, an adaptive program that was planned and implemented within one week [36, 37]. After initiation and initial feedback, the program quickly flexed from providing clinician-to-clinician consultation services to clinician-to-patient and family services through telehealth. This change was made after the team realized that frontline clinicians did not have the time necessary to include palliative care services in their essential patient care activities. The adaptation of the program required additional staff, and what began as two palliative care physicians providing consultative services to frontline providers increased to five clinicians providing direct patient and family services with medical students triaging telephone calls. Adaptive and novel, Mount Sinai's response to the COVID-19 pandemic is a prime example of the systems that were already in place that allowed the palliative care team to rapidly change how specialty palliative care was delivered and by whom.

## *Stuff*

During the COVID-19 pandemic, many hospitals reported shortages of medications used for relieving symptoms of patients with COVID-19, including medications to treat breathlessness, cough, and agitation, including opioids and benzodiazepines [36]. In response, hospitals, healthcare systems, and medical associations sent letters to governmental organizations, including the Drug Enforcement Administration and the Strategic National Stockpile, requesting additional medications and supplies. Healthcare systems also requested increases in national stockpiles to prepare for future escalations of infection and hospitalization rates [36]. The availability of supplies during the pandemic continues to be a pressing and unresolved issue after eight months and three waves of the COVID-19 pandemic in the U.S.

## *Staff*

In March and April 2020, the rapid acceleration of COVID-19 infection rates in New York City placed tremendous pressure on area hospitals responding to patient surges and increased demands for palliative care services [38, 39]. In response to this challenge, Mount Sinai's PATCH-24 program enlisted medical students and palliative care clinicians across the U.S. to triage palliative care telephone calls and to assist with palliative care consultations via telehealth. The palliative care team at Mount Sinai also used community health workers to provide care to patients with COVID-19 who were seriously ill but wished to stay home [37]. Other healthcare systems "repurposed" existing staff, detailing non-palliative care staff to palliative care tasks. For example, MedStar Health system serving Washington, D.C. and Baltimore, utilized physical and occupational therapists to act as advance care planning facilitators and to deliver advance care planning interventions via video telehealth visits to patients and families [37]. To address workforce shortages and to reinforce palliative skills for non-specialists engaging in primary palliative care, the creators of VitalTalk, a serious illness communication training program, developed a VitalTalk playbook for providers caring for COVID-19 patients [40, 41]. Online toolkits comprised of symptom management algorithms and other clinical resources for clinicians providing primary palliative care were also developed [42, 43].

### *Space*

Bed shortages, isolation needs, and the need for rooms equipped with appropriate filtering to protect healthcare providers from contracting COVID-19 limited the space available for in-person interactions between patients, families, and palliative care teams. Space limitations and preparations because of the COVID-19 pandemic necessitated a transition to telehealth for most routine, outpatient, or consultative healthcare interactions, including palliative care delivery [21, 37]. Palliative care teams utilizing telehealth during the COVID-19 pandemic have noted major benefits. These include a means of providing care during pandemic conditions [44, 45], reducing patient isolation in the intensive care unit and facilitating communication (e.g., patient-family, caregiver-provider) [23], and as a means to increase access to palliative care clinicians who can act as resources for other frontline clinicians [24, 25]. Disadvantages to telehealth include privacy concerns [46], technical issues and failures [34], lack of institutional leadership or resources for telehealth [31], challenges of establishing and maintaining a therapeutic relationship remotely [46], as well as challenges to cross-state licensure and reimbursement [30–32].

## Palliative Care for Patients with COVID-19: Preserving Patient-Centeredness During a Pandemic

Even with vetted frameworks, thoughtful preparation, and protocols in place before providers are immersed in a pandemic, the unfamiliar and alien nature of health care delivery during a pandemic may further add to the psychosocial stressors for members of healthcare teams. Patients with chronic pulmonary diseases may be particularly concerned about access to critical supplies like supplemental oxygen or breathing treatments routinely used to maintain their level of function. Patients may also feel disinclined to seek care during their own personal emergencies for fear of exposing themselves to greater risk of contracting a virus and/or concerns about being further isolated from their loved ones [34, 47, 48]. Through the lens of the COVID-19 pandemic, we provide an overview of a realignment to patient-centered care during a pandemic and identify areas that may require modifications.

### *What and How Things Changed During the COVID-19 Pandemic*

There has been a growing shift over the past several decades to prioritize patient and family engagement in and presence during the delivery of health care in the U.S., including during hospitalizations and intensive care unit admissions [49, 50]. This engagement promotes informed decision-making, fosters trust and enhances alignment between patients/surrogate decision makers (SDMs) and clinical providers and is associated with greater patient- and family-reported satisfaction [51, 52]. This type of involvement of family members has been a central tenet of palliative care to facilitate shared decision-making between patients/SDMs and clinical teams [33].

Practically overnight in March 2020, the COVID-19 pandemic upended the progress made to invite families/SDMs into acute care settings in the U.S. The initial surge affected the East Coast, New Orleans, and the Pacific Northwest and led healthcare facilities to severely restrict, if not completely eliminate, all family/SDM visits in hospitals and nursing homes. Patients entered hospital emergency departments alone, where they would remain isolated from their families/SDMs for days, weeks and even months until discharge, for those who survived the hospitalization. Developing rapport between families/SDMs and clinicians was limited to telephone or videoconference exchanges. Everything from routine updates to weighty goals-of-care conversations, often involving end-of-life decision-making, were conducted using telephone and/or video conferencing, if there were opportunities for them to take place at all. Families/SDMs relied on telephone or grainy video chats in attempts to comfort and support their loved one [53]. Further uncertainty and threats of scarce resources including symptom-targeted medications (opioids), mechanical ventilators and physical space for patients to be treated, hung over these impersonal exchanges during hospitalizations and nursing home stays [36, 54]. When decisions were made to forgo additional attempts to provide life-sustaining treatments, patients were routinely dying separated from their families. Medical teams were findings themselves substituting for families to provide support during the patient's final hours and minutes, while also providing end-of-life care [55–57].

## *Palliative Care as a Service to Promote Patient-Centered Care for Future Surges and Pandemics*

In response to these challenges, a multidisciplinary coalition of 35 organizations including clinicians, patient advocates, and other key stakeholders developed guidelines maintaining focus on patient-centered care, prioritizing high-quality relationship-building between patients/SDMs and clinicians during pandemics [53, 58]. The guidelines encouraged proactive communication by clinicians regarding visiting policies, and possible exceptions to those policies, in addition to frank discussions on patient condition and prognostic uncertainty (Table 18.4). The guidelines also expect families/SDMs to abide by visitation restrictions, hand hygiene, and mask policies in the interest of their loved one's safety, as well as in the interests of the hospital community at large.

In addition to these guidelines, palliative care principles also provide a framework for communication strategies and specific language for clinicians to use during the care of patients during a pandemic [40, 42, 59]. For several patients and families/SDMs requiring specialty care, palliative medicine specialists continue to

**Table 18.4** Guidelines for promoting family presence during pandemics [53]

| Principle | Considerations |
|---|---|
| Assess, and reassess restrictions based on facts | Community spread<br>Availability of personal protective equipment (PPE) |
| Minimize risk | Screen visitors<br>Assess patients' needs for family presence and consider lowest risk models possible |
| Proactive, compassionate communication | Clear, consistent and culturally-informed messaging |
| Establish compassionate exceptions | Timely decisions made on a case-by-case basis especially for circumstances such as pediatric patients, childbirth or end-of-life |
| Support meaningful connections when physical ones are not possible | Use of technology<br>Regular, dependable check-ins and updates |
| Inform and educate | Changing landscape for infection prevention, visitation, prognosis |
| Enlist families as members of the care team | Ensure protection for family members |
| Enhance discharge planning and follow up | Routine follow-up via telehealth and/or labs as indicated |

contribute invaluable support during the COVID-19 pandemic [56, 58, 60]. In addition to symptom control, goals of care conversations, and bereavement support, palliative experts may also assist in re-evaluating designated SDMs when initial designees find themselves unable or unwilling to continue to fulfill their role.

## Common Symptoms in Hospitalized COVID-19 Patients, Decedents and Survivors

Symptom assessment and management is essential throughout a patient's trajectory with COVID-19. Cough, dyspnea, agitation, delirium and fatigue are frequently reported among hospitalized patients with COVID-19 (Table 18.5), although prevalence varies with study design and the patient population of interest [36, 60–62, 64].

In addition to respiratory symptoms, neurologic symptoms may affect up to 80% of COVID-19 patients during their disease course and up to 93% of patients with severe disease [63]. Neurologic symptoms have been associated with poorer quality of life among survivors at hospital discharge [63]. In a case series of 101 patients from the United Kingdom, agitation and delirium were reported in 43% and 24%, respectively [60], of COVID-19 patients referred to palliative care. Agitation and delirium may be particularly difficult to manage due to risks to the patient, including compliance with respiratory support such as usual flow and high flow oxygen through nasal cannula, airway clearance treatment with nebulized medications, and non-invasive and invasive mechanical ventilation [62, 64]. Agitation and delirium also pose a significant risk to healthcare providers, as confused and agitated patients

**Table 18.5** Common distressing symptoms for hospitalized patients with COVID-19 [60–63]

| Symptom | General Prevalence (est.) | Prevalence in dying patients |
|---|---|---|
| Cough | 38–81% | 4–75% |
| Dyspnea | 18–71% | 84% |
| Fatigue/malaise | 21–70% | 9–20% |
| Agitation | 43–49% | 43% |
| Delirium | 24–77% | 24–77% |
| Diarrhea | 4–15% | 3–17% |
| Myalgias/pain | 12–52% | 10–23% |

may try to remove PPE from themselves or their providers, or may attempt to leave their isolation care setting. Management of symptoms in patients with COVID-19 appears to be responsive to usual doses of opioids and benzodiazepines to relieve dyspnea and agitation [58, 62], for example, but higher doses of antipsychotics may be required than typically used in older patients with multiple chronic diseases [64]. Reassuringly, end-of-life care for patients dying with COVID-19 does not appear to deviate from existing guideline-based practices for end-of-life care [65, 66].

Lingering symptom are increasingly reported among COVID-19 survivors. Symptoms most frequently reported include fatigue, and neurologic, and respiratory symptoms. In a phone survey of 120 COVID-19 survivors from France, fatigue, cough, and dyspnea were most frequently reported after more than 100 days from hospital admission for COVID-19 [64, 67]. Memory loss was reported by more than one-third of survivors, and sleep and attention disorders were also reported by 31% and 27% of survivors, respectively. Symptoms did not appear to vary with intensive care unit stays. Comprehensive assessments of symptom frequencies, intensities, effective treatments and long-term effects, beyond primary focus on symptom relief for those dying of COVID-19, are required as the pandemic persists, especially as the number of patients with prolonged COVID-19 recovery (sometimes referred to as “long-haulers”) grows.

While the evidence has increasingly found the benefits of earlier palliative care referral for patients with cancer as well as other conditions [68, 69], ongoing difficulty in the recognition of unmet palliative care needs and workforce limitations have contributed to late referrals to palliative care for most dying patients [70, 71]. As we might expect, these limitations to palliative care delivery in the setting of a global pandemic have remained or have been magnified. Unfortunately, palliative medicine consultants’ involvement is often relatively late, occurring in the last 2–3 days of life, a challenge to therapeutic relationship building between specialty palliative care teams and families/SDMs [62, 66].

Technology can facilitate shared decision-making and patient-centered care during a pandemic [72]. However such technology may also exacerbate disparities in vulnerable populations, including older persons and persons of color. For example, reliance on video-based teleconferencing may not be available for families without video-equipped devices (e.g., tablet computers, smart phones) or access to high-speed internet [73, 74].

### *Oxygen Use for Patients with Respiratory Diseases and COVID-19*

The role of supplemental oxygen in patients with breathlessness from chronic lung diseases has largely been reserved for patients only with sustained arterial partial pressure of oxygen less than 55 mm Hg or peripheral oxygen saturations less than 88% [75, 76]. For patients with respiratory failure due to COVID-19, guidelines suggest supplemental oxygen use for palliative purposes in patients with peripheral oxygen saturations less than 90%, although there have been varying opinions on targeted oxygenation levels and no specific evaluation of the needs for patients with chronic pulmonary diseases [77]. For patients transitioning to end-of-life care, supplemental oxygen should be identified as a life-sustaining treatment with indicated use only to maximize comfort, rather than to achieve normal oxygenation levels. This may be particularly relevant for patients who had been sustained on advanced oxygenation and/or ventilatory supports such as high-flow nasal oxygen or noninvasive or invasive mechanical ventilation, and explicit discussions acknowledging the down-titration of these supports to comfort only, with likely discontinuation of these life-sustaining treatments as comfort goals are achieved, are important to prepare patients and families/SDMs regarding end-of-life care.

## Ethical Considerations to Palliative Care during a Pandemic

Pandemics may shift ethical considerations and priorities in healthcare. For example, the impact of the COVID-19 pandemic threatened patient autonomy, a guiding ethical principle in medicine, while prioritizing the good the population. Clinicians may be tasked with attempting to save the most lives possible, while patient preferences are deprioritized during the crisis response. Standards of care shift from conventional, patient-centered provision of healthcare to contingency standards, where the usual standards of care are provided, but with modifications to their delivery, e.g., staffing and rooming expansion to increase capacity to care for more ventilated patients. In the direst public health emergencies, crisis standards of care may be deemed necessary by health system leadership and/or state governments. Under crisis standards of care, scarce resources are rationed according to unbiased triage grading and frameworks, ideally developed before the crisis (Fig. 18.2) [55, 78].

During the COVID-19 pandemic some communities were stretched close to or beyond their limits in terms of life-sustaining resources (e.g., mechanical ventilation, extracorporeal membrane oxygenation (ECMO)), requiring healthcare systems to consider fair, equitable, and transparent approaches to decide how to allocate limited resources to their patients [79]. Unilateral Do-Not-Resuscitate (DNR) orders were permitted during surge phases across multiple healthcare systems due to concerns over staff safety and practical barriers to timely initiation of cardiopulmonary

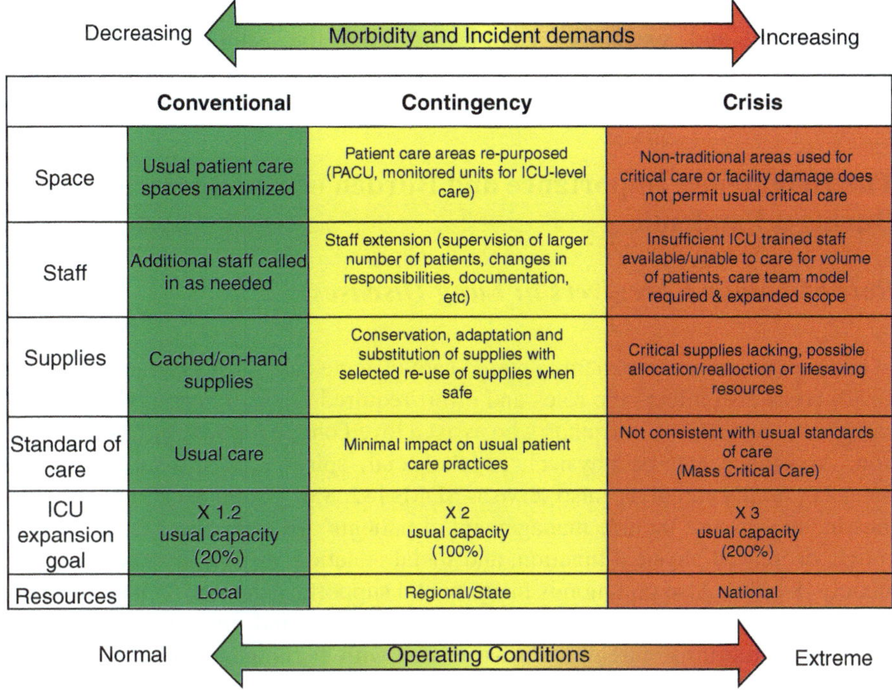


**Fig. 18.2** Adjustments health systems make as they respond to population needs under conventional, contingency, and crises standards of care during a pandemic. (With Permission from Elsevier [78]). COVID-19 coronavirus disease, CPR cardiopulmonary resuscitation, ICU intensive care unit

resuscitation (CPR) while requiring strict adherence to PPE use [80]. While existing guidelines for ethical and equitable approaches to managing scarcity during a pandemic were readily available [81], the real-time strains on clinicians as they struggled to implement triage and scarce resource allocation guidelines likely affected decision-making in unmeasurable ways for all patients in moments of peak surge, regardless of COVID-19 diagnosis. For example, a newly admitted patient with multiple chronic conditions including chronic pulmonary disease, who had repeated hospital and ICU stays in the prior months, presents with dyspneic crisis. Upon evaluating, triaging, and making treatment recommendations for the patient, a clinician practicing in a surge facility under strain, but not yet functioning under crisis standards of care, may frame prognosis and recommended goals of care towards end-of-life care rather than repeating the level of care provided to the patient during conventional care times. Without officially operating under crisis standards of care, recommendations and surrogate decision making may have been influenced by the existing system-level scarcity rather than individual patient's preferences. There remain unanswered and potentially unknowable aspects about the impact of the pandemic on goals of care counseling between health care providers and patients/

SDMs. These aspects of how care was delivered and decided may serve as additional burden and sources of complicated grief that family caregivers carry with them.

## The Heightened Importance and Burden of Family Caregivers During a Pandemic

### *Role of Family Caregivers in Lung Diseases*

In addition to strains on patient-centered care in acute care settings, responding to a health crisis also affects the roles and effort required of family caregivers. Family caregivers are relatives or friends who assist a loved one living with a serious condition. Assistance can be physical, psychosocial, spiritual, informational, and/or financial; family caregivers also serve as SDMs [82, 83]. Common caregiving activities in lung disease include management of patients' pain, fatigue, breathlessness, cough, decreased physical function, and social isolation, as well as depression and anxiety [84–86]. Also common is instrumental support, such as providing transportation and childcare, filling medication prescriptions, and preparing meals [83]. While often fulfilling, caregiving is associated with disrupted home and work routines, changes in family roles and relationships, economic burden and caregiver health concerns [82]. Caregiving also has a wide range of emotions associated with it, some positive (e.g., love, gratitude), and many negative (e.g., anxiety, burnout) [83, 87].

Possibly compounding family caregivers' distress that may be magnified during a pandemic is the lack of support from clinicians to perform and sustain their caregiving role [86]. The experiences of family caregivers often reflect those of patients in terms of fluctuating physical, psychosocial, and spiritual wellbeing, which may impact caregiving motivation and ability [88, 89]. Clinicians do not always recognize this interdependent relationship and may not consider the family caregiver-patient dyad when determining a therapeutic strategy or care planning [90–92]. Consequently, care plans may not be designed in a way that promotes successful implementation or maintenance [93]. In management of lung disease, and especially during a pandemic, care plans should address both family caregiver and patient support [89, 94].

### *Challenges of Family Caregiving in a Pandemic*

Under pandemic conditions, the role of family caregivers becomes even more critical [57], yet their ability to provide support is further stretched. Caregiving challenges may be heightened due to increased caregiving burden, financial insecurity, and as with COVID-19, isolation-related stress and mental and emotional strain [95]. These challenges affect families to varying degrees based on characteristics such as income level, mental health and/or special needs, experiences of racism or marginalization [95], experience and resilience as a caregiver, and health literacy [96]. Below we review these challenges.

***Caregiving burden*** Caregiving burden for family members of patients living with lung disease can increase for multiple reasons. For example, minimizing disruption to patients' essential treatments is a priority [97]. Thus, decisions about attending or postponing appointments are difficult to make and necessitate weighing exposure to infection in health care facilities with the risks of modifying or delaying treatment [98]. These are not straightforward decisions with an obvious "right" answer, and family caregivers may struggle as they attempt to make the best decisions with or for their loved ones [99]

Instrumental caregiving tasks (i.e., tasks related to day-to-day life) can likewise become more difficult during a pandemic. For example, connecting with a clinician by phone may take longer than usual due to higher call volume. Filling a prescription may become more complicated due to supply chain issues or the need to socially distance. For patients requiring hospitalization, family caregivers may not be permitted in the hospital and are thus unable to help care for patients and to serve as their advocates [100]. Additionally, family caregivers may not be able to fulfill their usual caregiving roles due to lack of PPE, inability to be physically present with the patient due to travel restrictions, being ill themselves, or being an essential worker with limited time for family caregiving [101].

***Financial insecurity*** Financial insecurity can also inhibit family caregivers' ability to provide support. During a pandemic, financial insecurity can occur due to job loss, reduced work hours, and increased cost of food, supplies, and services, among other reasons. In addition to increasing family caregivers' financial burden through reduced means to pay for health care, during the COVID-19 pandemic, financial concerns have been associated with worse mental health [102], which may also affect family caregivers' ability to provide care.

***Social isolation and changed routines*** Stressors related to isolation in the home include those related to crowding, loneliness, changed routines [95], adjustments to prior existing caregiving roles, and to compromised health routines [103]. Families may experience changes in terms of who is in the home, daily schedules, family rituals, and eating and sleeping behaviors. These shifts may negatively affect caregiving tasks as well as stamina for caregiving. The increased susceptibility to complications from an infectious disease among patients with lung diseases [97] necessitates vigilance and problem-solving around managing competing priorities between care delivered to a family member and self-care when isolation precautions are in place.

***Mental and emotional strain*** Feelings of anxiety, depression, and uncertainty that accompany life during a pandemic can be overwhelming and may inhibit family caregivers' ability to function optimally in their caregiving role. Such feelings may also exacerbate any pre-existing mental health issues [104], deepening mental and emotional strain. Reduced access to in-person mental health care and social services during the COVID-19 pandemic affects family caregivers' ability to obtain support and treatment, complicating self-care efforts and potentially the sustainability of the family caregiver role.

## *Opportunities for Support and Growth*

Any combination of the above challenges can increase overall caregiving burden. Table 18.6 summarizes recommendations to support family caregivers during the COVID-19 pandemic, which may also be helpful in future crises.

An important goal is to increase family caregivers' resilience to manage the challenges of caring for a loved one with lung disease as well as themselves amidst the added stress of a pandemic. Resilience is a constellation of behaviors that prompt individuals to persist and move forward despite adversity [105]. Behaviors include active problem-solving, seeking social support, sharing one's struggles with others, tolerating uncertainty, and generating hope for the future [106]. Resilience can be learned and is most strongly predicted by the cultivation of social support [107] and adaptive meaning making [106, 108]. With appropriate and ongoing support, family caregivers may experience "post-traumatic growth", meaning to thrive and not just survive amid the adversity of a pandemic [95].

To facilitate resilience, assessment of family caregivers' and patients' needs as a dyad should be routine practice for all palliative clinicians. Special consideration should be given to how the nature or degree of needs may change during a pandemic, as well as to the availability of resources and the feasibility of family caregivers' accessing

**Table 18.6** How to support family caregivers during COVID-19 [99]

| |
|---|
| Consider family caregivers in discussions of personal protective equipment (PPE) and provide guidance about its use and efficacy |
| Implement risk assessment questions or checklists to assess family caregiver capacity for care in the home before and after onset of COVID-19 (for patient, family caregiver or both) |
| Develop telehealth capacity to assess and treat patients and include family caregivers in these encounters |
| Encourage families to have difficult but necessary conversations with loved ones about their wishes for care if they become critically ill |
| Remind family caregivers of the extraordinary circumstances brought on by the pandemic, thank them, reassure them, and encourage them to leverage their social networks in helpful and safe ways |
| Familiarize family caregivers with guidance from major caregiving organizations on COVID-19 resources (e.g., the Center to Advance Palliative Care, the Family Caregiver Alliance, and the National Alliance for Caregiving) as well as with local organizations that may assist with resources such as meal delivery, resource navigation, and social support calls |

them. Communication and shared decision-making with patients and family caregivers can assist with identification of needs and creation of a care plan that addresses both patients and family caregivers and are activities that can inherently provide support.

## Palliative Communication and Shared Decision-Making Under Pandemic Conditions

Palliative communication challenges related to lung disease reflect the range of communication complexities in serious illness, including multidisciplinary communication around physical, psychosocial, and spiritual needs, and advanced care planning. These complexities may be amplified in lung disease due to potentially unclear prognoses, potential rapid decline, and the frequent delivery of bad news [109]. Continuous and coordinated communication is central to improving the quality of patients' and family caregivers' care experience [109, 110].

Foundational to palliative care [111], shared decision-making is a bi-directional exchange of information and discussion between a clinician and patient (and possibly others) that leads to a decision that reflects reasonable treatment options in the context of patients' preferences and priorities [112]. While there is some evidence that shared decision-making can contribute to higher patient satisfaction, less decisional conflict, and concordance between patients' values and treatment plans [113–115], evidence for shared decision-making in lung disease is still emerging [113, 116, 117]. Higher quality shared decision-making, including better prepared clinicians, more time allocated for shared-decision making, and use of decision aids, is needed [118, 119].

### *Obstacles to Palliative Communication During a Pandemic*

Pandemic conditions can inhibit quality communication and shared decision-making among patients, family caregivers, and clinicians for several reasons. These include patients' inability to communicate due to mechanical ventilation, dyspnea, delirium, hearing impairments or other barriers. Other conditions include the absence of family caregivers at the bedside, PPE that can impede rapport-building, isolation precautions that limit the occurrence or length of interpersonal interactions, reliance on telehealth, clinicians' lack of time to conduct comprehensive discussions due to high caseloads, and high anxiety and uncertainty that may curtail full engagement in a discussion [23, 120, 121]. Additionally, unreliable information about the pandemic, i.e., partial information, conflicting information, misinformation and disinformation [122], such as how the infectious disease may spread, who is affected, and how, complicates decision-making because it is difficult to make choices without accurate information.

## *Shared Decision-Making During a Pandemic: Magnification and Maximization*

During a pandemic, difficult decisions must be made while considering public health recommendations for disease containment and mitigation and allocation of resources, magnifying the imperative for shared decision-making [120]. Aligning patients' choices with their values and available effective therapies, reducing unnecessary and unwanted health care use, and promoting consistent practices among clinicians become paramount [123]. Ongoing values-based, patient-centered shared decision-making must be undertaken to ensure goal-concordant care and to inform choices around resource allocation [124]. Clinicians must acknowledge the limits of what is known about an infectious disease and must transparently share uncertainties with patients and families [125] to promote autonomy in decision-making. Such practices can assuage some of the difficulties of shared decision-making during a crisis.

Although established shared decision-making practices apply, a pandemic encourages re-evaluation of current practices [120] and challenges clinicians to innovate. Strategies to support shared decision-making informed by the COVID-19 pandemic include virtual shared decision-making using telehealth approaches and the use of shared decision-making to mitigate misinformation propagated by social media and informal, potentially unreliable sources of information [120]. Specialized guides to promote communication and shared decision-making during the COVID-19 pandemic have emerged quickly and have been disseminated, for example, communication strategies to use under crises standards of care (Table 18.7) [41,

**Table 18.7** Sample communication strategies to use under crisis standards of care

| CALMER: A Talking Map for COVID-Related Proactive Planning | SHARE: A Talking Map for Explaining Resource Allocation |
|---|---|
| **C**heck-In<br>*"How are you doing with all of this?"* | **S**how the guideline<br>*"Here's what our institution/system/region is doing for patients with this condition."* |
| **A**sk about COVID<br>*"What have you been thinking with COVID and your situation?"* | **H**eadline what it means for the patient's care<br>*"So for you, what this means is…"* |
| **L**ay out issues<br>*"Here is something I want us to be prepared for."* | **A**ffirm the care you will provide<br>*"We will be doing [the care plan], and we hope you will recover."* |
| **M**otivate them to choose a proxy and talk about what matters<br>*"Who is your backup person who helps us make decisions if you can't speak?"*<br>*"We're in an extraordinary situation. Given that, what matters to you?"* | **R**espond to emotion<br>*"I can see how it feels unfair."* |
| **E**xpect emotion<br>*"This can be hard to think about."* | **E**mphasize that the same rules apply to everyone<br>*"We are using the same rules with every other patient. We are not singling you out."* |
| **R**ecord the discussion<br>*"I'll write down what you said in the chart."* | |

Back et al. [127]

126, 127]. Strategies born within crises serve as trial-and-error exemplars to guide future response.

While palliative care specialists routinely assist with shared decision-making in the care of seriously ill patients during a pandemic, the strategic use of palliative care specialists [20, 25] as a limited resource must be considered. Palliative care specialists may be consulted to assist with shared decision-making around goals of care [25]. During the COVID-19 pandemic, telehealth approaches have supported such partnerships [34]. Expansion of palliative care resources through the training of non-palliative specialists in serious illness communication [25] has been another strategy to meet the overwhelming demand for complex patient care. Routine palliative care practices have been re-imagined, for example, with the honing of telehealth communication skills, helping to prepare healthcare systems with management of the increased demand for palliative care [19], and attending to clinician self-care under crisis conditions [24]. These innovations will reverberate in the post-COVID-19 world and will hopefully see healthcare systems better prepared for future pandemics.

## Conclusion

From the Bubonic plague to COVID-19, clinicians providing palliative care have lessened symptoms, eased suffering, and brought solace and comfort to patients and families. The lessons learned from these past and current pandemics are many, yet all emphasize the importance of timely palliative care, whether patients are in the hospital or at home, and either through in-person interactions or virtual technology. Pandemics force palliative care teams to adjust and adapt how palliative care is delivered. Moreover, providing palliative care during pandemics requires consideration of additional factors including barriers and opportunities to preserve patient-centeredness, symptom management considerations, ethical considerations, as well as alterations to the role of the family caregiver, palliative communication, and shared decision-making. Yet, some best practices remain relevant, including providing the highest-level care possible to our sickest and most vulnerable patients even amidst the most challenging of times.

## References

1. Carlson A, Riethman M, Gastañaduy P, Lee A, Leung J, Holshue M, et al. Notes from the field: community outbreak of measles—Clark County, Washington, 2018–2019. Morb Mortal Wkly Rep. 2019;68(19):446.
2. Killerby ME, Biggs HM, Midgley CM, Gerber SI, Watson JT. Middle East respiratory syndrome coronavirus transmission. Emerg Infect Dis. 2020;26(2):191–8.
3. Dong E, Du H, Gardner L. An interactive web-based dashboard to track COVID-19 in real time. Lancet Infect Dis. 2020;20(5):533–4.

4. Guilbeau C. End-of-life care in the Western world: where are we now and how did we get here? BMJ Support Palliat Care. 2018;8(2):136–44.
5. Patterson KD, Pyle GF. The geography and mortality of the 1918 influenza pandemic. Bull Hist Med. 1991;65(1):4–21.
6. Spreeuwenberg P, Kroneman M, Paget J. Reassessing the global mortality burden of the 1918 influenza pandemic. Am J Epidemiol. 2018;187(12):2561–7.
7. Jilani TN, Jamil RT, Siddiqui AH. H1N1 influenza (swine flu). StatPearls [Internet]. Treasure Island (FL): StatPearls Publishing; 2020 Jan.
8. Nickol ME, Kindrachuk J. A year of terror and a century of reflection: perspectives on the great influenza pandemic of 1918–1919. BMC Infect Dis. 2019;19(1):117.
9. Paul, W.E. 5th edition. Publisher is Lippincott Williams and Wilkins, Philidelphia, PA.
10. World Health Organization. Report of the review committee on the functioning of the international health regulations (2005) in relation to pandemic (H1N1) 2009. Sixty-fourth World Health Assembly: World Health Organization; 2011:49–50.
11. Chan-Yeung M, Xu RH. SARS: epidemiology. Respirology. 2003;8:S9–14.
12. Dawood FS, Iuliano AD, Reed C, Meltzer MI, Shay DK, Cheng P-Y, et al. Estimated global mortality associated with the first 12 months of 2009 pandemic influenza A H1N1 virus circulation: a modelling study. Lancet Infect Dis. 2012;12(9):687–95.
13. Centers for Disease Control and Prevention. First global estimates of 2009 H1N1 pandemic mortality released by CDC-led collaboration. Atlanta: Centers for Disease Control and Prevention; 2012.
14. Taubenberger JK, Morens DM. 1918 influenza: the mother of all pandemics. Emerg Infect Dis. 2006;12(1):15–22.
15. Taubenberger JK. The origin and virulence of the 1918 "Spanish" influenza virus. Proc Am Philos Soc. 2006;150(1):86–112.
16. Zhong N-S, Wong GW. Epidemiology of severe acute respiratory syndrome (SARS): adults and children. Paediatr Respir Rev. 2004;5(4):270–4.
17. Leong IY, Lee AO, Ng TW, Lee LB, Koh NY, Yap E, et al. The challenge of providing holistic care in a viral epidemic: opportunities for palliative care. Palliat Med. 2004;18(1):12–8.
18. Christian MD, Devereaux AV, Dichter JR, Geiling JA, Rubinson L. Definitive care for the critically ill during a disaster: current capabilities and limitations: from a Task Force for Mass Critical Care summit meeting. Chest. 2008;133(5):8S–17S.
19. Downar J, Seccareccia D. Palliating a pandemic: "all patients must be cared for". J Pain Symptom Manage. 2010;39(2):291–5.
20. Etkind SN, Bone AE, Lovell N, Cripps RL, Harding R, Higginson IJ, et al. The role and response of palliative care and hospice services in epidemics and pandemics: a rapid review to inform practice during the COVID-19 pandemic. J Pain Symptom Manage. 2020;60(1):e31–40.
21. Ankuda CK, Woodrell CD, Meier DE, Morrison RS, Chai E. A beacon for dark times: palliative care support during the coronavirus pandemic. NEJM Catalyst Innov Care Deliv; 2020.
22. Gesi C, Carmassi C, Cerveri G, Carpita B, Cremone IM, Dell'Osso L. Complicated grief: what to expect after the coronavirus pandemic. Front Psych. 2020;11:489.
23. Akgün KM, Shamas TL, Feder SL, Schulman-Green D. Communication strategies to mitigate fear and suffering among COVID-19 patients isolated in the ICU and their families. Heart Lung J Cardiopulmon Acute Care. 2020;49(4):344–5.
24. Akgün KM, Collett D, Feder SL, Shamas T, Schulman-Green D. Sustaining frontline ICU healthcare workers during the COVID-19 pandemic and beyond. Heart Lung J Cardiopulmon Acute Care. 2020;49(4):346–7.
25. Feder S, Akgün KM, Schulman-Green D. Palliative care strategies offer guidance to clinicians and comfort for COVID-19 patient and families. Heart Lung. 2020;49(3):227–8.
26. Sasangohar F, Jones SL, Masud FN, Vahidy FS, Kash BA. Provider burnout and fatigue during the COVID-19 pandemic: lessons learned from a high-volume intensive care unit. Anesth Analg. 2020;131:106–11.

27. Liu Q, Luo D, Haase JE, Guo Q, Wang XQ, Liu S, et al. The experiences of health-care providers during the COVID-19 crisis in China: a qualitative study. Lancet Glob Health. 2020;8:e790–8.
28. Unadkat S, Farquhar M. Doctors' wellbeing: self-care during the covid-19 pandemic. BMJ. 2020;368:m1150.
29. Dewey C, Hingle S, Goelz E, Linzer M. Supporting clinicians during the COVID-19 pandemic. American College of Physicians; 2020.
30. Calton BA, Rabow MW, Branagan L, Dionne-Odom JN, Parker Oliver D, Bakitas MA, et al. Top ten tips palliative care clinicians should know about telepalliative care. J Palliat Med. 2019;22(8):981–5.
31. Hancock S, Preston N, Jones H, Gadoud A. Telehealth in palliative care is being described but not evaluated: a systematic review. BMC Palliat Care. 2019;18(1):114.
32. Wynne B, LaRosa J. A tell-all on telehealth: where is congress heading next? Commonwealth Fund 2019;16.
33. Abbott J, Johnson D, Wynia M. Ensuring adequate palliative and hospice care during COVID-19 surges. JAMA. 2020;324(14):1393–4.
34. Ritchey KC, Foy A, McArdel E, Gruenewald DA. Reinventing palliative care delivery in the era of COVID-19: how telemedicine can support end of life care. Am J Hosp Palliat Care. 2020;37(11):992–7.
35. Lally K, Kematick BS, Gorman D, Tulsky J. Rapid conversion of a palliative care outpatient clinic to telehealth. JCO Oncol Pract. 2021;17(1):e62–7. 7.
36. Pettus K, Cleary JF, de Lima L, Ahmed E, Radbruch L. Availability of internationally controlled essential medicines in the COVID-19 pandemic. J Pain Symptom Manage. 2020;60(2):e48–51.
37. Hostetter M, Klein S, Tsega M. Palliative care: a vital component of COVID-19 care. Available from: http://features.commonwealthfund.org/palliative-care?utm_source=alert&utm_medium=email&utm_campaign=Delivery%20System%20Reform.
38. Moghadas SM, Shoukat A, Fitzpatrick MC, Wells CR, Sah P, Pandey A, et al. Projecting hospital utilization during the COVID-19 outbreaks in the United States. Proc Natl Acad Sci. 2020;117(16):9122–6.
39. Chidiac C, Feuer D, Naismith J, Flatley M, Preston N. Emergency palliative care planning and support in a COVID-19 pandemic. J Palliat Med. 2020;23(6):752–3.
40. Bowman BA, Back AL, Esch AE, Marshall N. Crisis symptom management and patient communication protocols are important tools for all clinicians responding to COVID-19. J Pain Symptom Manage. 2020;60(2):e98–e100.
41. Back A. COVID-ready communication skills: a playbook of vitaltalk tips. Available from: https://www.vitaltalk.org/guides/covid-19-communication-skills/.
42. deLima TJ, Leiter RE, Abrahm JL, Shameklis JC, Kiser SB, Gelfand SL, et al. Development of a palliative care toolkit for the COVID-19 pandemic. J Pain Symptom Manage. 2020;60(2):e22–e5.
43. Lai L, Sato R, He S, Ouchi K, Leiter R, deLima Thomas J, et al. Usage patterns of a web-based palliative care content platform (PalliCOVID) during the COVID-19 pandemic. J Pain Symptom Manage. 2020;60(4):e20–e7.
44. Rockwell KL, Gilroy AS. Incorporating telemedicine as part of COVID-19 outbreak response systems. Am J Manag Care. 2020;26(4):147–8.
45. Eccleston C, Blyth FM, Dear BF, Fisher EA, Keefe FJ, Lynch ME, et al. Managing patients with chronic pain during the COVID-19 outbreak: considerations for the rapid introduction of remotely supported (eHealth) pain management services. Pain. 2020;161(5):889–93.
46. Steindal SA, Nes AAG, Godskesen TE, Dihle A, Lind S, Winger A, et al. Patients' experiences of telehealth in palliative home care: scoping review. J Med Internet Res. 2020;22(5):e16218.
47. Sha Z, Chang K, Mi J, Liang Z, Hu L, Long F, et al. The impact of the COVID-19 pandemic on lung cancer patients. Ann Palliat Med. 2020;9(5):3373–8.

48. Lou E, Teoh D, Brown K, Blaes A, Holtan SG, Jewett P, et al. Perspectives of cancer patients and their health during the COVID-19 pandemic. PLoS One. 2020;15(10):e0241741.
49. Wiseman SM, Crump T, Cadesky E, Sutherland JM. Addressing the mental health of Canadians waiting for elective surgery: a potential positive post-pandemic legacy. Can J Surg. 2020;63(5):E393–E4.
50. Maurer M, Dardess P, Carman KL, Frazier K, Smeeding L (American Institutes for Research, Washington, DC). Guide to patient and family engagement: environmental scan report [Internet]. Rockville, Agency for Healthcare Research and Quality; 2012. Available from: http://www.ahrq.gov/qual/ptfamilyscan/ptfamilyscan.pdf.
51. The Joint Commission. Advancing effective communication, cultural competence, and patient-and family-centered care: a roadmap for hospitals. 2010. Available from: https://psnet.ahrq.gov/issue/advancing-effective-communication-cultural-competence-and-patient-and-family-centered-care.
52. Cypress BS. Family presence on rounds: a systematic review of literature. Dimens Crit Care Nurs. 2012;31(1):53–64.
53. Stricker KH, Kimberger O, Schmidlin K, Zwahlen M, Mohr U, Rothen HU. Family satisfaction in the intensive care unit: what makes the difference? Intensive Care Med. 2009;35(12):2051–9.
54. Frampton S, Agrawal S, Guastello S. Guidelines for family presence policies during the COVID-19 pandemic. JAMA Health Forum. 2020;1(7):e200807–e.
55. Wynne KJ, Petrova M, Coghlan R. Dying individuals and suffering populations: applying a population-level bioethics lens to palliative care in humanitarian contexts: before, during and after the COVID-19 pandemic. J Med Ethics. 2020;46(8):514–25.
56. Rao A, Kelemen A. Lessons learned from caring for patients with COVID-19 at the end of life. J Palliat Med. 2020. https://doi.org/10.1089/jpm.2020.0251. Epub ahead of print.
57. Hart JL, Turnbull AE, Oppenheim IM, Courtright KR. Family-centered care during the COVID-19 era. J Pain Symptom Manage. 2020;60(2):e93–e7.
58. Janssen DJA, Ekström M, Currow DC, Johnson MJ, Maddocks M, Simonds AK, et al. COVID-19: guidance on palliative care from a European Respiratory Society international task force. Eur Respir J. 2020;56:2002583.
59. Roberts B, Wright SM, Christmas C, Robertson M, Wu DS. COVID-19 pandemic response: development of outpatient palliative care toolkit based on narrative communication. Am J Hosp Palliat Care. 2020;37(11):985–7.
60. Carey I, Vora V, Marsh L, Higginson IJ, Prentice W, Edmonds P, Sleeman KE. Characteristics, symptom management, and outcomes of 101 patients with COVID-19 referred for hospital palliative care. J Pain Symptom Manage. 2020;60(1):e77–81. https://doi.org/10.1016/j.jpainsymman.2020.04.015. Epub 2020 Apr 20. PMID: 32325167; PMCID: PMC7169932.
61. Keeley P, Buchanan D, Carolan C, Pivodic L, Tavabie S, Noble S. Symptom burden and clinical profile of COVID-19 deaths: a rapid systematic review and evidence summary. BMJ Support Palliat Care. 2020 May 28:bmjspcare-2020-002368.
62. Hetherington L, Johnston B, Kotronoulas G, Finlay F, Keeley P, McKeown A. COVID-19 and Hospital Palliative Care - a service evaluation exploring the symptoms and outcomes of 186 patients and the impact of the pandemic on specialist Hospital Palliative Care. Palliat Med. 2020;34(9):1256–62.
63. Liotta EM, Batra A, Clark JR, Shlobin NA, Hoffman SC, Orban ZS, Koralnik IJ. Frequent neurologic manifestations and encephalopathy-associated morbidity in Covid-19 patients. Ann Clin Transl Neurol 2020. https://doi.org/10.1002/acn3.51210. Epub ahead of print.
64. Sanders BJ, Bakar M, Mehta S, Reid MC, Siegler EL, Abrams RC, et al. Hyperactive delirium requires more aggressive management in patients with COVID-19: temporarily rethinking "low and slow". J Pain Symptom Manage. 2020;60(2):e31–e2.
65. Jackson T, Hobson K, Clare H, Weegmann D, Moloughney C, McManus S. End-of-life care in COVID-19: an audit of pharmacological management in hospital inpatients. Palliat Med. 2020;34(9):1235–40.

66. Lovell N, Maddocks M, Etkind SN, Taylor K, Carey I, Vora V, et al. Characteristics, symptom management, and outcomes of 101 patients with COVID-19 referred for hospital palliative care. J Pain Symptom Manage. 2020;60(1):e77–81.
67. Oliosi E, Mallart E, Corre F, Zarrouk V, Moyer JD, Galy A, Honsel V, Fantin B, Nguyen Y. Post-discharge persistent symptoms and health-related quality of life after hospitalization for COVID-19. J Infect. 2020:S0163–4453(20)30562–4. https://doi.org/10.1016/j.jinf.2020.08.029. Epub ahead of print. PMID: 32853602; PMCID: PMC7445491.
68. Quinn KL, Shurrab M, Gitau K, Kavalieratos D, Isenberg SR, Stall NM, et al. Association of receipt of palliative care interventions with health care use, quality of life, and symptom burden among adults with chronic noncancer illness: a systematic review and meta-analysis. JAMA. 2020;324(14):1439–50.
69. Bakitas MA, Dionne-Odom JN, Ejem DB, Wells R, Azuero A, Stockdill ML, et al. Effect of an early palliative care telehealth intervention vs usual care on patients with heart failure: the ENABLE CHF-PC randomized clinical trial. JAMA Intern Med. 2020;180(9):1203–13. https://doi.org/10.1001/jamainternmed.2020.2861. PMID: 32730613; PMCID: PMC7385678.
70. Teno JM, Shu JE, Casarett D, Spence C, Rhodes R, Connor S. Timing of referral to hospice and quality of care: length of stay and bereaved family members' perceptions of the timing of hospice referral. J Pain Symptom Manage. 2007;34(2):120–5.
71. Teno JM, Gozalo P, Trivedi AN, Bunker J, Lima J, Ogarek J, et al. Site of death, place of care, and health care transitions among US Medicare beneficiaries, 2000–2015. JAMA. 2018;320(3):264–71.
72. Tran DL, Lai SR, Salah RY, Wong AY, Bryon JN, McKenna MC, et al. Rapid de-escalation and triaging patients in community-based palliative care. J Pain Symptom Manage. 2020;60(1):e45–e7.
73. Schumacher S, Kent N. 8 charts on internet use around the world as countries grapple with COVID-19. Pew Research Center Fact Tank. 2020. Available from: https://www.pewresearch.org/fact-tank/2020/04/02/8-charts-on-internet-use-around-the-world-as-countries-grapple-with-covid-19/.
74. Perrin A. Digital gap between rural and nonrural America persists. Pew Research Center Fact Tank. 2019. Available from: https://www.pewresearch.org/fact-tank/2019/05/31/digital-gap-between-rural-and-nonrural-america-.persists/#:~:text=Digital%20gap%20between%20rural%20and%20nonrural%20America%20persists.,Pew%20Research%20Center%20survey%20conducted%20in%20early%202019.
75. Continuous or nocturnal oxygen therapy in hypoxemic chronic obstructive lung disease: a clinical trial. Nocturnal Oxygen Therapy Trial Group. Ann Intern Med. 1980;93(3):391–8.
76. Ekström M, Ahmadi Z, Bornefalk-Hermansson A, Abernethy A, Currow D. Oxygen for breathlessness in patients with chronic obstructive pulmonary disease who do not qualify for home oxygen therapy. Cochrane Database Syst Rev. 2016;11(11):CD006429. https://doi.org/10.1002/14651858.CD006429.pub3. PMID: 27886372; PMCID: PMC6464154.
77. Janssen DJA, Spruit MA, Schols J, Wouters EFM. A call for high-quality advance care planning in outpatients with severe COPD or chronic heart failure. Chest. 2011;139(5):1081–8.
78. Hick JL, Einav S, Hanfling D, Kissoon N, Dichter JR, Devereaux AV, et al. Surge capacity principles: care of the critically ill and injured during pandemics and disasters: CHEST consensus statement. Chest. 2014;146(4 Suppl):e1S–e16S.
79. Antommaria AHM, Gibb TS, McGuire AL, Wolpe PR, Wynia MK, Applewhite MK, et al. Ventilator triage policies during the COVID-19 pandemic at U.S. hospitals associated with members of the association of bioethics program directors. Ann Intern Med. 2020;173(3):188–94.
80. Shamieh O, Richardson K, Abdel-Razeq H, Harding R, Sullivan R, Mansour A. COVID-19- impact on DNR orders in the largest cancer center in Jordan. J Pain Symptom Manage. 2020;60(2):e87–e9.
81. Altevogt BM, Stroud C, Hanson SL, Hanfling D, Gostin LO. Guidance for establishing crisis standards of care for use in disaster situations: a letter report. National Academy of Sciences; 2009.

82. Mosher CE, Bakas T, Champion VL. Physical health, mental health, and life changes among family caregivers of patients with lung cancer. Oncol Nurs Forum. 2013;40(1):53–61.
83. Schulz R, Eden J, Committee on Family Caregiving for Older Adults; Board on Health Care Services; Health and Medicine Division; National Academies of Sciences, Engineering, and Medicine, editors. Families caring for an aging America. Washington (DC): National Academies Press (US); November 8, 2016.
84. Sun V, Raz DJ, Erhunmwunsee L, Ruel N, Carranza J, Prieto R, et al. Improving family caregiver and patient outcomes in lung cancer surgery: study protocol for a randomized trial of the multimedia self-management (MSM) intervention. Contemp Clin Trials. 2019;83:88–96.
85. Iyer AS, Dionne-Odom JN, Ford SM, Crump Tims SL, Sockwell ED, Ivankova NV, et al. A formative evaluation of patient and family caregiver perspectives on early palliative care in chronic obstructive pulmonary disease across disease severity. Ann Am Thorac Soc. 2019;16(8):1024–33.
86. Dellon EP, Shores MD, Nelson KI, Wolfe J, Noah TL, Hanson LC. Family caregiver perspectives on symptoms and treatments for patients dying from complications of cystic fibrosis. J Pain Symptom Manage. 2010;40(6):829–37.
87. Ellis J. The impact of lung cancer on patients and carers. Chron Respir Dis. 2012;9(1):39–47.
88. Murray SA, Kendall M, Boyd K, Grant L, Highet G, Sheikh A. Archetypal trajectories of social, psychological, and spiritual wellbeing and distress in family care givers of patients with lung cancer: secondary analysis of serial qualitative interviews. BMJ. 2010;340:c2581.
89. Lal A, Bartle-Haring S. Relationship among differentiation of self, relationship satisfaction, partner support, and depression in patients with chronic lung disease and their partners. J Marital Fam Ther. 2011;37(2):169–81.
90. Plant H, Moore S, Richardson A, Cornwall A, Medina J, Ream E. Nurses' experience of delivering a supportive intervention for family members of patients with lung cancer. Eur J Cancer Care (Engl). 2011;20(4):436–44.
91. Grant M, Sun V, Fujinami R, Sidhu R, Otis-Green S, Juarez G, et al. Family caregiver burden, skills preparedness, and quality of life in non-small cell lung cancer. Oncol Nurs Forum. 2013;40(4):337–46.
92. Grey M, Schulman-green D, Knafl K, Reynolds NR. A revised self- and family management framework. Nurs Outlook. 2015;63:162–70.
93. Schulman-Green D, Jaser S, Martin F, Alonzo A, Grey M, McCorkle R, Redeker NS, Reynolds N, Whittemore R. Processes of self-management in chronic illness. J Nurs Scholarsh. 2012;44(2):136–44. https://doi.org/10.1111/j.1547-5069.2012.01444.x. Epub 2012 May 2. PMID: 22551013; PMCID: PMC3366425.
94. Göriş S, Klç Z, Elmal F, Tutar N, Takc Ö. Care burden and social support levels of caregivers of patients with chronic obstructive pulmonary disease. Holist Nurs Pract. 2016;30(4):227–35.
95. Prime H, Wade M, Browne DT. Risk and resilience in family well-being during the COVID-19 pandemic. Am Psychol. 2020;75(5):631–43.
96. Schulman-Green D, Jaser SS, Park C, Whittemore R. A metasynthesis of factors affecting self-management of chronic illness. J Adv Nurs. 2016;72:1469–89.
97. Passaro A, Addeo A, Von Garnier C, Blackhall F, Planchard D, Felip E, et al. ESMO management and treatment adapted recommendations in the COVID-19 era: lung cancer. ESMO Open. 2020;5(Suppl 3):e000820.
98. Burki TK. Cancer guidelines during the COVID-19 pandemic. Lancet Oncol. 2020;21(5):629–30.
99. Kent EE, Ornstein KA, Dionne-Odom JN. The family caregiving crisis meets an actual pandemic. J Pain Symptom Manage. 2020;60(1):e66–e9.
100. Schlaudecker JD. Essential family caregivers in long-term care during the COVID-19 pandemic. J Am Med Dir Assoc. 2020;21(7):983.
101. Stokes JE, Patterson SE. Intergenerational relationships, family caregiving policy, and COVID-19 in the United States. J Aging Soc Policy. 2020;32(4–5):416–24.

102. Wilson JM, Lee J, Fitzgerald HN, Oosterhoff B, Sevi B, Shook NJ. Job insecurity and financial concern during the COVID-19 pandemic are associated with worse mental health. J Occup Environ Med. 2020;62(9):686–91.
103. Martinez-Ferran M, de la Guía-Galipienso F, Sanchis-Gomar F, Pareja-Galeano H. Metabolic impacts of confinement during the COVID-19 pandemic due to modified diet and physical activity habits. Nutrients. 2020;12(6):1549.
104. Choi KR, Heilemann MV, Fauer A, Mead M. A second pandemic: mental health spillover from the novel coronavirus (COVID-19). J Am Psychiatr Nurses Assoc. 2020;26(4):340–3.
105. Masten AS. Resilience theory and research on children and families: past, present, and promise. J Fam Theory Rev. 2018;10(1):12–31.
106. PeConga EK, Gauthier GM, Holloway A, Walker RSW, Rosencrans PL, Zoellner LA, et al. Resilience is spreading: mental health within the COVID-19 pandemic. Psychol Trauma. 2020;12(S1):S47–S8.
107. Ozer EJ, Best SR, Lipsey TL, Weiss DS. Predictors of posttraumatic stress disorder and symptoms in adults: a meta-analysis. Psychol Bull. 2003;129(1):52–73.
108. Burton MS, Cooper AA, Feeny NC, Zoellner LA. The enhancement of natural resilience in trauma interventions. J Contemp Psychother. 2015;45(4):193–204.
109. Villalobos M, Siegle A, Hagelskamp L, Jung C, Thomas M. Communication along milestones in lung cancer patients with advanced disease. Oncol Res Treat. 2019;42(1–2):41–6.
110. Villalobos M, Coulibaly K, Krug K, Kamradt M, Wensing M, Siegle A, et al. A longitudinal communication approach in advanced lung cancer: a qualitative study of patients', relatives' and staff's perspectives. Eur J Cancer Care (Engl). 2018;27(2):e12794.
111. Bakitas M, Kryworuchko J, Matlock DD, Volandes AE. Palliative medicine and decision science: the critical need for a shared agenda to foster informed patient choice in serious illness. J Palliat Med. 2011;14(10):1109–16.
112. Truglio-Londrigan M, Slyer JT. Shared decision-making for nursing practice: an integrative review. Open Nurs J. 2018;12:1–14.
113. Tanner NT, Banas E, Yeager D, Dai L, Hughes Halbert C, Silvestri GA. In-person and telephonic shared decision-making visits for people considering lung cancer screening: an assessment of decision quality. Chest. 2019;155(1):236–8.
114. Kew KM, Malik P, Aniruddhan K, Normansell R. Shared decision-making for people with asthma. Cochrane Database Syst Rev. 2017;10(10):CD012330.
115. Allen LA, McIlvennan CK, Thompson JS, Dunlay SM, LaRue SJ, Lewis EF, et al. Effectiveness of an intervention supporting shared decision making for destination therapy left ventricular assist device: the DECIDE-LVAD randomized clinical trial. JAMA Intern Med. 2018;178(4):520–9.
116. Dobler CC. Shared decision making rarely happens for lung cancer screening. JAMA Intern Med. 2019;179(1):122.
117. George M, Bender B. New insights to improve treatment adherence in asthma and COPD. Patient Prefer Adherence. 2019;13:1325–34.
118. Brenner AT, Malo TL, Margolis M, Elston Lafata J, James S, Vu MB, et al. Evaluating shared decision making for lung cancer screening. JAMA Intern Med. 2018;178(10):1311–6.
119. Sassen B, Kok G, Schepers J, Vanhees L. Supporting health care professionals to improve the processes of shared decision making and self-management in a web-based intervention: randomized controlled trial. J Med Internet Res. 2014;16(10):e211.
120. Abrams EM, Shaker M, Oppenheimer J, Davis RS, Bukstein DA, Greenhawt M. The challenges and opportunities for shared decision making highlighted by COVID-19. J Allergy Clin Immunol Pract. 2020;8(8):2474–80 e1.
121. Houchens N, Tipirneni R. Compassionate communication amid the COVID-19 pandemic. J Hosp Med. 2020;15(7):437–9.
122. Larson HJ. A call to arms: helping family, friends and communities navigate the COVID-19 infodemic. Nat Rev Immunol. 2020;20(8):449–50.

123. Forner D, Noel CW, Densmore R, Goldstein DP, Corsten M, Pieterse AH, et al. Shared decision making for surgical care in the era of COVID-19. Otolaryngol Head Neck Surg. 2020;164:297–9. 194599820954138.
124. Simpson N, Milnes S, Steinfort D. Don't forget shared decision-making in the COVID-19 crisis. Intern Med J. 2020;50(6):761–3.
125. Barreto-Filho JAS, Veiga A, Correia LC. COVID-19 and uncertainty: lessons from the front-line for promoting shared decision making. Arq Bras Cardiol. 2020;115(2):149–51.
126. Gaur S, Pandya N, Dumyati G, Nace DA, Pandya K, Jump RLP. A structured tool for communication and care planning in the era of the COVID-19 pandemic. J Am Med Dir Assoc. 2020;21(7):943–7.
127. Back A, Tulsky JA, Arnold RM. Communication skills in the age of COVID-19. Ann Intern Med. 2020;172(11):759–60. https://doi.org/10.7326/M20-1376. Epub 2020 Apr 2. PMID: 32240282; PMCID: PMC7143152.

# Index




K. O. Lindell, S. K. Danoff (eds.), *Palliative Care in Lung Disease*, Respiratory Medicine, https://doi.org/10.1007/978-3-030-81788-6

GPSR Compliance

*The European Union's (EU) General Product Safety Regulation (GPSR) is a set of rules that requires consumer products to be safe and our obligations to ensure this.*

*If you have any concerns about our products, you can contact us on ProductSafety@springernature.com*

In case Publisher is established outside the EU, the EU authorized representative is:

Springer Nature Customer Service Center GmbH
Europaplatz 3
69115 Heidelberg, Germany

**Batch number: 10370708**

Printed by Printforce, the Netherlands